Pediatric Endoscopy

Editor

CATHARINE M. WALSH

GASTROINTESTINAL ENDOSCOPY CLINICS OF NORTH AMERICA

www.giendo.theclinics.com

Consulting Editor
CHARLES J. LIGHTDALE

April 2023 • Volume 33 • Number 2

ELSEVIER

1600 John F. Kennedy Boulevard • Suite 1800 • Philadelphia, Pennsylvania, 19103-2899

http://www.theclinics.com

GASTROINTESTINAL ENDOSCOPY CLINICS OF NORTH AMERICA Volume 33, Number 2
April 2023 ISSN 1052-5157, ISBN-13: 978-0-323-93913-3

Editor: Kerry Holland
Developmental Editor: Jessica Cañaberal

Gastrointestinal Endoscopy Clinics of North America (ISSN 1052-5157) is published quarterly by Elsevier Inc., 360 Park Avenue South, New York, NY 10010-1710. Months of issue are January, April, July, and October. Business and Editorial Offices: 1600 John F. Kennedy Blvd., Suite 1800, Philadelphia, PA, 19103-2899. Periodicals postage paid at New York, NY and additional mailing offices. Subscription prices are $381.00 per year for US individuals, $703.00 per year for US institutions, $100.00 per year for US and Canadian students/residents, $419.00 per year for Canadian individuals, $830.00 per year for Canadian institutions, $501.00 per year for international individuals, $830.00 per year for international institutions, and $245.00 per year for international students/residents. To receive student/resident rate, orders must be accompanied by name of affiliated institution, date of term, and the *signature* of program/residency coordinator on institution letterhead. Orders will be billed at individual rate until proof of status is received. Foreign air speed delivery is included in all *Clinics* subscription prices. All prices are subject to change without notice. **POSTMASTER:** Send address change to *Gastrointestinal Endoscopy Clinics of North America*, Elsevier Health Sciences Division, Subscription Customer Service, 3251 Riverport Lane, Maryland Heights, MO 63043. **Customer Service: 1-800-654-2452 (US). From outside the United States, call 1-314-447-8871. Fax: 1-314-447-8029. E-mail: JournalsCustomerService-usa@elsevier.com (for print support) or JournalsOnlineSupport-usa@elsevier.com (for online support).**

Reprints. For copies of 100 or more, of articles in this publication, please contact the Commercial Reprints Department, Elsevier Inc., 360 Park Avenue South, New York, NY 10010-1710. Tel. 212-633-3874; Fax: 212-633-3820; E-mail: reprints@elsevier.com.

Gastrointestinal Endoscopy Clinics of North America is covered in *Excerpta Medica, MEDLINE/PubMed (Index Medicus), and MEDLINE/MEDLARS.*

Contributors

CONSULTING EDITOR

CHARLES J. LIGHTDALE, MD
Professor of Medicine, Division of Digestive and Liver Diseases, Columbia University Medical Center, New York, New York, USA

EDITOR

CATHARINE M. WALSH, MD, MEd, PhD
Associate Professor, Division of Gastroenterology, Hepatology and Nutrition, and the SickKids Research and Learning Institutes, The Hospital for Sick Children, Department of Paediatrics, and The Wilson Centre, Temerty Faculty of Medicine, University of Toronto, Toronto, Ontario, Canada

AUTHORS

THOMAS M. ATTARD, MD
Associate Professor, Division of Gastroenterology, Hepatology and Nutrition, Children's Mercy Hospital, Professor of Pediatrics, The University of Missouri in Kansas City School of Medicine, Kansas City, Missouri, USA

MONIQUE T. BARAKAT, MD, PhD
Assistant Professor, Division of Pediatric Gastroenterology, Lucile Packard Children's Hospital, Division of Gastroenterology, Stanford University Medical Center, Stanford, California, USA

LEE M. BASS, MD
Professor of Pediatrics, Director of Endoscopy, Division of Gastroenterology, Hepatology and Nutrition, Ann & Robert H. Lurie Children's Hospital of Chicago, Northwestern University Feinberg School of Medicine, Chicago, Illinois, USA

NICHOLAS CARMAN, MD
Division of Gastroenterology, Hepatology and Nutrition, Department of Paediatrics, CHEO Inflammatory Bowel Disease Centre, Children's Hospital of Eastern Ontario, University of Ottawa, Ottawa, Ontario, Canada; Division of Gastroenterology, Hepatology and Nutrition, Department of Paediatrics, SickKids Inflammatory Bowel Disease Centre, The Hospital for Sick Children, University of Toronto, Toronto, Ontario, Canada

SHLOMI COHEN, MD
Associate Professor, Pediatric Gastroenterology Institute, Dana-Dwek Children's Hospital, Tel Aviv Sourasky Medical Center, Affiliated to the Sackler Faculty of Medicine, Tel Aviv University, Tel Aviv, Israel

JASBIR DHALIWAL, MBBS, MSc
Division of Pediatric Gastroenterology, Hepatology and Nutrition, Cincinnati Children's Hospital Medical Center, University of Cincinnati, Cincinnati, Ohio, USA

CAROL DURNO, MSc, MD
Pediatric Gastroenterologist, Associate Professor of Pediatrics, Familial Gastrointestinal Cancer Registry, Department of Surgery, Mount Sinai Hospital, Division of Gastroenterology, Hepatology and Nutrition, The Hospital for Sick Children, Scarborough Health Network, Scarborough Centenary Hospital, University of Toronto, Ontario, Canada

DOUGLAS S. FISHMAN, MD
Department of Pediatrics, Baylor College of Medicine, Division of Pediatric Gastroenterology, Hepatology, and Nutrition, Texas Children's Hospital, Houston, Texas, USA

AMIT S. GROVER, MD
Division of Gastroenterology, Hepatology and Nutrition, Boston Children's Hospital, Boston, Massachusetts, USA

ROBERTO GUGIG, MD
Division of Pediatric Gastroenterology, Lucile Packard Children's Hospital, Stanford University Medical Center, Stanford, California, USA

GIRISH HIREMATH, MD, MPH
Division of Pediatric Gastroenterology, Hepatology, and Nutrition, Monroe Carell Jr. Children's Hospital at Vanderbilt, Vanderbilt University Medical Center, Nashville, Tennessee, USA

JEANNIE S. HUANG, MD, MPH, F-NASPGHAN
Professor, Department of Pediatrics, University of California, San Diego, La Jolla, California, USA; Division of Pediatric Gastroenterology, Rady Children's Hospital San Diego, San Diego, California, USA

JULIE KHLEVNER, MD, AGAF
Division of Pediatric Gastroenterology, Hepatology and Nutrition, Columbia University Vagelos College of Physicians and Surgeons, Associate Professor of Pediatrics, Columbia University Medical Center, Director, Gastrointestinal Motility Center, NewYork-Presbyterian Morgan Stanley Children's Hospital, New York, New York, USA

AMORNLUCK KRASAELAP, MD
Assistant Professor of Pediatrics, University of Missouri-Kansas City School of Medicine, Division of Pediatric Gastroenterology, Hepatology and Nutrition, Children's Mercy Hospital, Kansas City, Missouri, USA

KRISTINA LEINWAND, DO
Section of Pediatric Gastroenterology, Hepatology and Nutrition, Northwest Permanente, Department of Pediatric Gastroenterology, Hepatology, and Nutrition, Doernbecher Children's Hospital, Oregon Health and Science University, Portland, Oregon, USA

DIANA G. LERNER, MD
Associate Professor of Pediatrics, Division of Pediatric Gastroenterology, Department of Pediatrics, Hepatology and Nutrition, Medical College of Wisconsin, Milwaukee, Wisconsin, USA

JENIFER R. LIGHTDALE, MD, MPH
Associate Chief, Division of Gastroenterology, Hepatology and Nutrition, Boston Children's Hospital, Boston, Massachusetts, USA

LISA B. MAHONEY, MD
Division of Gastroenterology, Hepatology and Nutrition, Boston Children's Hospital, Boston, Massachusetts, USA

MICHAEL A. MANFREDI, MD
Associate Professor of Pediatrics University of Pennsylvania, Division of Gastroenterology, Hepatology and Nutrition, Children's Hospital of Philadelphia, Philadelphia, Pennsylvania, USA

PRIYA NARULA, MD
Department of Paediatric Gastroenterology, Sheffield Children's NHS Foundation Trust, Sheffield, Sheffield, United Kingdom

KENNETH NG, DO
Division of Pediatric Gastroenterology, Hepatology, and Nutrition, Johns Hopkins Children's Center, Assistant Professor of Pediatrics, Johns Hopkins School of Medicine, Baltimore, Maryland, USA

NATHALIE NGUYEN, MD
Gastrointestinal Eosinophilic Diseases Program, Section of Pediatric Gastroenterology, Hepatology and Nutrition, Digestive Health Institute, Children's Hospital Colorado, University of Colorado School of Medicine, Aurora, Colorado, USA

INNA NOVAK, MD
Associate Professor, Department of Pediatrics, Division of Pediatric Gastroenterology, Hepatology and Nutrition, Children's Hospital at Montefiore, Albert Einstein College of Medicine, Bronx, New York, USA

SALVATORE OLIVA, MD, PhD
Assistant Professor of Pediatrics, Maternal and Child Health Department, Pediatric Gastroenterology and Liver Unit, Sapienza - University of Rome, Rome, Italy

DHIREN PATEL, MBBS, MD
Division of Pediatric Gastroenterology, Hepatology and Nutrition, Associate Professor, Department of Pediatrics, St Louis University, Cardinal Glennon Children's Medical Center, St Louis University School of Medicine, Medical Director, Neurogastroenterology and Motility, SSM Cardinal Glennon Children's Medical Center, St Louis, Missouri, USA

JOSEPH A. PICORARO, MD
Division of Pediatric Gastroenterology, Hepatology and Nutrition, Columbia University Irving Medical Center, NewYork-Presbyterian Morgan Stanley Children's Hospital, New York, New York, USA

LEONEL RODRIGUEZ, MD, MS
Section Chief of Pediatric Gastroenterology, Hepatology and Nutrition, Division of Pediatric Gastroenterology, Hepatology and Nutrition, Department of Pediatrics, Yale New Haven Children's Hospital, Yale School of Medicine, New Haven, Connecticut, USA

WENLY RUAN, MD
Department of Pediatrics, Baylor College of Medicine, Division of Pediatric Gastroenterology, Hepatology, and Nutrition, Texas Children's Hospital, Houston, Texas, USA

RAMY SABE, MBBCh
Division of Pediatric Gastroenterology, Hepatology, and Nutrition, Rainbow Babies and Children's Hospitals, Case Western Reserve University School of Medicine, Cleveland, Ohio, USA

RAJITHA D. VENKATESH, MD
Division of Pediatric Gastroenterology, Hepatology, and Nutrition, Nationwide Children's Hospital, Department of Pediatrics, The Ohio State University College of Medicine, Columbus, Ohio, USA

CATHARINE M. WALSH, MD, MEd, PhD
Associate Professor, Division of Gastroenterology, Hepatology and Nutrition, and the SickKids Research and Learning Institutes, The Hospital for Sick Children, Department of Paediatrics, and The Wilson Centre, Temerty Faculty of Medicine, University of Toronto, Toronto, Ontario, Canada

JESSICA L. YASUDA, MD
Assistant Professor of Pediatrics, Harvard Medical School, Division of Gastroenterology, Hepatology and Nutrition, Boston Children's Hospital, Boston, Massachusetts, USA

Contents

Sedation for pediatric endoscopy has evolved from an endoscopist-administered component of procedures to an almost entirely anesthesiologist-supported endeavor. Nevertheless, there are no ideal endoscopist or anesthesiologist-administered sedation protocols, and wide practice variation exists in both models. Furthermore, sedation for pediatric endoscopy, whether administered by endoscopists or anesthesiologists, remains the highest risk to patient safety. This underscores the importance of both specialties identifying best sedation practices together that can safeguard patients while maximizing procedural efficiency and minimizing costs. In this review, the authors discuss specific levels of sedation for endoscopy and the risks and benefits of various regimens.

 Video content accompanies this article at http://www.giendo. theclinics.com.

Pediatric endoscopists are at risk of work-related injuries from overuse and repetitive motions during endoscopy. Recently, there has been increasing appreciation for the importance of ergonomics education and training to help build long-term habits that prevent injury. This article reviews the epidemiology of endoscopy-related injuries in pediatric practice, describes methods for controlling exposures in the workplace, discusses key ergonomic principles that can be used to mitigate injury risk, and outlines tips for integrating education on endoscopy ergonomics during training.

Upskilling in ileocolonoscopy is an important aspect of pediatric endoscopic practice as it enables endoscopists to learn additional skills through education and training to improve outcomes. With the advent of technologies, endoscopy is continuously evolving. Many devices can be applied to improve endoscopy quality and ergonomics. In addition, techniques such as dynamic position change can be employed to increase procedural efficiency and completeness. Key to upskilling is enhancing endoscopists' cognitive, technical and nontechnical skills and the concept of "training the trainer" to ensure trainers have the requisite skills to teach endoscopy effectively. This chapter details aspects of upskilling pediatric ileocolonoscopy.

Quality indicators and standards for pediatric endoscopy have recently been developed by the inaugural working group of the international Pediatric Endoscopy Quality Improvement Network (PEnQuIN). Currently available electronic medical record (EMR) functionalities can enable real-time capture of quality indicators to support continuous quality measurement and improvement within pediatric endoscopy facilities. Ultimately, EMR interoperability and cross-institutional data sharing can serve to validate PEnQuIN standards of care and permit benchmarking across endoscopy services, in the pursuit of elevating the quality of endoscopic care for children everywhere.

The application of artificial intelligence (AI) has great promise for improving pediatric endoscopy. The majority of preclinical studies have been undertaken in adults, with the greatest progress being made in the context of colorectal cancer screening and surveillance. This development has only been possible with advances in deep learning, like the convolutional neural network model, which has enabled real-time detection of pathology. Comparatively, the majority of deep learning systems developed in inflammatory bowel disease have focused on predicting disease severity and were developed using still images rather than videos. The application of AI to pediatric endoscopy is in its infancy, thus providing an opportunity to develop clinically meaningful and fair systems that do not perpetuate societal biases. In this review, we provide an overview of AI, summarize the advances of AI in endoscopy, and describe its potential application to pediatric endoscopic practice and education.

Unsedated transnasal endoscopy (TNE) is a feasible, safe, and cost-effective procedure for pediatric patients. TNE provides direct visualization of the esophagus and enables acquisition of biopsy samples while eliminating the risks associated with sedation and anesthesia. TNE should be considered in the evaluation and monitoring of disorders of the upper gastrointestinal tract, particularly in diseases such as eosinophilic esophagitis that often require repeated endoscopy. Setting up a TNE program requires a thorough business plan as well as training of staff and endoscopists.

Eosinophilic esophagitis (EoE) is a chronic allergen-mediated clinicopathologic condition that currently requires esophagogastroduodenoscopy with biopsies and histologic evaluation to diagnose and monitor its progress. This state-of-the art review outlines the pathophysiology of EoE, reviews the application of endoscopy as a diagnostic and therapeutic tool, and discusses potential complications related to therapeutic endoscopic interventions. It also introduces recent innovations that can enhance the endoscopist's ability to diagnose and monitor EoE with minimally invasive procedures and perform therapeutic maneuvers more safely and effectively.

The endoscopist plays a critical role in the management of patients with congenital esophageal defects. This review focuses on esophageal atresia and congenital esophageal strictures and, in particular, the endoscopic management of comorbidities related to these conditions, including anastomotic strictures, tracheoesophageal fistulas, esophageal perforations, and esophagitis surveillance. Practical aspects of endoscopic techniques for stricture management are reviewed including dilation, intralesional steroid injection, stenting, and endoscopic incisional therapy. Endoscopic surveillance for mucosal pathology is essential in this population, as patients are at high risk of esophagitis and its late complications such as Barrett's esophagus.

Children and adolescents are increasingly impacted by pancreatic disease. Interventional endoscopic procedures, including endoscopic retrograde cholangiopancreatography) and endoscopic ultrasonography, are integral to the diagnosis and management of many pancreatic diseases in the adult population. In the past decade, pediatric interventional endoscopic procedures have become more widely available, with invasive surgical procedures now being replaced by safer and less disruptive endoscopic interventions.

 Video content accompanies this article at http://www.giendo. theclinics.com.

Although pediatric neurogastroenterology and motility (PNGM) disorders are prevalent, often debilitating, and remain challenging to diagnose and treat, this field has made remarkable progress in the last decade. Diagnostic and therapeutic gastrointestinal endoscopy emerged as a valuable tool in the management of PNGM disorders. Novel modalities such as functional lumen imaging probe, per-oral endoscopic myotomy, gastric-POEM, and electrocautery incisional therapy have changed the diagnostic and therapeutic landscape of PNGM. In this review, the authors highlight the emerging role of therapeutic and diagnostic endoscopy in esophageal, gastric, small bowel, colonic, and anorectal disorders and disorders of gut and brain axis interaction.

Upper gastrointestinal bleeding (UGIB) in children has many causes, with its prevalence varying by age. Often presenting as hematemesis or melena, the initial treatment is stabilization of the patient, including protection of the airway, fluid resuscitation, and a transfusion hemoglobin threshold of 7 g/L. Endoscopy should be performed with the goal of using combinations of therapies to treat a bleeding lesion, generally involving epinephrine injection along with either cautery, hemoclips, or hemospray. This review discusses the diagnosis and treatment of variceal and non-variceal gastrointestinal bleeding in children with a focus on current advances in the treatment of severe UGIB.

Small bowel evaluation has been transformed by capsule endoscopy and advances in small bowel imaging, which provide reliable and noninvasive means for assessing the mucosal surface. Device-assisted enteroscopy has been critical for histopathological confirmation and endoscopic therapy for a wide range of small bowel pathology that conventional endoscopy cannot reach. The purpose of this review is to provide a comprehensive overview of the indications, techniques, and clinical applications of capsule endoscopy; device-assisted enteroscopy; and imaging studies for small bowel evaluation in children.

Endoscopic characterization of pediatric inflammatory bowel disease (IBD) has developed in accordance with advances in treatment and improved understanding of disease progression and complications. Reliable and consistent endoscopic reporting practices and tools continue to evolve. The roles of endoscopic ultrasonography, capsule endoscopy, and deep enteroscopy in the care of children and adolescents with IBD are beginning to be clarified. Opportunities for therapeutic intervention with endoscopy in pediatric IBD, including endoscopic balloon dilation and electroincision therapy, require further study. This review discusses the current utility of endoscopic assessment in Pediatric Inflammatory Bowel Disease, as well as emerging and evolving techniques to improve patient care.

Polypectomy is the most common therapeutic endoscopic intervention in children. Management of sporadic juvenile polyps is limited to polypectomy to resolve symptoms, whereas polyposis syndromes pose a multidisciplinary challenge with broader ramifications. In preparation for polypectomy, there are key patient, polyp, endoscopy unit, and provider characteristics that factor into the likelihood of success. Younger age and multiple medical comorbidities increase the risk of adverse outcomes, classified as intraoperative, immediate postoperative, and delayed postoperative complications. Novel techniques, including cold snare polypectomy, can significantly decrease adverse events but a more structured training process for polypectomy in pediatric gastroenterology is needed.

GASTROINTESTINAL ENDOSCOPY CLINICS OF NORTH AMERICA

SERIES OF RELATED INTEREST

Gastroenterology Clinics
(www.gastro.theclinics.com)
Clinics in Liver Disease
(www.liver.theclinics.com)

THE CLINICS ARE AVAILABLE ONLINE!
Access your subscription at:
www.theclinics.com

Foreword

Pediatric Gastrointestinal Endoscopy Continues to Grow and Progress

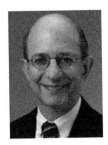

Charles J. Lightdale, MD
Consulting Editor

Swiftly flow the years. The North American Society for Gastroenterology, Hepatology, and Nutrition celebrated its 50th anniversary in 2022. Back in the 1970s, if a pediatrician needed an endoscopy for a patient, it often involved obtaining valuable time in an operating room. If that wasn't enough of a hurdle, the only available endoscopist was probably trained in adult internal medicine and gastroenterology. Fifty years and some three generations later, the new pediatric gastrointestinal (GI) fellows would have little awareness of this inauspicious early landscape. Pediatric GI endoscopy is firmly in the mainstream now, and pediatricians have their own well-trained corps of GI endoscopists, including a growing cadre skilled in advanced therapeutic procedures, working in dedicated pediatric endoscopy rooms.

I am very grateful that Dr Catharine M. Walsh agreed to be Editor for this issue of the *Gastrointestinal Endoscopy Clinics of North America* dedicated to Pediatric GI Endoscopy. Dr Walsh is widely recognized as a deeply thoughtful leader in pediatric gastroenterology with a broad interest in the progress of endoscopy in the management of illness in children from infants to adolescents. She has brought together a remarkable group of experts in the field to cover key topics in pediatric endoscopy. There is an emphasis on training and quality improvement that permeates throughout. Dr Walsh has authored or coauthored three articles, all with a pediatric focus on hot issues in modern GI endoscopy: ergonomics, artificial intelligence, and the electronic medical record.

Other articles cover important contributions to the growth of pediatric GI endoscopy, including the critical evolution of sedation, and the development of thinner endoscopes made possible by smaller and smaller powerful charge-coupled device sensors and camera technologies as the instruments metamorphosed from fiberoptic to digital.

Gastrointest Endoscopy Clin N Am 33 (2023) xiii–xiv
https://doi.org/10.1016/j.giec.2023.01.001
1052-5157/23/© 2023 Published by Elsevier Inc.

Transnasal endoscopy performed with thin instruments and without sedation is discussed in detail. Articles describing the impact of diagnostic and therapeutic endoscopy in the management of common diseases seen by pediatric gastroenterologists include eosinophilic esophagitis, small intestinal disease, inflammatory bowel disease, polyps and polyposis syndromes, motility disorders, congenital esophageal defects, pancreatitis, and GI bleeding.

This is a terrific issue of the *Gastrointestinal Endoscopy Clinics of North America* with a thorough state-of-the-art review and strong nod to the future. The issue is a testament to the amazing progress in pediatric GI endoscopy and should be of great interest to all pediatric gastroenterologists.

Charles J. Lightdale, MD
Department of Medicine
Columbia University Medical Center
161 Fort Washington Avenue
New York, NY 10032, USA

E-mail address:
CJL18@columbia.edu

Preface

Pediatric Endoscopy

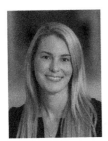

Catharine M. Walsh, MD, MEd, PhD
Editor

In 2022, the North American Society for Pediatric Gastroenterology, Hepatology and Nutrition celebrated its 50th anniversary. Just as the field of pediatric gastroenterology has expanded over the last five decades, pediatric endoscopy has grown exponentially since its beginnings as fiberoptic endoscopy in the early 1970s. Thanks to reductions in instrument diameters, technological improvements, and progress in sedation and anesthetics, endoscopy in infants, children, and adolescents has become easier and safer. The number of pediatric endoscopies performed has grown steadily, and practice patterns have changed with expanding diagnostic and therapeutic indications and the shift to performing endoscopy outside of the general operating room.

Pediatric endoscopy has flourished in recent years, with more individuals seeking training in advanced procedures and an expanded appreciation for endoscopy quality. Reflective of the needs of pediatric patients and their families and the unique nature of pediatric endoscopy, the international Pediatric Endoscopy Quality Improvement Network recently identified quality standards and indicators for pediatric endoscopy, which will be crucial in guiding future quality assurance and improvement initiatives. There is also increasing recognition of the importance of high-quality endoscopy education and the value of trained trainers who are not only competent in performing pediatric endoscopy themselves but also successful in imparting the knowledge, skills, and attitudes to their trainees in an effective manner. This focus on quality and training will serve to support the next generation of pediatric endoscopists who will continue to expand the role of pediatric endoscopy and lead the provision of high-quality, patient- and family-centered endoscopic care.

I feel extremely fortunate to have worked with a talented and passionate group of colleagues and thought-leaders to assemble state-of-the-art reviews on important topics in the field of pediatric endoscopy, including transnasal endoscopy, quality improvement, and small bowel endoscopy. This issue of *Gastrointestinal Endoscopy Clinics of North America* also covers emerging technologies, such as artificial

Gastrointest Endoscopy Clin N Am 33 (2023) xv–xvi
https://doi.org/10.1016/j.giec.2022.12.003
1052-5157/23/© 2022 Published by Elsevier Inc.

intelligence and endoscopy ergonomics, and we will undoubtedly see further development in their applications in pediatric endoscopy moving forward. Whether it's here and now, or on the bright horizon of the future, I hope readers find these articles useful in advancing pediatric endoscopic practice and education for the benefit of patients and their families. I also encourage pediatric endoscopy researchers and innovators to address some of the many knowledge gaps raised in this issue and continue to dedicate their work to advancing the evidence for what we do.

I would like to express my sincere thanks to the contributing authors for their generosity in sharing their time and knowledge as well as to Jessica Cañaberal from Elsevier, who coordinated the production of this issue. I would also like to thank Dr Charles Lightdale for the opportunity to serve as guest editor for this exciting issue of *Gastrointestinal Endoscopy Clinics of North America*.

Since the inception of pediatric endoscopy over 50 years ago, advances in diagnostic and therapeutic applications of pediatric endoscopy have been nothing short of transformational, with resultant positive effects on the health of infants, children, and adolescents. It will be important for the next generation of pediatric endoscopists to build on this progress and continue to innovate and advance the field moving forward.

Catharine M. Walsh, MD, MEd, PhD
Division of Gastroenterology
Hepatology and Nutrition
SickKids Research and Learning Institutes
The Hospital for Sick Children
Department of Paediatrics and the Wilson Centre
Temerty Faculty of Medicine
University of Toronto
Toronto M5G 1X8, Canada

E-mail address:
catharine.walsh@utoronto.ca

The Evolution of Sedation for Pediatric Gastrointestinal Endoscopy

Lisa B. Mahoney, MD, Jenifer R. Lightdale, MD, MPH*

KEYWORDS

- Sedation • Pediatrics • Procedural sedation • General anesthesia • Sedatives
- Endoscopy • Gastrointestinal • Gastrointestinal procedures

KEY POINTS

- No ideal sedative regimen has been established for pediatric gastrointestinal endoscopy procedures, regardless of whether procedural sedation is being administered by endoscopists or anesthesiologists.
- Adverse events related to sedation remain the most common patient safety risks of gastrointestinal endoscopy, even when anesthesiologists administer sedation.
- Over the past two decades, propofol-based anesthesiologist-administered sedation has become the most widely used regimen for pediatric endoscopy.
- Broadly speaking, general anesthesia with endotracheal intubation is not necessary for routine pediatric upper endoscopy or ileocolonoscopy and may increase patient risks as well as decrease procedural efficiency.
- An open dialogue between pediatric endoscopists and anesthesiologists is imperative to identifying best sedation practices for children undergoing gastrointestinal endoscopy procedures.

INTRODUCTION

The role of endoscopy in the diagnosis and treatment of digestive diseases of childhood has grown steadily over the past 50 years.[1] Over that time, sedation as a fundamental component of pediatric gastrointestinal endoscopic procedures has evolved from endoscopist-administered regimens to the almost universal employment of anesthesiologists. Although sedation in both models is appropriately viewed as essential to performing safe, comfortable, and technically successful endoscopic procedures in children, optimal sedative regimens for either have not been established. In addition, there may be unwarranted variation among anesthesiologists providing sedation for

Division of Gastroenterology, Hepatology and Nutrition, Boston Children's Hospital, 300 Longwood Avenue, Boston, MA 02115, USA
* Corresponding author.
E-mail address: jenifer.lightdale@childrens.harvard.edu

Gastrointest Endoscopy Clin N Am 33 (2023) 213–234
https://doi.org/10.1016/j.giec.2022.10.001
giendo.theclinics.com

pediatric endoscopy that may be ripe for analysis of best practices and standardization.[2]

In general, the types of providers primarily responsible for administering procedural sedation have shifted in recent years across all pediatric disciplines, and pediatric endoscopy is no exception.[3] Whereas many pediatric endoscopy facilities previously provided endoscopist-administered sedatives to children undergoing procedures, most now rely on a staff of anesthesiologists. With this evolution, anesthesia providers have been required to gain knowledge about various gastrointestinal procedures and evolving evidence for best endoscopic sedation practices. Nevertheless, it has remained incumbent on endoscopists who perform procedures in children to also be knowledgeable about sedation, as well as to maintain familiarity with sedation-based educational curricula and endoscopy guidelines, to optimally work with their anesthesia colleagues to meet patient needs.[4,5]

Most procedural sedation for pediatric endoscopy involves intravenous (IV) medications and ideally maintains a child's ability to breathe spontaneously with adequate airway reflexes. From a regulatory standpoint, either an endoscopist or an anesthesiologist can administer procedural sedation that aims for moderate levels of consciousness that assure airway protection. When an anesthesiologist is involved, it may be acceptable to aim for deep levels of sedation that may verge into general anesthesia and involve the loss of protective airway reflexes.[6] In the absence of an anesthesiologist, it is important that endoscopists be familiar with moderate sedation regimens and know how to rescue patients should the level of sedation become deeper than expected.[4]

Given that many children undergoing stressful and uncomfortable procedures can be agitated, it has become common to plan for deep levels of sedation or general anesthesia for pediatric patients undergoing diagnostic endoscopy.[7,8] Nevertheless, most anesthesiologists and endoscopists agree that sedation plans that call for general anesthesia with endotracheal intubation are generally not necessary for routine pediatric endoscopic procedures.[2] Instead, protocols which seek to achieve general anesthesia necessitating endotracheal intubation can be reserved for therapeutic cases or for children with medical complexity or conditions that may be associated with increased procedural or sedation risks.

Patient safety should and does remain paramount. In this regard, it has become clear that the use of procedural sedation to achieve all levels of consciousness (minimal, moderate, deep, and general anesthesia) represents the most common risk factor for adverse events related to endoscopy.[9–11] Adverse events due to sedation, regardless of who has administered it, have been consistently documented to occur more commonly during pediatric endoscopy than adverse events related to technical aspects of the procedures, such as bleeding or perforation.[12–15] Furthermore, recent evidence has suggested that lengthy or repeated exposures to sedatives and anesthetics, including those used routinely in pediatric gastrointestinal endoscopy, may affect neurocognitive development in young children.[16]

In short, the intersection between performance of gastrointestinal endoscopic procedures in children, efficiency, costs, patient safety, and sedation remains a topic of great interest among pediatric gastroenterologists.[12,17,18] In recent years, the topic of sedation for pediatric endoscopy has also gained interest within the field of anesthesia. Anesthesiologists are increasingly recognizing that best approaches for sedating children for endoscopy may be quite different from those of other pediatric procedures as well as from sedation of adults for gastrointestinal endoscopic procedures.[11] These realities underscore why all endoscopists should understand the myriad of implications of sedation choices inherent to performing endoscopic procedures in children.[4,7] **Box 1** lists patient risk factors for adverse events during procedural sedation and anesthesia that should be discussed by endoscopists working with anesthesiologists to perform sedated endoscopy in children.

This state-of-the art review broadly outlines various sedative regimens for pediatric gastrointestinal endoscopy, with a focus on their benefits, limitations and pitfalls, and opportunities to minimize patient risk while optimizing procedural efficiency. The authors also have emphasized the importance of engaging in open dialogue with

---

Box 1
Patient risk factors for sedation/anesthesia adverse events during pediatric gastrointestinal endoscopic procedures

Patient age

Planned procedure

High body mass index

Relevant comorbidities
- Anxiety
- Cardiac disease
- Diabetes
- Reactive airways
- Seizure disorder
- Psychiatric disorders

Aspiration risk factors
- Achalasia
- Emergency procedures
- Food/foreign body impaction
- Full-column gastroesophageal reflux (by clinical history)

Concerns for difficult airways
- Congenital abnormalities
  - Pierre Robin syndrome
  - Treacher Collins' syndrome
  - Laryngeal atresia
  - Craniofacial abnormalities
- Anatomic variations
  - Large tongue
  - Highly arched or narrow palate
  - Short, thick neck
  - Prominent overbite
  - Limited range of motion of neck

Relevant medications
- Cardiopulmonary
- Anti-seizure
- Psychotropic
- Analgesics
  - Benzodiazepines
  - Opioids

History of recreational drug use

Known social considerations
- Limitations of parental presence/right to consent
- Legal guardian information

Consideration of these factors and others should be communicated before the procedure by endoscopists to all providers, including anesthesiologists, involved in administering sedation.

anesthesiologists, who are increasingly being called on to gain familiarity with best sedation practices for pediatric endoscopy.

SEDATION AS A COMPONENT OF HIGH-QUALITY ENDOSCOPY IN CHILDREN

Quality standards, indicators, and reporting elements for all aspects of high-quality pediatric endoscopy, including sedation, have only recently been established through an international consensus process sponsored by the North American and European Societies for Pediatric Gastroenterology, Hepatology and Nutrition (NASPGHAN and ESPGHAN).[1,19] Specifically, a working group called the Pediatric Endoscopy Quality Improvement Network (PEnQuIN), composed of 33 endoscopists from 31 centers in 11 countries across North America and Europe, was formed to review and synthesize evidence for best endoscopic practices, including those concerning sedation.[1] In their recently published guidelines that have now been endorsed by the American Society for Gastrointestinal Endoscopy (ASGE) and the Canadian Association of Gastroenterology (CAG), PEnQuIN identified a number of sedation-related metrics deemed essential to providing high-quality endoscopic care in children (**Table 1**).[20] It is now incumbent upon both endoscopists and anesthesiologists to know these metrics, as well as the body of evidence that supports them.

The PEnQuIN working group also recognized that provider role clarity is central to the discussion of pediatric endoscopy quality. In understanding the landscape, the PEnQuIN group reviewed a 2005 NASPGHAN survey that was felt to contrast dramatically with present day sedation practices.[21] The 2005 NASPGHAN sedation survey (32% response rate) found wide practice variation in types of sedation, with 31% of respondents using endoscopist-administered sedation and 48% using anesthesiologist-administered sedation. Indeed, a 2022 informal electronic survey of the PEnQuIN working group (66% response rate) suggests that more than 90% of endoscopists today use anesthesiology-administered propofol-based sedation (**Fig. 1**). These recent survey results illustrate the remarkable evolution in sedation trends for pediatric endoscopy.[22]

Patient safety has been cited as a driving factor toward anesthesiologist-administered regimens, despite a number of studies that have found that adverse event rates related to sedation are similar whether anesthesiologists or endoscopists are responsible for its provision.[12–15] Another often cited factor may be efforts to improve procedural efficiency.[10] However, single-center studies showing marked variation in sedation practices, including the use of endotracheal intubation, again suggest this motivation may not be supported by actual experience.[2] Further research is now needed to understand whether real life experiences support these and other presumed reasons that anesthesiologist-administered sedation protocols are now commonly used for pediatric endoscopy, as well as what best practices in the future might optimize patient, provider, and facility experience assuming this trend continues.

PROCEDURE LOCATION

Procedure location is another important discussion point when surveying the evolving landscape of sedation for pediatric endoscopy. The universal employment of anesthesiologists, especially in operating room settings, for relatively brief procedures that do not require patients to be fully immobile, may involve unnecessary use of health care resources.[9,17,23] Although only 10% of respondents in the 2005 NASPGHAN survey of sedation practices reported using general anesthesia for all procedures, a full third reported mostly performing procedures with general anesthesia in hospital operating

Table 1
Sedation-related Pediatric Endoscopy Quality Improvement Network standards and indicators for pediatric gastrointestinal endoscopic procedures

Sedation-Related Standards		Sedation-Related Indicators	
1. Facility-Related Standards			
S4	Endoscopy facilities where pediatric procedures are performed should implement and monitor adherence to *preprocedure* policies that ensure best practice in pediatric care. [evidence: very low]	I2	Rate with which a preprocedure history and directed physical examination is performed.
		I3	Rate of appropriate prophylactic antibiotic administration in accordance with accepted guidelines.
		I4	Rate with which a preprocedural team pause is conducted.
		I5	Rate with which sedation-related fasting guidelines are followed.
S12	Endoscopy facilities where pediatric procedures are performed should monitor their rate of serious adverse events from pediatric endoscopic procedures and anesthesia using a reliable system and report the results to the appropriate institutional or facility oversight committee. [evidence: very low]	I7	Rate of documented intraprocedural adverse events.
		I8	Rate of documented immediate postprocedural adverse events.
		I9	Rate of documented late adverse events.
		I10	Rate of adverse events.
S20	Endoscopy facilities where pediatric procedures are performed should ensure availability of pediatric-specific monitoring and resuscitation equipment. [evidence: moderate]		
2. Procedure-Related Standards			
S30	For all endoscopic procedures, the sedation/anesthetic plan should be documented along with a standardized measure of patient complexity. [evidence: low]	I20	Rate with which the sedation/anesthetic plan is documented.
		I21	Rate with which ASA status is documented.
S31	Appropriate sedation/anesthesia should be provided to ensure patient cooperation, comfort, and safety in line with best practices and consistent with evidence-based guidelines, when available. [evidence: low]	I22	Rate with which patient monitoring during sedation/anesthesia is performed.
		I23	Rate with which the dose and route of administration of all medications used during the procedure are documented.
		I24	Rate with which intraoperative patient comfort is documented.
		I25	Rate with which reversal agents are used.
		I26	Rate with which the procedure is interrupted and/or prematurely terminated due to a sedation/anesthesia-related issue.

(continued on next page)

Table 1 (continued)			
Sedation-Related Standards		**Sedation-Related Indicators**	
S39	All patients and/or caregivers, on discharge, should be given written information regarding potential symptoms that may indicate a procedure-related adverse event and instructions on what to do should these symptoms develop. [evidence: very low]	I38	Rate with which patients/ caregivers receive written postprocedure instructions on discharge.

Walsh, Catharine M. et al. Overview of the Pediatric Endoscopy Quality Improvement Network Quality Standards and Indicators for Pediatric Endoscopy: A Joint NASPGHAN/ESPGHAN Guideline. Journal of Pediatric Gastroenterology and Nutrition: March 2022 - Volume 74 - Issue S1 - p S3-S15 doi: 10.1097/MPG.0000000000003262.

rooms.[21] Another third of respondents performed most of their procedures with anesthesiologist-administered propofol in a dedicated endoscopy facility, outside of main operating rooms. Today, the performance of pediatric endoscopy outside of the main operating room has become standard practice in many institutions.[7,9] In the 2022 survey of the PEnQuIN working group, over 95% of respondents performed at least some of their endoscopic procedures with anesthesiologist-administered sedation outside of the operating room.

GOALS AND LEVELS OF SEDATION FOR PEDIATRIC ENDOSCOPIC PROCEDURES

The primary goal of sedation for pediatric endoscopy is to perform procedures safely, with minimal emotional and physical discomfort. Secondary goals may include achieving periprocedural amnesia, maximizing procedural efficiency, minimizing recovery times, and maintaining cost-effectiveness. Although some gastrointestinal procedures may be preferentially performed without sedation, almost all will require some sedation to ensure patient cooperation.

The depth of sedation can generally be classified into one of four levels—minimal, moderate, deep, and general anesthesia—and should be considered a continuum without discrete boundaries (**Table 2**).[24] The four levels of sedation are defined by a patient's responsiveness to stimulation (verbal, tactile, or painful stimuli) and cardiorespiratory function. Minimally sedated patients retain the ability to respond voluntarily to vocal commands (ie, "take a deep breath" or "turn on your back") and their protective airway reflexes. Moderate sedation describes a depth of sedation where patients can tolerate unpleasant procedures while maintaining adequate cardiorespiratory function, protective airway reflexes, and the ability to react to verbal or tactile stimulation. Deep sedation is used to describe a medically controlled state of depressed consciousness from which the patient is not easily aroused but may respond purposefully to painful stimulation. Deeply sedated patients may require assistance in protecting their airway and for ventilation. General anesthesia describes the deepest level of sedation where the patient is unconscious, with reduced responses to stimuli, and with an unprotected airway that may require ventilatory support.

Targeted depths of sedation may vary depending on the procedure. In upper endoscopy, a major goal of sedation may be to avoid gagging and increase patient cooperation; in ileocolonoscopy, the goal of sedation is often to avoid visceral pain associated with looping of the colonoscope. Child anxiety levels may also vary by

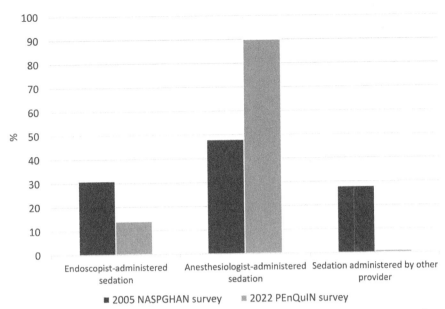

Fig. 1. Results from 2005 survey of North American Society of Pediatric Gastroenterology, Hepatology, and Nutrition (NASPGHAN) members and the 2022 survey of Pediatric Endoscopy Quality Improvement Network (PEnQuIN) working group.

developmental stage and for different procedures. For upper endoscopy, premedication with topical sprays and oral sedatives has been shown to independently improve pediatric patient tolerance and satisfaction.[25,26]

Generally speaking, the depth of sedation is directly related to cardiovascular stability; the deeper the level of sedation, the greater the risk of cardiopulmonary events (**Fig. 2**). During all sedated gastrointestinal procedures, even those being conducted with anesthesiologist assistance, pediatric endoscopists must be familiar with the fine line between achieving adequate procedural sedation and creating the potential for a child to become deeply sedated.[27] For instance, deep sedation may develop in minimally sedated patients due to delayed drug absorption or a secondary decrease in painful stimuli common to procedures (ie, after successful navigation of the hepatic flexure during ileocolonoscopy).[28,29]

Over the past two decades, it has become standard to work with an anesthesiologist to achieve deep sedation verging into general anesthesia. To some extent, this is the most reliable level of sedation to assure tolerance of the procedure without signs of distress that may include vocalization and disruptive movements. Many endoscopists who previously may have performed procedures with endoscopist-administered moderate sedation have recognized the benefits of being assured that a child is deeply sedated. However, it is important to balance these benefits with potential drawbacks, including the potential for adverse events associated with deeper sedation, longer procedure and recovery times, and greater challenges in achieving optimal patient positioning.

UNSEDATED ENDOSCOPIC PROCEDURES

Unsedated transnasal endoscopy (TNE) is increasing being used in pediatric centers in the diagnostic evaluation of a variety of upper gastrointestinal disorders.[30] During

Table 2
Depth of sedation for pediatric gastrointestinal endoscopy

	Minimal Sedation	Moderate Sedation	Deep Sedation	General Anesthesia
Response to stimuli	Normal response to verbal stimulation	Purposeful response to verbal or light tactile stimulation	Purposeful response to painful stimulation	Not arousable, even with painful stimulation
Airway reflexes	Unaffected	Adequate	May be impaired	Impaired
Spontaneous ventilation	Unaffected	Adequate	May require support	Requires support
Cardiovascular function	Unaffected	Usually maintained	Usually maintained	May be impaired

From Continuum of Depth of Sedation: Definition of General Anesthesia and Levels of Sedation/Analgesia. American Society of Anesthesiologists. Updated October 23, 2019. Accessed July 30, 2022. https://www.asahq.org/standards-and-guidelines/continuum-of-depth-of-sedation-definition-of-general-anesthesia-and-levels-of-sedationanalgesia.

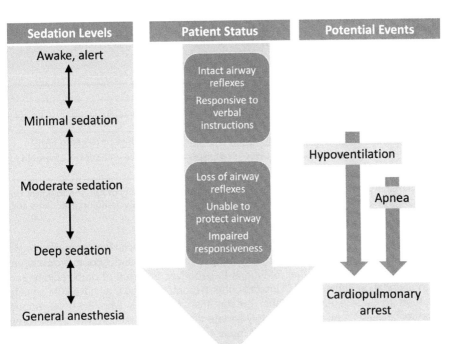

Fig. 2. Commonly used terms to describe sedation, their relationship to the continuum of sedation levels, as well as their relationship to potential adverse events.

this procedure, an ultrathin endoscope (outer diameter 2.8–6 mm; length 600–1100 mm) is inserted into the nare of an upright awake patient, and advanced through the esophagus to as far as the duodenum. Biopsies can be taken during the procedure for histologic analysis. This approach is particularly advantageous for surveillance in conditions that require repeated endoscopic assessment such as eosinophilic esophagitis (EoE), and technical success rates over 98% have been reported in pediatric EoE populations.[31] When compared with traditional upper endoscopy, TNE is associated with lower costs, fewer adverse events, and shorter recovery times.[31] An additional benefit may be the ability to perform TNE in an office setting, similar to how flexible laryngoscopies can be performed in otolaryngology clinics. Currently, widespread implementation of TNE has been limited by technical challenges and patient selection criteria. Active research into clinical strategies that improve accessibility and patient tolerance, such as that afforded by disposable equipment and intraprocedural virtual reality goggles, may ultimately make unsedated TNE more common in the future.[32]

PATIENT RISK STRATIFICATION AND AIRWAY ASSESSMENT

Sedation for pediatric gastrointestinal endoscopic procedures should be tailored to a patient's physical status, in accordance with guidelines from the American Society of Anesthesiologists (ASA) (**Table 3**).[33] Accounting for a patient's age and developmental status when choosing a sedation regimen may also improve procedural success. Data suggest that the smallest and youngest pediatric patients with the highest ASA classifications are at greatest risk for adverse events during endoscopic procedures.[11,14,34]

Table 3
American Society of Anesthesiologists classification of patients' physical status

ASA Class	Physical Status
1	A normal healthy patient
2	A patient with mild systemic disease
3	A patient with severe systemic disease
4	A patient with severe systemic disease that is a constant threat to life
5	A moribund patient who is not expected to survive without the emergent procedure

Adapted from ASA Physical Status Classification System. American Society of Anesthesiologists. Updated December 13, 2020. Accessed July 30, 2022. https://www.asahq.org/standards-and-guidelines/asa-physical-status-classification-system.

It has also been noted that age, personality, and psychosocial development stages may vary widely among children undergoing gastrointestinal endoscopic procedures, which may greatly impact their reactions to sedatives in terms of both rapidity and depth of sedation achieved.[35,36] Infants under 6 months of age may have little anxiety and tend to sedate easily. Infants greater than 6 months who have developed "stranger anxiety" may more smoothly sedate if parents remain present in the room during induction. School-aged children (ages 4–11 years) manifest "concrete thinking" and may have higher anxiety levels than may be appreciated, which can translate into the need for larger doses of sedatives.[37,38] Adolescents may be composed during preprocedure preparations and then become disinhibited and exhibit strong anxiety with initial doses of sedatives.

Engaging children in a preprocedure discussion of what to expect during endoscopy has been shown to decrease anxiety levels and may even lower procedure duration and sedative doses required for procedure completion.[36,39] Information should be imparted early in the process and include explanations about IV-line insertions. Children with greater distress during IV placement have been shown to experience significantly greater distress and pain throughout the rest of the procedure.[40] The use of topical local anesthetics for IV insertion can reduce pain and distress. Preprocedural oral, inhalational, or intranasal anxiolytics, such as midazolam, lorazepam, or nitrous oxide, are commonly used, although it is unclear if this practice objectively lowers stress levels in children.[26,40,41] Listening to music in the perioperative period has also been shown to reduce anxiety and pain in children undergoing endoscopy.[42]

Regardless of the sedation regimen used, it is also essential to perform preprocedure airway assessments. Attention to a patient's potential safety risks due to their airway should be taken at the time of scheduling a procedure and while performing it. Standardized grading scales (eg, the Mallampati score) are commonly used to assess airway risk.[43]

Currently, the decision as to which children are appropriate for endoscopist-administered procedural sedation versus anesthesiologist-administered sedation outside of the operating room often depends on a particular institution's facilities and resources.[17] To a certain extent, it may be prudent for ambulatory endoscopy centers to have stricter patient and airway criteria than academic or community hospitals, where emergency care resources may be more readily available.

Patient assessments for endoscopy in settings far from emergency care resources should also include an understanding of underlying gastrointestinal and extraintestinal disorders that may place them at high risk for adverse events.[44] In particular, patients with upper gastrointestinal bleeds, anatomic or physiologic obstruction of the upper gastrointestinal tract, recent ingestion of blood or food, and septic patients, particularly those who may need common bile duct clearance, are all at higher risk for adverse events both from the procedure and the sedation.[45] In addition, premature infants, as well as underweight, overweight, or obese older children may also be at increased sedation risks.[46] Such patients should undergo procedures in facilities that have timely access to critical care teams (eg, code teams).[19]

PATIENT POSITIONING

All patients undergoing diagnostic upper and lower endoscopic procedures with sedation should be placed in the left lateral decubitus position to start the procedure. This is because patients who are placed in the supine position are more susceptible to pooling of secretions in oral pharynx and risk upper airway obstruction or laryngospasm. As the procedure progresses, patient positioning can be adjusted to aid with scope advancement and visualization. However, it is important for all providers to realize that changing patient positioning can be more challenging when patients are more deeply sedated, or as well as in those who are receiving general anesthesia with endotracheal intubation. Patients undergoing endoscopic retrograde cholangiopancreatography may require the prone or prone-oblique position with advanced airway monitoring.

USE OF A LARYNGEAL MASK AIRWAY

A laryngeal mask airway (LMA) is a supraglotic airway device that is positioned in the hypopharynx, providing a seal over the larynx to allow spontaneous respiration while under deep sedation or general anesthesia.[47] An LMA does not protect the airway from pulmonary aspiration and is not a substitute for endotracheal intubation when indicated. The use of an LMA for upper endoscopy in children has been associated with decreased procedure times and decreased hospital times when compared with procedures done with endotracheal intubation.[48] On the other hand, deeper levels of anesthesia may be required to prevent airway stimulation caused by the LMA compared with a spontaneous breathing technique.

PATIENT MONITORING

Although visual assessments are considered to be as important as electronic monitoring for ensuring patient safety, oxygen desaturation is also a standard means of detecting poor respiratory effort in sedated children. Even if a provider has not detected suboptimal ventilation by clinical assessment, she or he will often intervene to stimulate patient respiration if a pulse oximeter detects minor desaturation. Nevertheless, it is important to recognize that oxygen desaturation is a relatively late sign of suboptimal ventilation and patients may experience significant ventilatory compromise in the setting of normal oxygen saturations.[49] Over the past 2 decades, aspiration flow technology has improved to allow capnography monitoring, with accurate real-time graphic display of ventilatory waveforms in non-intubated patients of end-tidal carbon dioxide (EtCO$_2$).[49,50] Using capnography in the pediatric endoscopy setting has revealed that abnormal ventilation occurs during procedures in children at rates higher than expected, and can be used to prompt intervention before apnea occurs.[51] Capnography may also reveal carbon dioxide (CO$_2$) retention, although ventilatory compromise during endoscopy is more likely to be reflected in abnormal capnograms than in elevated levels of CO$_2$. Capnography is now recommended as standard patient monitoring for pediatric endoscopic procedures.[19] Both endoscopists and anesthesiologists using capnography should also be mindful that the use of CO_2 for insufflation during endoscopic procedures can be associated with transient spikes in $EtCO_2$ of unclear clinical significance.[52]

COMMON SEDATIVES USED FOR CHILDREN UNDERGOING ENDOSCOPY

Several sedation regimens have been reported to be safe and relatively efficacious for children undergoing procedures.[53] **Table 4** lists commonly used sedatives for pediatric gastrointestinal endoscopic procedures and their recommended dosages. In general, the most common moderate procedural sedation regimens used for pediatric endoscopy combine a narcotic analgesic (eg, meperidine or fentanyl), which offers the benefit of analgesia, with a benzodiazepine (eg., diazepam or midazolam), which provides anxiolysis and amnesia. There are also some reports of the use of ketamine to achieve moderate sedation for pediatric endoscopy, which renders patients immobile and mute, while still having awareness of the procedure.[54] Most deep sedation regimens and general anesthesia for endoscopy currently use propofol as a mainstay sedative. Propofol is an ultra-short-acting anesthetic that can be used to induce and maintain a spectrum of sedation levels, ranging from moderate sedation to general anesthesia.

Table 5 lists drug-specific side-effects associated with various sedatives and rescue agents. Regardless of regimen used, it is imperative that pediatric endoscopists respect the potential for oversedation, and its risks of morbidity and mortality. In particular, it is a key to understand that all sedatives have the potential to significantly depress the central nervous system. This may compromise airway protective reflexes, increasing the risk for aspiration, as well as ventilatory responses to CO_2. In turn, patients may develop apnea, which can progress to CO_2 retention and hypoxemia. Ultimately, the body may develop tissue ischemia and significant cardiovascular compromise.

Fentanyl

As a fat-soluble narcotic that rapidly penetrates the blood brain barrier, fentanyl is considerably more potent and fast acting than both morphine and meperidine. Its onset of action is about 30 seconds, and its opioid effects last about 30 to 45 minutes. Fentanyl should always be given to children via slow IV push, as its rapid administration has been associated with dangerous side effects of chest wall and glottic rigidity.[55] Fentanyl is variably metabolized by the liver, especially in young children, and is most safely administered to children in small increments allowing for several minutes between each dose. Several studies have suggested that fentanyl may not represent an ideal sedative for infants. In particular, it has been associated with significant apnea in infants less than 3 months of age.[56] Also, delayed fentanyl excretion has been reported in neonates with compromised hepatic blood flow.[57]

Midazolam

Midazolam is 3 to 6 times more potent than diazepam, with an onset of action of 1 to 5 minutes, and peak effect achieved at about 30 minutes to 1 hour. Several pharmacokinetic studies have suggested that midazolam may be metabolized and excreted more rapidly in children than adults.[26,58,59] In addition, midazolam is relatively unique among benzodiazepines in that its clearance seems to be dose-related, with increased clearance with increased dosage.[60] Both metabolic facts may explain why pediatric gastroenterologists have reported the need to give larger weight-

Table 4

Recommendations for dosages of drugs commonly used for intravenous sedation for pediatric gastrointestinal endoscopic procedures, including reversal agents for benzodiazepines and opioids

Sedatives	Route	Maximum Dose (mg/kg)	Time to Onset (min)	Duration of Action (min)
Benzodiazepines				
Diazepam	IV	0.1–0.3	1–3	15–30
	Rectal	0.2–0.3	2–10	15–30
Midazolam	Oral	0.5–0.75	15–30	60–90
	IV	0.05–0.15	2–3	45–60
	Rectal	0.5–0.75	10–30	60–90
Opioids				
Meperidine	IV	1–3	<5	2–4
	IM	1–3	10–15	2–3
Fentanyl	IV	0.001–0.005 (1–5 μgm/kg in 0.5–1.0 μgm/kg increments)	2–3	30–60
Ketamine	IV	1–3	1	15–60
	IM	2–10	3–5	15–150

Reversal Agents	Route	Maximum Dose (mg/kg)	Time to Onset (min)	Duration of Action (min)
For Benzodiazepines				
Flumazenil	IV	3 mg/h	1–2	<60
For Opioids				
Naloxone	IV	0.1	2–5	20–60
	IM	0.1	2–5	20–60

Table 5
Common agents for procedural sedation in endoscopy and their side effects

Class/Name	Potential Side Effects/Complications
Topical	
Benzocaine	Methemoglobinemia
Lidocaine	Potential for systemic absorption and toxicity
Benzodiazepines	
Diazepam	Respiratory depression; apnea; thrombophlebitis
Midazolam	Respiratory depression; apnea
Opioids	
Meperidine	Respiratory and central nervous system depression; seizures; nausea; vomiting
Fentanyl	Apnea, bradycardia; chest wall and glottic rigidity
Ketamine	Emergence delirium; increased airway secretions; laryngospasm
Propofol	Rapid progression to general anesthesia; impaired gastrointestinal contractility
Antagonists	
Flumazenil	Short duration of action; resedation
Naloxone	Catecholamine release, tachyarrhythmias, sudden death

adjusted doses to their patients than adult gastroenterologists to achieve similar levels and duration of sedation.[61]

Ketamine

Ketamine is a dissociative agent that largely spares upper airway muscular tone and laryngeal reflexes. It is contraindicated in patients less than 3 months of age, as well as those with histories of airway instability, tracheal abnormalities, active pulmonary disease, cardiovascular disease, head injury, central nervous system masses, hydrocephalus, porphyria, and thyroid disease.[62] Ketamine is also contraindicated in patients with a history of psychosis, as its traditional main drawback has been its association with hallucinogenic emergence reactions in some children.[63] Ketamine has been associated with increased airway secretions and increased incidence of postoperative nausea and vomiting and has also been highly associated with laryngospasm during both upper and lower gastrointestinal endoscopic procedures.[23,54,64,65]

Propofol

Having a patient breathe spontaneously, without endotracheal intubation, while under a propofol-based general anesthetic, is perhaps the most common approach to sedating children for pediatric endoscopy. A wide spectrum of sedation levels can be targeted with propofol, and it has been shown in multiple studies to be highly effective at inducing sedation in children who are undergoing both upper and lower endoscopy.[9,66,67] Propofol may be administered either as a total IV anesthetic or in combination with inhalational agents.[68]

Children who receive propofol have shorter induction times than children who received midazolam and fentanyl. Nevertheless, evidence does not show that this faster induction time leads to improved procedural efficiency in pediatric endoscopy units.[10] The disconnect between shorter induction time and procedural efficiency may be in large part secondary to indisputable variation in anesthesiology practice regarding endotracheal intubation for airway protection during propofol sedation for pediatric endoscopic procedures.[2] Although endotracheal intubation may be necessary during therapeutic procedures, most children do not require endotracheal intubation to perform routine diagnostic endoscopy.[2,9]

Indications for endotracheal intubation with administration of propofol

Determining if a patient requires endotracheal intubation is a major decision that should be made in open dialogue between endoscopists and anesthesiologists during sedation planning. Children at known risk for pulmonary aspiration, or with underlying issues that increase their risk of airway obstruction, require endotracheal intubation. Procedures that are longer and more invasive have the potential to cause greater airway stimulation, and thus intubation should be considered. Although many anesthesiology practitioners routinely intubate infants and toddler aged children to prevent airway adverse events, there is no evidence that intubation increases patient safety, or is advantageous in other ways, in this specific age group.

Propofol infusion without endotracheal intubation for pediatric endoscopy

It is important to recognize that it is possible and perhaps preferable, to use a propofol-based regimen for pediatric endoscopic procedures without performing endotracheal intubation. In these cases, patients typically receive a mask anesthetic induction with a volatile anesthetic gas for IV catheter placement, if not already present. An IV induction dose of propofol of 1 to 2 mg/kg is then administered, followed by initiation of a propofol infusion intended to maintain anesthesia. Generally speaking, high doses in the range of 100 to 300 mcg/kg/min are required to provide ideal conditions for endoscopic procedures in pediatric patients. Pharmacokinetic studies of children who have received propofol demonstrate that average total propofol doses per kilogram of body weight to achieve targeted plasma propofol concentrations are higher in younger children.[69]

Of course, an important pharmacologic disadvantage of propofol is its relatively narrow therapeutic range, characterized by a very small difference between an ideal depth of anesthesia and respiratory depression. For this reason, providing a bolus of propofol for inadequate anesthesia may result in apnea, which has been reported in up to 20% of pediatric patients receiving anesthesiologist administered propofol for upper endoscopy.[67]

Propofol sedation for pediatric upper endoscopy

Once an appropriate level of anesthesia is attained, any anesthetic gas can be discontinued, a nasal cannula or mask equipped with CO_2 monitoring should be taped into place, a pediatric bite block inserted. If possible, the patient is ideally placed in the lateral decubitus position to minimize risks of aspiration. In situations involving a total intraveous anesthetic (TIVA) regimen, the patient can be placed into this position prior to administering the propofol. Assistance by the anesthesiology provider in extending the patient's neck can then help facilitate passage of the endoscope during upper endoscopy. Maintaining a manual jaw thrust during the entire procedure may be appropriate to keep the airway patent, and for many anesthesiologists, the provision of active airway management by using jaw thrusts or chin tilts has become a standard component of sedation care during pediatric endoscopy.

Topical lidocaine before propofol sedation

It is helpful to anticipate that insertion of the endoscope will typically be the most stimulating part of an upper endoscopy for a sedated patient. In turn, a common clinical practice is to use topical lidocaine as a local anesthetic before the start of the procedure. With the patient in a sitting position, a tongue depressor is used, and the patient is instructed to phonate "ahh" to expose the posterior oral pharynx and base of the tongue. The first spray is straight back into the oral pharynx. The second spray is directed 90° downward to anesthetize the hypopharynx and the glottic structures. Staying within maximal mg/kg lidocaine doses and avoiding the routine use of benzocaine in children can avoid the toxicity of local anesthetics.

Propofol sedation for pediatric ileocolonoscopy

A propofol-based regimen for a spontaneously breathing patient intended to provide deep sedation verging on general anesthesia is well suited for lower endoscopic procedures.[70] In ileocolonoscopy, the risk of airway compromise still exists, but it is greatly reduced compared with upper endoscopy as the airway is not being stimulated. On the other hand, ileocolonoscopy may be more painful than upper endoscopy. Loop formation of the scope in the colon, as well as loop reduction maneuvers, may cause pain and patient movement, leading to increased sedation requirements.

For this reason, propofol sedation for ileocolonoscopy can be optimized by standard use of an opioid, typically fentanyl 0.5 mcg/kg, as opposed to using propofol alone, which may require high doses to keep patients from reacting to pain, thus increasing risk of respiratory depression and apnea.[71] A balanced sedation/anesthetic with propofol and an opioid ideally will maximize the benefits of a combination of agents while minimizing the unwanted side effects of specific agents. Of course, opioids themselves can cause hypoventilation in a dose-dependent way, but careful weight-based dosing and titration in children should result in the desired balanced effect. The use of IV lidocaine administered in conjunction with propofol has also been described to reduce the propofol requirement and improve pain management during pediatric ileocolonoscopy.[72]

Emergence from propofol sedation

Propofol infusions for endoscopic procedures are commonly stopped approximately 5 to 10 minutes before complete withdrawal of the scope. The child is kept in the lateral decubitus position until the endoscope is withdrawn, and bite block removed. Assuming a spontaneous breathing technique was used (ie, no endotracheal intubation was performed), the patient can then be transported to the postanesthetic care unit (PACU) with supplemental oxygen while still asleep. In many respects, the fact that no extubation or emergence is required in the procedure room is one of the efficiency benefits of using the spontaneously breathing technique. Once in the PACU, the patient can continue to slowly emerge from their sedated state.

Propofol with endotracheal intubation

Endotracheal intubation is indicated during propofol sedation regimens in patients at risk for aspiration. Patients with airway abnormalities that predispose to obstruction should also have their airways secured with an endotracheal tube. Patients that require endotracheal intubation for non-aspiration indications can be induced and intubated using standard anesthetic techniques. Children with the potential for full-esophageal column reflux during procedural sedation, as well as those who may require procedures despite likely esophageal or gastric contents (ie, patients with achalasia, or those who require emergency button battery removal, and so forth) may be appropriate candidates for a rapid sequence induction to minimize the risk of pulmonary aspiration with the induction of general anesthesia.[22,73]

Propofol for very small pediatric patients

Given the potential for increased anesthetic risk, many experienced pediatric practitioners choose to routinely intubate infants and toddlers.[11] The decision to intubate very small pediatric patients should be weighed against risks of instrumenting the airway, potentially causing inflammation or trauma, and possibly increasing the incidence of postoperative airway adverse events. There is no consensus among pediatric anesthesiologists concerning an age cutoff to routinely intubate patients. Rather, it is important to recognize that the routine intubation of all children, including very young children, undergoing upper endoscopic procedures is not supported in the anesthesia literature.[74] In addition, it can make patient position changes, to aid with scope advancement or visualization, more difficult.

Non-anesthesiologist administered propofol for children
Non-anesthesiologist Administered Propofol Sedation (NAAPS) is an acronym used to describe the administration of propofol under the direction of a physician by an appropriately qualified registered nurse or physician who has not been trained as an anesthesiologist.[74] In NAAPS, propofol may be used either alone or in combination with one or more other agents, and a level of moderate-to-deep sedation is targeted. A growing body of recent literature has described experiences with NAAPS in pediatric endoscopy, where propofol is administered either by pediatric endoscopists or hospitalists as part of a sedation team.[75,76]

RESCUE STRATEGIES FOR SEDATION-RELATED ADVERSE EVENTS

The depth of sedation occurs along a continuum, and clinicians providing sedation must be prepared for children transitioning into a state of sedation that is deeper than originally intended. A fundamental skill in providing sedation is the ability to recognize and rescue patients from its related adverse events. Reversal agents are available for benzodiazepines and narcotics and should be used in cases of oversedation due these agents. There are no reversal agents for other sedatives routinely used for pediatric endoscopy, including ketamine and propofol. **Table 4** lists reversal agents and their recommended dosages for children. Of note, reversal effects are nearly always shorter than the effects of the sedatives being reversed. As such, most endoscopy guidelines stipulate that patients who receive a dose of a reversal agent should be monitored for an extended period and should be administered repeat doses if necessary.

Regardless of type of sedation used, or anesthesiologist presence, emergency airway equipment should be immediately and easily accessible wherever gastrointestinal endoscopic procedures are performed.[19] In particular, all pediatric sizes of LMAs and endotracheal tubes, bag valve masks for delivering positive pressure ventilation, laryngoscopes, nasopharyngeal and oropharyngeal tubes, and suction equipment should be stocked. Finally, all pediatric endoscopists should ideally be trained in emergency patient ventilation techniques.[4]

SUMMARY

Sedation is a fundamental component of pediatric endoscopy that has evolved dramatically over the past 5 decades, as gastrointestinal endoscopic procedures have become more commonly performed in children around the world. Although patient safety must be always be prioritized, there has also been growing imperatives to consider efficiencies and costs in various sedation practices. The undeniable shift over the past 20 years to providing propofol-based anesthesiologist-administered sedation for pediatric endoscopy is evident in international surveys of endoscopic practice. However, this trend has not led to increased patient safety. Instead, it is important for pediatric endoscopists to recognize that employment of anesthesiologists to provide endoscopic sedation does not excuse them from remaining comfortable with fundamental sedation principles and common regimens, or from engaging in open dialogue with their anesthesiology colleagues about best sedation practices. It is equally critical that anesthesiologists become knowledgeable about various types of pediatric endoscopic procedures, and avoid unwarranted variations in anesthesia care that can detract from procedural quality and compromise patient safety. Both pediatric endoscopists and anesthesiology providers should know the benefits and risks associated with various sedation regimens for pediatric gastrointestinal endoscopic procedures and strive to work together to optimize patient outcomes.

CLINICS CARE POINTS

- Anesthesiologist-administered propofol sedation has become the most widely used sedative regimen for pediatric endoscopy.
- General anesthesia with endotracheal intubation is generally not necessary for routine diagnostic pediatric endoscopic procedures.
- Adverse events related to sedation, regardless of whether the sedation is administered by an endoscopist or anesthesiologist, occur more commonly during pediatric endoscopy than adverse events related to technical aspects of procedures.
- The depth of sedation occurs along a continuum, ranging from minimal sedation to general anesthesia; the deeper the sedation, the greater the potential for cardiorespiratory compromise.
- Clinicians providing sedation for pediatric endoscopy must be prepared both for children transitioning into a level of sedation deeper than originally intended, and to recognize and be able to rescue patients from sedation-related adverse events.
- Open communication between endoscopists and anesthesiologists about sedation planning for pediatric gastrointestinal procedures continues to be essential to identify best sedation practices and optimize patient outcomes.

DISCLOSURE

J.R. Lightdale: Mead-Johnson (advisory board), Perrigo (advisory board), Sanofi (advisory board); L.B. Mahoney: Nothing to disclose.

REFERENCES

1. Walsh CM, Lightdale JR, Mack DR, et al. Overview of the pediatric endoscopy quality improvement network quality standards and indicators for pediatric endoscopy: a joint NASPGHAN/ESPGHAN guideline. J Pediatr Gastroenterol Nutr 2022;74(S1):S3–15.
2. Hartjes KT, Dafonte TM, Lee AF, et al. Variation in pediatric anesthesiologist sedation practices for pediatric gastrointestinal endoscopy. Front Pediatr 2021;9: 709433.
3. Kamat PP, McCracken CE, Simon HK, et al. Trends in outpatient procedural sedation: 2007–2018. Pediatrics 2020;145(5):e20193559.
4. AASLD, ACG, AGA, et al. Multisociety sedation curriculum for gastrointestinal endoscopy. Gastrointest Endosc 2012;76(1):e1–25.
5. ASGE Standards of Practice Committee, Early DS, Lightdale JR, et al. Guidelines for sedation and anesthesia in GI endoscopy. Gastrointest Endosc 2018;87(2): 327–37.

6. Sheahan CG, Mathews DM. Monitoring and delivery of sedation. BJA Br J Anaesth 2014;113(suppl_2):ii37–47.

7. ASGE Standards of Practice Committee, Lightdale JR, Acosta R, et al. Modifications in endoscopic practice for pediatric patients. Gastrointest Endosc 2014; 79(5):699–710.

8. Lightdale JR, Valim C, Mahoney LB, et al. Agitation during procedural sedation and analgesia in children. Clin Pediatr 2010;49(1):35–42.

9. van Beek EJAH, Leroy PLJM. Safe and effective procedural sedation for gastrointestinal endoscopy in children. J Pediatr Gastroenterol Nutr 2012;54(2):171–85.

10. Lightdale JR, Valim C, Newburg AR, et al. Efficiency of propofol versus midazolam and fentanyl sedation at a pediatric teaching hospital: a prospective study. Gastrointest Endosc 2008;67(7):1067–75.

11. Biber JL, Allareddy V, Allareddy V, et al. Prevalence and predictors of adverse events during procedural sedation anesthesia-outside the operating room for esophagogastroduodenoscopy and colonoscopy in children. Pediatr Crit Care Me 2015;16(8):e251–9.

12. Ament ME, Christie DL. Upper gastrointestinal fiberoptic endoscopy in pediatric patients. Gastroenterology 1977;72(6):1244–8.

13. Gilger MA, Jeiven SD, Barrish JO, et al. Oxygen desaturation and cardiac arrhythmias in children during esophagogastroduodenoscopy using conscious sedation. Gastrointest Endosc 1993;39(3):392–5.

14. Thakkar K, El-Serag HB, Mattek N, et al. Complications of pediatric EGD: a 4-year experience in PEDS-CORI. Gastrointest Endosc 2007;65(2):213–21.

15. Mamula P, Markowitz JE, Neiswender K, et al. Safety of intravenous midazolam and fentanyl for pediatric GI endoscopy: prospective study of 1578 endoscopies. Gastrointest Endosc 2007;65(2):203–10.

16. The U.S. Food and Drug Administration. FDA Drug Safety Communication: FDA review results in new warnings about using general anesthetics and sedation drugs in young children and pregnant women. 2017. Available at: https://www. fda.gov/drugs/drug-safety-and-availability/fda-drug-safety-communication-fda-review-results-new-warnings-about-using-general-anesthetics-and.   Accessed February 15, 2023.

17. Orel R, Brecelj J, Dias JA, et al. Review on sedation for gastrointestinal tract endoscopy in children by non-anesthesiologists. World J Gastrointest Endosc 2015;7(9):895–911.

18. Lightdale JR. Sedation for pediatric endoscopy. Tech Gastrointest Endosc 2013; 15(1):3–8.

19. Lightdale JR, Walsh CM, Narula P, et al. Pediatric endoscopy quality improvement network quality standards and indicators for pediatric endoscopy facilities: a joint NASPGHAN/ESPGHAN guideline. J Pediatr Gastroenterol Nutr 2022; 74(S1):S16–29.

20. Walsh CM, Lightdale JR. Pediatric endoscopy quality improvement network (PEnQuIN) quality standards and indicators for pediatric endoscopy: an ASGE-endorsed guideline. Gastrointest Endosc 2022;96(4):593–602.

21. Lightdale JR, Mahoney LB, Schwarz SM, et al. Methods of sedation in pediatric endoscopy: a survey of NASPGHAN members. J Pediatr Gastroenterol Nutr 2007;45(4):500–2.

22. Chung HK, Lightdale JR. Sedation and monitoring in the pediatric patient during gastrointestinal endoscopy. Gastrointest Endosc Clin N Am 2016;26(3):507–25.

23. Miqdady MIS, Hayajneh WA, Abdelhadi R, et al. Ketamine and midazolam sedation for pediatric gastrointestinal endoscopy in the Arab world. World J Gastroentero 2011;17(31):3630–5.

24. American Society of Anesthesiologists. Continuum of depth of sedation: definition of general anesthesia and levels of sedation/analgesia. Available at: https://www.asahq.org/standards-and-guidelines/continuum-of-depth-of-sedation-definition-of-general-anesthesia-and-levels-of-sedationanalgesia. Accessed February 15, 2023.

25. Fox V. Upper gastrointestinal endoscopy. Walker W.A.Durie P.R.Hamilton J.R. et. al.Pediatric gastrointestinal disease: pathophysiology, diagnosis, management. St Louis, MO: Mosby; 2000. p. 1514–32.

26. Liacouras CA, Mascarenhas M, Poon C, et al. Placebo-controlled trial assessing the use of oral midazolam as a premedication to conscious sedation for pediatric endoscopy. Gastrointest Endosc 1998;47(6):455–60.

27. American Society of Anesthesiologists. Distinguishing Monitored Anesthesia Care ("MAC") from Moderate Sedation/Analgesia (Conscious Sedation). Available at: https://www.asahq.org/standards-and-guidelines/distinguishing-monitored-anesthesia-care-mac-from-moderate-sedationanalgesia-conscious-sedation. Accessed February 15, 2023.

28. Mahoney LB, Lightdale JR. Sedation of the pediatric and adolescent patient for GI procedures. Curr Treat Options Gastroenterol 2007;10(5):412–21.

29. Dial S, Silver P, Bock K, et al. Pediatric sedation for procedures titrated to a desired degree of immobility results in unpredictable depth of sedation. Pediatr Emerg Care 2001;17(6):414–20.

30. Venkatesh RD, Leinwand K, Nguyen N. Pediatric unsedated transnasal endoscopy. Gastrointest Endosc Clin N Am 2023;33(2):267–79.

31. Nguyen N, Mark J, Furuta GT. Emerging role of transnasal endoscopy in children and adults. Clin Gastroenterol H 2021;20(3):501–4.

32. Nguyen N, Lavery WJ, Capocelli KE, et al. Transnasal endoscopy in unsedated children with eosinophilic esophagitis using virtual reality video goggles. Clin Gastroenterol H 2019;17(12):2455–62.

33. American Society of Anesthesiologists. ASA physical status classification system. Available at: https://www.asahq.org/standards-and-guidelines/asa-physical-status-classification-system. Accessed February 15, 2023.

34. Peck J, Brown J, Fierstein JL, et al. Comparison of general endotracheal anesthesia vs. sedation without endotracheal intubation during initial PEG insertion for infants: a retrospective cohort study. Pediatr Anesth 2022;32(12):1310–9.

35. Kupietzky A. Treating very young patients with conscious sedation and medical immobilization: a Jewish perspective. Alpha Omegan 2005;98(4):33–7.

36. Gilger MA. Conscious sedation for endoscopy in the pediatric patient. Gastroenterol Nurs 1993;16(2):75–9.

37. Squires RH, Morriss F, Schluterman S, et al. Efficacy, safety, and cost of intravenous sedation versus general anesthesia in children undergoing endoscopic procedures. Gastrointest Endosc 1995;41(2):99–104.

38. Choi YJ, Park EJ, Lee YM, et al. Effects of anxiety on sedation among pediatric patients undergoing esophagogastroduodenoscopy. Clin Child Psychol P 2022;27(3):793–803.

39. Volkan B, Bayrak NA, Ucar C, et al. Preparatory information reduces gastroscopy-related stress in children as confirmed by salivary cortisol. Saudi J Gastroenterol 2019;25(4):262–7.

40. Claar RL, Walker LS, Barnard JA. Children's knowledge, anticipatory anxiety, procedural distress, and recall of esophagogastroduodenoscopy. J Pediatr Gastroenterol Nutr 2002;34(1):68–72.
41. Chennou F, Bonneau-Fortin A, Portolese O, et al. Oral lorazepam is not superior to placebo for lowering stress in children before digestive endoscopy: a double-blind, randomized, controlled trial. Pediatr Drugs 2019;21(5):379–87.
42. Bay C, Henriquez R, Villarroel L, et al. Effect of music on pediatric endoscopic examinations: a randomized controlled trial. Endosc Int Open 2021;09(04): E599–605.
43. Mallampati SR, Gatt SP, Gugino LD, et al. A clinical sign to predict difficult tracheal intubation; a prospective study. Can Anaesth Soc J 1985;32(4):429–34.
44. Lightdale JR, Liu QY, Sahn B, et al. Pediatric endoscopy and high-risk patients: a clinical report from the NASPGHAN endoscopy committee. J Pediatr Gastroenterol Nutr 2019;68(4):595–606.
45. Beach ML, Cohen DM, Gallagher SM, et al. Major adverse events and relationship to nil per os status in pediatric sedation/anesthesia outside the operating room. Anesthesiology 2016;124(1):80–8.
46. Najafi N, Veyckemans F, Vanhonacker D, et al. Incidence and risk factors for adverse events during monitored anaesthesia care for gastrointestinal endoscopy in children: a prospective observational study. Eur J Anaesth 2019;36(6): 390–9.
47. Lopez-Gil M, Brimacombe J, Diaz-Reganon G. Anesthesia for pediatric gastroscopy: a study comparing the ProSeal laryngeal mask airway with nasal cannulae. Pediatr Anesth 2006;16(10):1032–5.
48. Acquaviva MA, Horn ND, Gupta SK. Endotracheal intubation versus laryngeal mask airway for esophagogastroduodenoscopy in children. J Pediatr Gastroenterol Nutr 2014;59(1):54–6.
49. Vargo JJ, Zuccaro G, Dumot JA, et al. Automated graphic assessment of respiratory activity is superior to pulse oximetry and visual assessment for the detection of early respiratory depression during therapeutic upper endoscopy. Gastrointest Endosc 2002;55(7):826–31.
50. Colman Y, Krauss B. Microstream capnograpy technology: a new approach to an old problem. J Clin Monit Comput 1999;15(6):403–9.
51. Lightdale JR, Goldmann DA, Feldman HA, et al. Microstream capnography improves patient monitoring during moderate sedation: a randomized, controlled trial. Pediatrics 2006;117(6):e1170–8.
52. Dike CR, Rahhal R, Bishop WP. Is carbon dioxide insufflation during endoscopy in children as safe and as effective as we think? J Pediatr Gastroenterol Nutr 2020; 71(2):211–5.
53. Tolia V, Peters JM, Gilger MA. Sedation for pediatric endoscopic procedures. J Pediatr Gastroenterol Nutr 2000;30(5):477–85.
54. Lightdale JR, Mitchell PD, Fredette ME, et al. a pilot study of ketamine versus midazolam/fentanyl sedation in children undergoing GI endoscopy. Int J Pediatr 2011;2011:623710.
55. Arandia HY, Patil VU. Glottic closure following large doses of fentanyl. Anesthesiology 1987;66(4):574–5.
56. Balsells F, Wyllie R, Kay M, et al. Use of conscious sedation for lower and upper gastrointestinal endoscopic examinations in children, adolescents, and young adults: a twelve-year review. Gastrointest Endosc 1997;45(5):375–80.
57. Koehntop DE, Rodman JH, Brundage DM, et al. Pharmacokinetics of Fentanyl in Neonates. Anesth Analg 1986;65(3):227.

58. Tolia V, Brennan S, Aravind MK, et al. Pharmacokinetic and pharmacodynamic study of midazolam in children during esophagogastroduodenoscopy. J Pediatr 1991;119(3):467–71.
59. Salonen M, Kanto J, Iisalo E, et al. Midazolam as an induction agent in children: a pharmacokinetic and clinical study. Anesth Analg 1987;66(7):625.
60. Jacobsen J, Flachs H, Dich-Nielsen JO, et al. Comparative plasma concentration profiles after I.V., I.M. and rectal administration of pethidine in children. BJA Br J Anaesth 1988;60(6):623–6.
61. Gremse DA, Kumar S, Sacks AI. Conscious sedation with high-dose midazolam for pediatric gastrointestinal endoscopy. Southampt Med J 1997;90(8):821–5.
62. Green SM, Nakamura R, Johnson NE. Ketamine sedation for pediatric procedures: part 1, a prospective series. Ann Emerg Med 1990;19(9):1024–32.
63. Motamed F, Aminpour Y, Hashemian H, et al. Midazolam-ketamine combination for moderate sedation in upper GI endoscopy. J Pediatr Gastroenterol Nutr 2012;54(3):422–6.
64. Gilger MA, Spearman RS, Dietrich CL, et al. Safety and effectiveness of ketamine as a sedative agent for pediatric GI endoscopy. Gastrointest Endosc 2004;59(6):659–63.
65. Green SM, Klooster M, Harris T, et al. Ketamine sedation for pediatric gastroenterology procedures. J Pediatr Gastroenterol Nutr 2001;32(1):26–33.
66. Khoshoo V, Thoppil D, Landry L, et al. Propofol versus midazolam plus meperidine for sedation during ambulatory esophagogastroduodenoscopy. J Pediatr Gastroenterol Nutr 2003;37(2):146–9.
67. Kaddu R, Bhattacharya D, Metriyakool K, et al. Propofol compared with general anesthesia for pediatric GI endoscopy: Is propofol better? Gastrointest Endosc 2002;55(1):27–32.
68. Elitsur Y, Blankenship P, Lawrence Z. Propofol sedation for endoscopic procedures in children. Endoscopy 2000;32(10):788–91.
69. Schüttler J, Ihmsen H. Population pharmacokinetics of propofol: a multicenter study. Anesthesiology 2000;92(3):727–38.
70. Cohen S, Glatstein MM, Scolnik D, et al. Propofol for pediatric colonoscopy: the experience of a large, tertiary care pediatric hospital. Am J Ther 2013;21(6):509–11.
71. VanNatta ME, Rex DK. Propofol alone titrated to deep sedation versus propofol in combination with opioids and/or benzodiazepines and titrated to moderate sedation for colonoscopy. Am J Gastroenterol 2006;101(10):2209–17.
72. Yao W, Zhang L, Lu G, et al. Use of intravenous lidocaine for dose reduction of propofol in paediatric colonoscopy patients: a randomised placebo-controlled study. Bmc Anesthesiol 2021;21(1):299.
73. Engelhardt T, Weiss M. A child with a difficult airway: what do I do next? Curr Opin Anesthesio 2012;25(3):326.
74. Rajasekaran S, Hackbarth RM, Davis AT, et al. The safety of propofol sedation for elective nonintubated esophagogastroduodenoscopy in pediatric patients. Pediatr Crit Care Me 2014;15(6):e261–9.
75. Khalila A, Shavit I, Shaoul R. Propofol sedation by pediatric gastroenterologists for endoscopic procedures: a retrospective analysis. Front Pediatr 2019;7:98.
76. Lee FC, Queliza K, Chumpitazi BP, et al. Outcomes of non-anesthesiologist-administered propofol in pediatric gastroenterology procedures. Front Pediatr 2021;8:619139.

Enhancing Ergonomics in Pediatric Endoscopy Training and Practice

Catharine M. Walsh, MD, MEd, PhD

KEYWORDS

- Ergonomics • Pediatric endoscopy • Musculoskeletal injury • Endoscopy unit
- Injury prevention • Occupational safety • Personal protective equipment
- Gastrointestinal endoscopy

KEY POINTS

- Performing endoscopy places unique strains on the body which are known risk factors for workplace injuries.
- Ergonomics is the science of designing a job to fit the breadth of workers so that work is safer and more efficient, rather than obliging individuals to fit themselves to a job.
- Incorporation of ergonomic principles into pediatric endoscopic training and practice is essential to minimize risks to the endoscopist, patients, and the entire endoscopy team.
- Institutions can foster a culture of safety by implementing policies and practices which promote injury prevention, such as mandating a pre-procedure ergonomic time-out, and by proactively maintaining equipment to ensure it is functioning optimally.
- To optimize endoscopist interactions with their work environment, an endoscopy suite should be adjustable, including the bed, video monitor, and endoscopy tower.
- At the endoscopist level, personal controls that can be used to mitigate the risk of endoscopy-related injuries include the use of ergonomically favorable technique, being mindful of positioning during endoscopy, maintenance of physical fitness, and personal accessories such as compression stockings.

 Video content accompanies this article at http://www.giendo.theclinics.com.

INTRODUCTION

Performing endoscopy places unique strains on the body, which are known risk factors for work-related injuries. Incorporation of ergonomic principles into pediatric endoscopic training and practice is essential to minimize risk to the endoscopist,

Division of Gastroenterology, Hepatology and Nutrition and the SickKids Research and Learning Institutes, The Hospital for Sick Children, Department of Paediatrics and The Wilson Centre, Temerty Faculty of Medicine, University of Toronto, 555 University Avenue, Toronto, ON M5G 1X8, Canada
E-mail address: catharine.walsh@utoronto.ca

Gastrointest Endoscopy Clin N Am 33 (2023) 235–251
https://doi.org/10.1016/j.giec.2022.12.002
1052-5157/23/© 2022 Elsevier Inc. All rights reserved.

patients, and the entire endoscopy team. Ergonomics, as applied to pediatric endoscopy, can be defined as the study of endoscopists' interactions with elements of their work environment, including the endoscope and endoscopy unit, and how these can be intentionally designed to minimize the risk of endoscopy-related musculoskeletal injury (ERI), optimize endoscopist well-being, and maximize overall system performance.[1,2] Ergonomics focuses on devising a job to fit the breadth of workers so that work is safer and more efficient, rather than obliging individuals to fit themselves to a job.

This state-of-the-art review outlines the scope of ERIs in pediatric practice, describes risk factors for ERIs including design flaws of the endoscope and system-based contributors to injury, and discusses key ergonomic principles that can be used to mitigate injury risk. It also outlines tips for integrating education on endoscopy ergonomics during training, with the aim of promoting the development of safe and effective technique at the beginning of endoscopists' careers to enhance endoscopist safety and help extend career lifespans.

EPIDEMIOLOGY

Endoscopy makes up a significant part of many pediatric gastroenterologists' clinical practice, with the majority of pediatric gastroenterologists performing more than four procedures per week.[3] Endoscopy is a complex, physically demanding skill that requires prolonged periods of standing, repetitive movements, sustained high right-thumb pinch forces and non-neutral body positioning, all of which place the endoscopist at high risk of musculoskeletal injury.[4] In particular, the combination of repetition along with potential high forces on the forearms, wrists, and thumbs during manipulation of the dials and insertion tube and on the neck and back from looking at the monitor can lead to strain, microtrauma, and overuse injuries.[4–6]

ERIs are common among pediatric endoscopists. A recent survey-based study of 146 pediatric gastroenterologists who attended the 2019 North American Society of Pediatric Gastroenterology, Hepatology, and Nutrition annual meeting reported a high prevalence of endoscopy-related musculoskeletal pain and injury, with 36.5% (35/95) of faculty and 30.0% (15/29) trainees reporting an injury attributable to endoscopy.[3] These rates are only slightly lower than those reported in the adult survey-based literature, which indicates that between 39% and 95% of practicing adult endoscopists[7–9] and 20%–54.8% of trainees[10–12] have experienced musculoskeletal injuries. Similar to adult endoscopists, the most common sites of injury reported by pediatric endoscopists with an ERI were the neck and upper back, thumb, hands and fingers, and lower back.[3]

Risks factors for endoscopy-related injury that have been noted in the adult literature include higher procedure volumes, specifically more than 20 cases or greater than 16 hours of procedures per week, and cumulative time performing endoscopy.[7,8,13] In the recent pediatric study, no relationship was found between injury and number of years performing endoscopy, procedure volume, or duration.[3] These findings likely reflect the overall lower procedural volumes in pediatrics. One adult study also found that prior injury is a risk factor for subsequent injury, which speaks to the importance of preventative care and identifying issues before they become problematic.[14]

Research examining the relationship between gender and injury risk in adult practice has yielded mixed results.[7,15] The most recent and largest study of 1277 adult endoscopists found no difference in the overall prevalence of ERI between men and women.[7] Alternatively, gender was found to be associated with ERI among pediatric gastroenterologists (43.4% of men vs. 23.4% of women; $P = 0.013$).[3] Among both pediatric and adult gastroenterologists, gender-based differences in injury location have been noted. Female pediatric endoscopists were significantly more likely to report pain in their hands, fingers and shoulders compared with their male counterparts.[3] Similar results have been seen in adult-based studies, with women reporting more upper extremity and upper back ERI.[7,12]

Although the reasons underlying gender-based variations in ERIs have not been evaluated systematically, differences in hand size and grip and pinch force may require female endoscopists to exert more effort to generate equivalent force.[6,16] Individuals with smaller hand sizes report greater difficulty in learning endoscopy.[17] In addition, a recent survey of 332 adult gastroenterology fellows and attendings looking at gender-specific factors influencing careers in advanced endoscopy found that fewer women decide to pursue advanced endoscopy training and one of the deterring factors reported was a lack of ergonomically designed equipment for women (ie, gender-adjusted ergonomic equipment).[18] It is important for both training programs and pediatric endoscopy services to acknowledge and mitigate gender-based differences, when possible, given the potential negative impacts on productivity, career longevity, and willingness to pursue advanced endoscopy.

RISK MANAGEMENT STRATEGIES

Given the high prevalence of ERIs among practicing endoscopists and trainees and their potential to jeopardize career longevity and quality of life, risk mitigation strategies are essential to use to help prevent injuries, instead of reacting to injuries when they occur. Related to ergonomics, there is a framework called the *hierarchy of controls,* developed by the National Institute for Occupational Safety and Health (NIOSH), which outlines methods for controlling exposures in the workplace and mitigating the risk of work-related injury that can be applied to endoscopy.[19,20] In thinking about how to use the principles of ergonomics to improve the endoscopy workplace, it is important to prioritize those interventions that are most effective. Despite a tendency for strategies to focus on individuals and what they can do to prevent injury, it is important to recognize that personal strategies are at the bottom of the hierarchy of effective methods for reducing risk, whereas strategies that focus on "prevention through design" are most effective (**Fig. 1**).

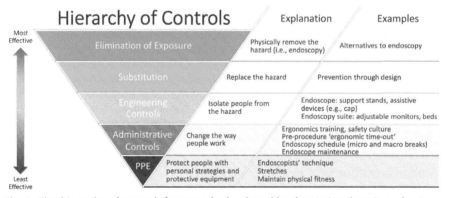

Fig. 1. The *hierarchy of controls* framework, developed by the National Institute for Occupational Safety and Health, can be applied to endoscopy as a means to think about methods for controlling exposures in the workplace and mitigating the risk of work-related injury.[19,20]

The most effective methods for reducing risk to endoscopists are *elimination of exposure* and *substitution*.[19,20] *Elimination* removes the hazard, for example, through the development of non-invasive diagnostic tests as an alternative to endoscopy. *Substitution* focuses on replacing the hazard with another design that carries less risk. This type of prevention through design requires engagement and buy-in from endoscope and device companies to adopt a user-centered design process, whereby designers focus on the end-users and their needs during each phase of an iterative product design process, with the goal to develop safer and more user-friendly endoscopes and devices.[21] In line with an important ergonomic design principle, endoscopes and devices should ideally accommodate the breadth of endoscopists ranging from the 5th percentile female to the 95th percentile male in terms of anthropometric measurements (eg, standing height, standing eye height, hand span).[22]

Until the introduction of more ergonomic endoscope designs, the next most effective solutions in the hierarchy are *engineering controls*, which aim to reduce or prevent hazards from coming into contact with individuals.[19,20] Such controls encompass modifications to the tools, the operator–tool interactions or the work environment, which remove the exposure at the source.[20] Examples of devices that aim to optimize endoscopist interactions with the endoscope include support stands which lessen the static load of the endoscope,[23] angulation dial adaptors which extend the width of the dial and permit easier access for endoscopists with smaller hand spans (ie, <19 cm) who have difficulty reaching the dials,[24] and devices such as caps[25,26] that decrease the time required for cecal intubation. This level also includes tools that optimize endoscopist interactions with their work environment, such as adjustable monitors and beds which facilitate neutral upper body postures during the performance of endoscopy.[20]

The next most effective method to mitigate risk on the NIOSH hierarchy is *administrative controls*, which are policies and procedures that aim to change the way people work.[19,20] Examples include adjustments in procedural scheduling. Schedule templates often focus on efficiency and are not typically designed with injury prevention in mind. Daily schedules that allow for breaks between procedures to promote muscle recovery and spacing out shifts over a week may help to alleviate the risk of ERI.[20] Training is also essential to ensure all endoscopy team members are aware of ergonomic principles and how they can be applied to mitigate injury risk.[27] In addition, policies can be implemented to encourage behaviors which foster a safe working environment, such as a mandated pre-procedure ergonomic time-out. Furthermore, endoscope maintenance programs are critical to ensure endoscopes are performing at the manufacturer-recommended specifications so that endoscopists are not having to apply greater than normal force to the dials to achieve the same degree of tip deflection.[20]

The final level in the hierarchy of controls—the least effective, but often the last line of defense and the most readily available—is *personal protective equipment* and other personal controls that seek to protect workers from the hazard or control exposure.[19,20] This includes endoscopist positioning, ergonomically favorable technique, personal strategies such as maintenance of physical fitness and personal accessories, such as compression stockings and anti-fatigue mats and insoles.

OPTIMIZING ERGONOMICS DURING ENDOSCOPY

To facilitate integration into training and practice, endoscopists can think about ergonomic principles that can be applied to mitigate ERI risk as they pertain to the three key phases of endoscopy: (1) pre-endoscopy; (2) intra-endoscopy; and (3) post-endoscopy.[28,29]

Pre-Endoscopy: Room Setup and Time-Out

Thoughtful design and adjustment of the endoscopy suite is crucial as this is where endoscopists are at highest risk of acquiring ERIs. An ergonomic endoscopy suite is adjustable and enables an ergonomic stance during endoscopy. The endoscopist's body should be square to the monitor, with a neutral neck, back, and shoulder position without hyperextension or flexion, their feet hip width apart, and equal weight distribution on both legs. The video monitor should be adjusted to maintain a vertical neutral neck position, with the center of the screen directly in front of the endoscopist at a resting eye angle, 15°–25° below the horizon (**Fig. 2**).[2,30–32] Depending on the monitor specifications, the monitor should be 52 and 182 cm away from the endoscopist to avoid eye strain.[33] Within the anthropometric range, a monitor should be adjustable between 93 and 162 cm from the floor.[2] The bed should be positioned at optimal height between elbow height and 10 cm below elbow height, allowing for a neutral back and shoulder posture and a working range of both forearms from 0°–10° below the elbows. To accommodate neutral body positions for individuals of various heights, the bed should be height adjustable from 85 to 120 cm from the floor.

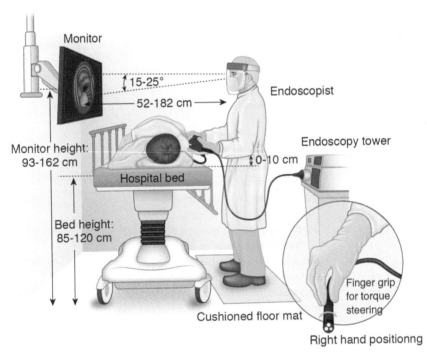

Fig. 2. Recommended positioning of the monitor, bed, patient, endoscope, processer, and endoscopist for optimal ergonomics during endoscopy. The bed and monitor should be adjustable to accommodate a wide range of individuals from the 5th percentile female to 95th percentile male height. It is suggested to hold the endoscope shaft in the right hand using a finger grip (vs fist grip) to enhance the endoscopist's ability to feel resistance and enable precise torque control (inset). (*From* Walsh CM, Qayed E, Aihara H, et al. Core curriculum for ergonomics in endoscopy. Gastrointest Endosc. 2021;93(6):1222-1227.)

The endoscopy tower should be positioned directly behind the endoscopist such that the insertion of the endoscope into the tower is in line with the orifice to be intubated (ie, anorectum for ileocolonoscopy, mouth for upper endoscopy).[2,27] When possible, a cushioned anti-fatigue floor mat, which causes slight instability of the legs, should be used to improve blood flow and decrease discomfort and fatigue associated with prolonged standing.[34–36] Cushioned insoles can similarly provide a supportive interface between the endoscopist's feet and the floor to optimize body weight distribution,[35] and compression stockings can be used to prevent venous pooling.[37,38] Cords and tubing should be bundled, and ideally covered, to help prevent injury related to tripping over exposed cords.[39,40] The use of ceiling-mounted plugs can also help to decrease exposed wiring. Floor pedals should be easily accessible, positioned in front of the endoscopist and within reach to avoid awkward movements and the need to look downward during the procedure. Typically, the non-dominant foot controls the water pump which leaves the dominant foot free to control the electrosurgical unit pedals, if required.

Endoscopy teams should be encouraged to perform an *ergonomic time-out* prior the start of the procedure, as a prompt for all team members to check their posture, the monitor and bed height encourage communication of ergonomic-related concerns and highlight other elements of proper ergonomics. This time-out can be augmented by an endoscopy *ergonomic checklist* which can serve to initiate, guide, and formalize communication among team members in the pre-endoscopy workflow (**Fig. 3**).[39,41,42]

Pre-Endoscopy Ergonomic Time-Out Checklist

- **Monitor:** directly in front, 15–25° below eye height
- **Bed:** positioned between elbow height and 10 cm below elbow height
- **Endoscopy tower:** endoscope insertion in line with orifice to be intubated (i.e., patient's anorectum or mouth)
- **Foot pedal:** in front of body
- **Cords and wires:** contained on the floor
- **Cushioned floor mat:** in place
- **Led apron (if applicable):** 2-piece
- **Endoscopist position:** neutral posture (back, upper and lower extremities in neutral position and square to the monitor), feet hip-width apart
- **Endoscope positioning (lower endoscopy):** horizontal positioning of endoscope control head, shaft in 'C position', finger grip 15–30 cm from patient's anorectum
- **Communication:** encourage team members to raise any ergonomic-related concerns

Fig. 3. An ergonomic checklist that can be used during a pre-endoscopy time-out to guide and formalize communication among team members related to ergonomics.

Intra-Endoscopy: Technique and Teamwork

Although no uniform endoscope handling technique exists, several elements from the recently published American Society for Gastrointestinal Endoscopy's (ASGE) Core Curriculum for Ergonomics in Endoscopy are suggested to promote efficiency and minimize risk of injury.[27] Endoscopists should begin the procedure in a neutral body posture with the positions of the monitor, bed, and endoscopy tower optimized, as described above. In addition, it is important to adjust the monitor, bed, and tower positions dynamically throughout the procedure, to ensure the setup remains ergonomic, as required (eg, between upper and lower endoscopy, if the endoscopist performing the procedure changes).

The core elements of an ergonomically favorable technique include adoption of a neutral grip and use of a one-handed technique with facilitated torque steering. For upper endoscopy, it is suggested to hold the endoscope control head such that the umbilicus (ie, universal cord) is located on the inside of the endoscopist's forearm. This position enables the use of left arm and/or body movements throughout the procedure to apply torque along the longitudinal shaft of the endoscope (ie, insertion tube), without having to twist the shaft with the right hand.[43]

Alternatively, for colonoscopy, a "C position" is recommended, wherein the control head of the colonoscope is held horizontally in the left hand to form a "C" shape, the shaft is supported on the bed and held by the right hand 15–30 cm from the anus, and the umbilicus is located on the outside of the endoscopist's left forearm (**Fig. 4**).[27,44] This positioning enables a more balanced colonoscope control head and shaft and facilitates application of torque when the endoscope shaft is straight.[27,44] In addition, it permits easier access to the angulation control dials as they tilt toward the thumb when the control head is held horizontally, a factor which is particularly important for individuals with smaller hands. Although the "C" technique has not been systematically evaluated, it additionally enables the use of the larger muscles of the left arm to help with torque steering (Video 1). The use of a one-handed steering technique is recommended for ileocolonoscopy, such that the right hand holds the shaft held between the thumb and fingers (ie, finger grip or "cigar-rolling" technique), 15–30 cm from the anus, and steering is primarily accomplished with the up-down wheel and rotational torque of the shaft. A finger grip, in addition to the "C" technique, can prevent

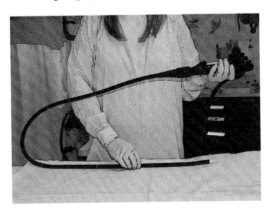

Fig. 4. Use of a "C position" during ileocolonoscopy can facilitate the use of the larger muscles of the left arm to help with torque steering. The control head of the colonoscope is held horizontally in the left hand to form a "C" shape. The shaft is supported on the bed and held by the right hand using a finger-grip, 15–30 cm from the anus. The umbilicus is located on the outside of the endoscopist's left forearm.

excessive wrist angulation and permits the shaft to rotate more than 360°, compared with a maximum of 180° of rotation achieved by wrist-twist.[27,44] A finger grip also makes it easier for the endoscopist to feel resistance caused, for example, by a bend or loop. It is important for endoscopists to use different strategies (eg, patient position change, water-assisted endoscopy) to maintain a short and straight endoscope to ensure the tip remains responsive to wheel angulation and torque steering.[27]

Patient repositioning can be used during pediatric endoscopy to aid with colonoscope advancement and visualization. To decrease the risk of ERIs, endoscopy team members should be encouraged to rotate responsibilities, avoid lifting beyond their capabilities, and use proper lift techniques, including the use of hips and knees, a wide base and minimizing forward flexion to reduce back strain. The use of abdominal pressure should be reserved for specific situations where it has been shown to be most beneficial (eg, preventing U-loop formation with a transverse "lift").[45]

If lead aprons are required for procedures using fluoroscopy, team members should be encouraged to wear two-piece lead aprons. As compared with one-piece aprons, these distribute the weight of the apron more evenly across the spine and pelvis, decreasing the force on the endoscopist's neck, shoulders, and lower back.[46–48] In addition, two monitors are often required for fluoroscopy, necessitating the endoscopist to turn their head frequently during the procedure. Placement of the endoscopy and fluoroscopy monitors close together can help to prevent neck torsion, decrease eye strain, and reduce fluoroscopy time.[49,50]

Post-Endoscopy: Recovery

Endoscopists should be encouraged to take 1–2-minute micro-breaks during procedures which have been shown to alleviate pain and improve performance in surgery.[51] In addition, short, scheduled breaks between cases can help to improve muscle recovery. Stretching exercises can be incorporated in between procedures and at completion of an endoscopist's list. Although the effect of stretching on ERI has not been evaluated, advantages demonstrated in other domains include injury prevention and maintenance of flexibility and strength.[52] Video-based resources such as those published by the ASGE VideoGIE journal (https://www.videogie.org/)[53] and American College of Gastroenterology Universe (https://universe.gi.org/)[54] are available, which illustrate stretches for the wrists, fingers, shoulders, and back. Endoscopists should also think about how their week is scheduled. Half instead of full-day endoscopy blocks may be considered, and spacing out endoscopy sessions over the week, as opposed to having them on back-to-back days, can permit additional recovery time.[52]

It is important for institutions to foster a culture of safety and support endoscopy teams through the development of policies and practices which promote a safety culture (eg, mandating ergonomic time-outs, ergonomically minded scheduling incorporating breaks between endoscopy procedures and spacing out endoscopy sessions, promotion of stretching and physical fitness) and by maintaining equipment to ensure it is functioning optimally.[52] Educational programs that formally assess ergonomics and ERI risk and implement personalized strategies for improvement have been shown to reduce subjective musculoskeletal complaints among endoscopists with baseline ERIs and foster ergonomically-minded habits that are valuable throughout endoscopists' careers.[55]

INTEGRATING ERGONOMICS DURING TRAINING

Despite the prevalence of injury and the recognized importance of education on endoscopy ergonomics, studies have demonstrated that endoscopists lack proper education and training on ergonomics. Only 20.9% of pediatric gastroenterologists report having received any formal training, whereas 41.2% report receiving informal bedside teaching on ERI prevention during fellowship.[3] The importance of education is highlighted by research which indicates that injury rates are higher among gastroenterology fellows who have not received education[11] and that ergonomics education can improve ergonomic-related behaviors.[41,56] In addition, a recent survey-based study found that gastroenterologists had a lower likelihood of injury after incorporating ERI prevention strategies.[7] Furthermore, in the trainee population, an ergonomics curriculum was associated with decreased ERI injury risk as assessed using validated ergonomic risk-assessment tools.[41]

Across both pediatric and adult studies, endoscopists report being motivated to implement practice changes to prevent ERI and perceive ergonomics training as important.[3,10,11] The ASGE Core Curriculum for Ergonomics in Endoscopy identifies core knowledge and skills related to endoscopy ergonomics, including cognitive skills (eg, identify ERI risk factors), technical skills (eg, adjust room setup to maintain neutral body posture), and non-technical skills (eg, support team members to adopt ergonomic principles and avoid injury).[27] The ASGE curriculum is intended to be used by endoscopy training directors, endoscopists involved in teaching endoscopy, as well as by endoscopy trainees, and to guide ergonomics education during fellowship training. Ideally, by integrating the ASGE ergonomics curriculum into training programs, endoscopists can build foundational long-term habits that prevent injury, enhance well-being, and improve efficiency and performance over the duration of their careers.

Ergonomics-focused educational initiatives should emphasize key ergonomic principles and should ideally be team-based to improve overall ergonomic awareness and enable the entire endoscopy team to become part of the solution. Training outside of the endoscopy suite can incorporate small-group sessions, online education, videos, reading materials, and simulation-based training.[41,55,57] This asynchronous education that is away from patient care may be optimal for focusing on the cognitive aspects of ergonomics in endoscopy, including ERI injury prevalence and risk factors, technical skills such as neutral body positioning, endoscopy room setup, and other ergonomic principles which can be applied to mitigate injury risk. It can also address non-technical elements including situational awareness and a team-based approach to ergonomics, as illustrated by the use of the ergonomic time-out and checklist described earlier.[27,41]

In the clinical setting, there are several things endoscopy trainers can do to foster a focus on ergonomics.[42] Before the procedure, alignment of agendas between the trainer and trainee with achievable and realistic goals for the training session helps to minimize cognitive load and the physical loading that can occur due to suboptimal technique.[44,58,59] In setting objectives, ergonomic aspects of endoscopy should be incorporated. The trainer should also empower the trainee to perform an ergonomic time-out, with the goal of ensuring that the physical setup of the endoscopy suite enables the trainee to assume an ergonomic stance during endoscopy. The use of a targeted time-out has shown benefit within the simulation-based setting.[41]

During procedures, endoscopy trainers should position themselves at the foot of the bed opposite the monitor to ensure they have a good view of the monitor, the endoscope, and the trainee's hands (**Fig. 5**).[44,58,59] This viewpoint can help trainers identify when trainees are having difficulty in maintaining a neutral posture.[27] Furthermore, by focusing on the trainee's positioning, as well as the patient and monitor, the trainer is better able to recognize when progression during an endoscopy is being impeded by ergonomic factors or endoscope handling skills. In providing instruction during the procedure, trainers should also strive to highlight non-technical aspects of

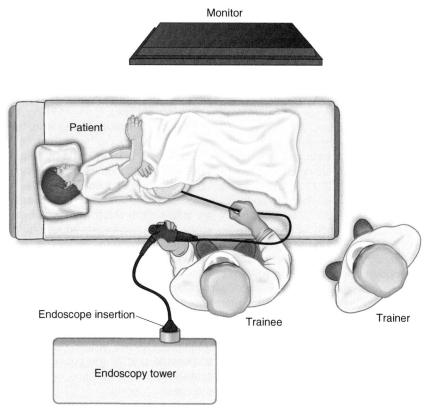

Fig. 5. Recommended setup of the endoscopy room for training to optimize the trainer's visualization of the patient's face, the video monitor, and the trainee's hands. (*From* Walsh CM, Qayed E, Aihara H, et al. Core curriculum for ergonomics in endoscopy. Gastrointest Endosc. 2021;93(6):1222-1227.)

ergonomics. This will help to ensure trainees develop the situational awareness, teamwork, communication, leadership, and decision-making skills necessary to create a healthy working environment.[60,61] Trainers should lead by example, supporting team members to adopt ergonomic principles and encouraging others to not only recognize their own limitations in performing activities related to endoscopy (eg, repositioning patients) but also to effectively communicate these limitations to other team members. In addition, trainers can help trainees remain attentive and mindful throughout the procedure, thereby ensuring adequate ergonomics for everyone (eg, encouraging assistants to rotate responsibilities, letting an assistant know when abdominal pressure can be released).

Intra-procedural teaching should be augmented with dedicated post-procedure performance enhancing feedback on trainee's performance that is specific and goal-directed with the aim to foster reflection and increase trainee's self-awareness.[44,58,59] Feedback should focus on observable behaviors and specific suggestions related to ergonomics should be highlighted. Feedback from trainers that is focused on improving trainee technique will also enhance ergonomics. In addition, an ergonomic checklist (see **Fig. 3**) can be used to help structure teaching, facilitate real-time optimization of ergonomics both before and during procedures, promote trainee self-reflection, and help frame feedback provision that guides future learning.[27,41]

ADDITIONAL CONSIDERATIONS
Performance of Endoscopy While Pregnant

Given increasing rates of female pediatric gastroenterologists of childbearing age, it is important to consider the physical demands of performing procedures while pregnant. Pregnancy is known to impact ERI risk, with a large adult study reporting that 80% of women experience new-onset ERI and 70% experience worsening of existing ERIs during pregnancy.[7] Endoscopists face additional musculoskeletal challenges during pregnancy due to physiological and anatomical changes, including increased joint laxity, a shifted center of gravity, fluid retention, and a predisposition to carpal tunnel syndrome, De Quervain's tenosynovitis, and syncope.[62-69] Endoscopy-related postural demands, such as standing for prolonged periods of time, exacerbates many of these issues.[39]

Risk mitigation strategies related to pregnancy include workplace ergonomic interventions and individual endoscopist interventions. At an institutional level, measures can be introduced to minimize occupational exposures that place pregnant endoscopists at risk, including working hours, physical workloads, lifting, and standing.[70] Daily schedules can be adjusted to decrease procedural loads in the third trimester, and endoscopists should be afforded sufficient time between procedures to eat, rehydrate, sit down, and stretch as needed. Policies can be implemented to ensure recommended weight limits for lifting at work during pregnancy are followed.[71] The endoscopy suite should be adjustable, including the bed, monitor, and endoscopy tower, to optimize endoscopist positioning. In addition, equipment should be provided, as required, to mitigate ERI risk. This includes stools with lower back rests to facilitate seated endoscopy, cushioned anti-fatigue floor mats, and footrests to enable alternate raising of one of the lower extremities to help reduce low back pain and avoid static postures with prolonged standing.[72]

To facilitate informed decision-making, all endoscopists should be provided with radiation safety protocols that specifically address modifications for pregnancy. If women perform fluoroscopic procedures while pregnant, maternity lead aprons should be provided to afford supplementary coverage against radiation exposure and enable complete adjustability throughout pregnancy.[73] Fetal dosimeters, which are worn in the abdominal area underneath the lead garment to monitor fetal radiation exposure, should be considered for pregnant interventional endoscopy care providers who perform fluoroscopic procedures regularly.

At the endoscopist level, simple measures can also be taken to help minimize ERI risk during pregnancy, such as making use of personal support items including pelvic braces for stability, wrist splints to keep the joints neutral, and compression stockings to enhance venous return.[39,70] It is also important for pregnant women to stretch between procedures and stay well hydrated.

Impact of Endoscopy-Related Injuries

It is important for pediatric endoscopists to recognize that ERIs can have a significant impact on their careers and related financial stability. Although only 8.0% of pediatric endoscopists report taking time off from performing endoscopy due to an ERI, 24.0% report receiving treatment for an injury and over a third adjust their practice.[3] Adult research has shown similar results.[7,8,30] Occupational injuries also affect endoscopy team members, with one study revealing that injured endoscopy personnel had a mean of 6.1 lost workdays.[74]

Financial protection against potential ERIs is important, and disability insurance should be strongly considered. It is important to think about disability insurance early in one's career and seek expertise to help guide decision-making. An understanding of the terminology used in disability insurance and the potential add-on options (ie, riders) will also aid in choosing the appropriate policy. Issues to consider include the definition of disability (ie, "own occupation" vs "any occupation"), the benefit amount, the waiting period, and inclusion of a residual benefit to cover a partial loss of income, cost of living adjustments, and future purchase options that enable one to increase future coverage as their income grows, regardless of health.[75,76] Also of note, a gender gap exists in policy rates, with women being charged higher premiums as they are considered to be at increased risk for developing a disabling condition.[75,77] Women should, therefore, seek out plans with unisex or gender neutral policy rates. Even if disability insurance is provided through one's employer, it is important to obtain private coverage unrelated to an employer-based policy to help assure sufficient coverage.

SUMMARY

Ergonomics is an essential component of safe endoscopic practice. Significant rates of occupational injuries are reported among both practicing pediatric endoscopists and trainees, related to overuse, repetitive motions, and non-neutral postures during endoscopy. Methods for controlling exposures in the workplace and mitigating injury risk can be applied at multiple levels, ranging from equipment and endoscopy suite design to regulation of the work environment, to the endoscopist. A multifaceted approach will have the greatest and long-lasting impact.

It is essential for endoscopists to recognize the risks of ERIs and learn how to optimize their work environment and technique to help preserve their health and well-being. In addition, if an injury occurs, it is important for endoscopists to acknowledge musculoskeletal symptoms, even if they seem mild, seek treatment, and adjust their practice as required, to prevent long-term injury. At the institutional level, workplace policies and practices can be adapted to help promote safe ergonomic practices, and endoscopy suites should be designed with adjustability in mind to ensure they accommodate the breadth users. At a broader level, the pediatric endoscopy community needs to work with industry to design safer and more user-friendly endoscopes and endoscopy equipment.

Education and training is an effective vehicle for behavior change. Endoscopy training programs should strive to incorporate formal ergonomics training into their curricula, with a focus on team-based initiatives to promote a culture of safety during all facets of patient care. Successful training in ergonomics also requires endoscopy trainers who are capable of providing performance enhancing instruction and feedback with a focus on ergonomics to help trainees develop ergonomically favorable technique as well as the non-technical skills necessary to create a healthy working environment. Incorporating ergonomic principles during both training and practice can help to mitigate risks for musculoskeletal injuries, improve productivity, and enhance well-being, benefiting the endoscopist, patients, and the entire endoscopy team.

CLINICS CARE POINTS

- Ergonomics training should include team-based activities to promote a culture of safety that benefits the entire endoscopy team.

- Ergonomically minded scheduling that incorporates breaks between endoscopy procedures and spaces out endoscopy sessions is essential to promote muscle recovery and help mitigate the risk of endoscopy-related injuries.
- A pre-endoscopy ergonomic time-out can be used to prompt all team members to check their posture and the room setup and to encourage communication of ergonomic-related concerns.
- To ensure the endoscopy suite setup remains ergonomic, it is important for endoscopists to adjust the video monitor, bed, and endoscopy tower positions dynamically throughout the procedure, if required.
- Endoscopy trainers can foster a focus on ergonomics in setting relevant learning objectives, providing instruction during procedures to promote the development of ergonomically favorable technique and highlighting specific suggestions related to ergonomics when providing post-procedure performance enhancing feedback.

FUNDING/SUPPORT

C.M. Walsh holds an Early Researcher Award from the Ontario Ministry of Research and Innovation. The funders had no role in the design and conduct of the review, decision to publish and preparation, review, or approval of the article.

DISCLOSURE

The author has nothing to disclose.

SUPPLEMENTARY DATA

Supplementary data related to this article can be found online at https://doi.org/10.1016/j.giec.2022.12.002.

REFERENCES

1. Carnahan H, Dubrowski A, Walsh C, et al. Where is the learner in ergonomics? J Ergon 2012;2:1000e108.
2. Shergill AK, McQuaid KR. Ergonomic endoscopy: An oxymoron or realistic goal? Gastrointest Endosc 2019;90:966–70.
3. Ruan W, Walsh CM, Pawa S, et al. Musculoskeletal injury and ergonomics in pediatric gastrointestinal endoscopic practice. Surg Endosc 2023;37:248–54.
4. Rempel D, Harrison R, Barnhart S. Work-related cumulative trauma disorders of the upper extremity. Am J Ind Med 1992;267:838–42.
5. Shergill AK, Asundi KR, Barr A, et al. Pinch force and forearm-muscle load during routine colonoscopy: a pilot study. Gastrointest Endosc 2009;69:142–6.
6. Shergill AK, Rempel D, Barr A, et al. Biomechanical risk factors associated with distal upper extremity musculoskeletal disorders in endoscopists performing colonoscopy. Gastrointest Endosc 2021;93:704–11.e3.
7. Pawa S, Banerjee P, Kothari S, et al. Are all endoscopy-related musculoskeletal injuries created equal? Results of a national gender-based survey. Am J Gastroenterol 2021;116:530–8.
8. Yung DE, Banfi T, Ciuti G, et al. Musculoskeletal injuries in gastrointestinal endoscopists: A systematic review. Expert Rev Gastroenterol Hepatol 2017;11:939–47.
9. Kamani L, Kalwar H. Ergonomic injuries in endoscopists and their risk factors. Clin Endosc 2021;54:356–62.

10. Austin K, Schoenberger H, Sesto M, et al. Musculoskeletal injuries are commonly reported among gastroenterology trainees: Results of a national survey. Dig Dis Sci 2019;64:1439–47.

11. Villa E, Attar B, Trick W, et al. Endoscopy-related musculoskeletal injuries in gastroenterology fellows. Endosc Int Open 2019;07:E808–12.

12. Pawa S, Martindale SL, Gaidos JKJ, et al. Endoscopy-related injury among gastroenterology trainees. Endosc Int Open 2022;10:E1095–104.

13. Ridtitid W, Coté GA, Leung W, et al. Prevalence and risk factors for musculoskeletal injuries related to endoscopy. Gastrointest Endosc 2015;81:294–302.e4.

14. Edelman KM, Zheng J, Erdmann A, et al. Endoscopy-related musculoskeletal injury in AGA gastroenterologists is common while training in ergonomics is rare. Gastroenterology 2017;152:S217.

15. Morais R, Vilas-Boas F, Pereira P, et al. Prevalence, risk factors and global impact of musculoskeletal injuries among endoscopists: A nationwide European study. Endosc Int Open 2020;08:E470–80.

16. Leyk D, Gorges W, Ridder D, et al. Hand-grip strength of young men, women and highly trained female athletes. Eur J Appl Physiol 2007;99:415–21.

17. Cohen DL, Naik JR, Tamariz LJ, et al. The perception of gastroenterology fellows towards the relationship between hand size and endoscopic training. Dig Dis Sci 2008;53:1902–9.

18. David YN, Dixon RE, Kakked G, et al. Gender-specific factors influencing gastroenterologists to pursue careers in advanced endoscopy: Perceptions vs reality. Am J Gastroenterol 2021;116:539–50.

19. The National Institute for Occupational Safety and Health (NIOSH). Hierarchy of controls. Centers Dis. Control Prev. 2022. Available at: https://www.cdc.gov/niosh/topics/hierarchy/default.html. Accessed February 15, 2023.

20. Shergill AK, Harris Adamson C. Failure of an engineered system: The gastrointestinal endoscope. Tech Gastrointest Endosc 2019;21:116–23.

21. Norman D. The design of everyday things: revised and exapanded edition. New York, New York: Basic Books; 2013.

22. The Eastman Kodak Company. Kodak's ergonomic design for people at work. 2nd edition. Hoboken, New Jersey: John Wiley and Sons; 2004.

23. Shergill AK, Barr A, Harris-Adamson C. Tu1041 Ergonomic evaluation of an endoscope support stand during simulated colonoscopies. Gastrointest Endosc 2018;87:AB506.

24. Akerkar G, McQuaid K, Terdiman J, et al. An angulation dial adapter to facilitate endoscopy. Gastrointest Endosc 1999;49:AB120.

25. Rex DK, Repici A, Gross SA, et al. High-definition colonoscopy versus Endocuff versus EndoRings versus full-spectrum endoscopy for adenoma detection at colonoscopy: a multicenter randomized trial. Gastrointest Endosc 2018;88:335–44.e2.

26. Ngu WS, Bevan R, Tsiamoulos ZP, et al. Improved adenoma detection with Endocuff Vision: The ADENOMA randomised controlled trial. Gut 2019;68:280–8.

27. Walsh CM, Qayed E, Aihara H, et al. Core curriculum for ergonomics in endoscopy. Gastrointest Endosc 2021;93:1222–7.

28. Walsh CM, Lightdale JR, Mack DR, et al. Overview of the Pediatric Endoscopy Quality Improvement Network quality standards and indicators for pediatric endoscopy: A joint NASPGHAN/ESPGHAN guideline. J Pediatr Gastroenterol Nutr 2022;74:S3–15.

29. Walsh CM, Lightdale JR. Pediatric Endoscopy Quality Improvement Network (PEnQuIN) quality standards and indicators for pediatric endoscopy: An ASGE-endorsed guideline. Gastrointest Endosc 2022;96:593–602.
30. Shergill AK, McQuaid KR, Rempel D. Ergonomics and GI endoscopy. Gastrointest Endosc 2009;70:145–53.
31. Matern U, Faist M, Kehl K, et al. Monitor position in laparoscopic surgery. Surg Endosc Other Interv Tech 2005;19:436–40.
32. Haveran LA, Novitsky YW, Czerniach DR, et al. Optimizing laparoscopic task efficiency: The role of camera and monitor positions. Surg Endosc Other Interv Tech 2007;21:980–4.
33. El Shallaly G, Cuschieri A. Optimum view distance for laparoscopic surgery. Surg Endosc Other Interv Tech 2006;20:1879–82.
34. Speed G, Harris K, Keegel T. The effect of cushioning materials on musculoskeletal discomfort and fatigue during prolonged standing at work: A systematic review. Appl Ergon 2018;70:300–14.
35. King PM. A comparison of the effects of floor mats and shoe in-soles on standing fatigue. Appl Ergon 2002;33:477–84.
36. Redfern MS, Cham R. The influence of flooring on standing comfort and fatigue. AIHAJ 2000;61:700–8.
37. Benigni J, Sadoun S, Allaert F, et al. Efficacy of Class 1 elastic compression stockings in the early stages of chronic venous disease. A comparative study. Int Angiol 2003;22:383–92.
38. Kraemer WJ, Volek JS, Bush JA, et al. Influence of compression hosiery on physiological responses to standing fatigue in women. Med Sci Sports Exerc 2000;32:1849–58.
39. Lipowska AM, Shergill AK. Ergonomics in the unit: Modeling the environment around the endoscopist. Tech Innov Gastrointest Endosc 2021;23:256–62.
40. Cappell MS. Injury to endoscopic personnel from tripping over exposed cords, wires, and tubing in the endoscopy suite: A preventable cause of potentially severe workplace injury. Dig Dis Sci 2010;55:947–51.
41. Khan R, Scaffidi MA, Satchwell J, et al. Impact of a simulation-based ergonomic training curriculum on work-related musculoskeletal injury risk in colonoscopy. Gastrointest Endosc 2020;92:1070–80.e3.
42. Khan R, Faggen A, Shergill A, et al. Integrating ergonomics into endoscopy training: A guide for faculty and fellows. Clin Gastroenterol Hepatol 2023;14. S1542-3565(23)00083-6.
43. Sugimoto K, Osawa S. 'Four-position method' makes beginner endoscopists aware of spatial positioning of the left hand to master upper gastrointestinal endoscopy. Endosc Int Open 2020;08:E1225–30.
44. Anderson JT. Optimizing ergonomics during endoscopy training. Tech Gastrointest Endosc 2019;21:143–9.
45. Choy MC, Matharoo M, Thomas-Gibson S. Diagnostic ileocolonoscopy: Getting the basics right. Frontline Gastroenterol 2020;11:484–90.
46. Pedrosa MC, Farraye FA, Shergill AK, et al. Minimizing occupational hazards in endoscopy: Personal protective equipment, radiation safety, and ergonomics. Gastrointest Endosc 2010;72:227–35.
47. Khalil T, Abdel-Moty E, Rosomoff H. Ergonomics in back pain: Guide to prevention and rehabilitation. New York, New York: Van Nostrand; 1993.
48. Ross AM, Segal J, Borenstein D, et al. Prevalence of spinal disc disease among interventional cardiologists. Am J Cardiol 1997;79:68–70.

49. O'Sullivan S, Bridge G, Ponich T. Musculoskeletal injuries among ERCP endoscopists in Canada. Can J Gastroenterol 2002;16:369–74.
50. Jowhari F, Hopman W, Hookey L. A simple ergonomic measure reduces fluoroscopy time during ERCP: a multivariate analysis. Endosc Int Open 2017;05: E172–8.
51. Park AE, Zahiri HR, Hallbeck MS, et al. Intraoperative 'micro breaks' with targeted stretching enhance surgeon physical function and mental focus a multicenter cohort study. Ann Surg 2017;265:340–6.
52. Lipowska AM, Shergill AK. Ergonomics of endoscopy. Gastrointest Endosc Clin N Am 2021;31:655–69.
53. Chang MA, Mitchell J, Abbas Fehmi SM. Optimizing ergonomics after endoscopy. VideoGIE 2017;2:171.
54. Zibert K, Singla M, Young PE. Using ergonomics to prevent injuries for the endoscopist. Am J Gastroenterol 2019;114:541–3.
55. Markwell SA, Garman KS, Vance IL, et al. Individualized ergonomic wellness approach for the practicing gastroenterologist (with video). Gastrointest Endosc 2021;94:248–59.e2.
56. Ali MF, Samarasena J. Implementing ergonomics interventions in the endoscopy suite. Tech Gastrointest Endosc 2019;21:159–61.
57. Sussman M, Sendzischew-Shane MA, Bolanos J, et al. Assurance for endurance? Introducing a novel ergonomics curriculum to reduce pain and enhance physical well-being among GI fellows. Dig Dis Sci 2020;65:2756–8.
58. Walsh CM, Anderson JT, Fishman DS. Evidence-based approach to training pediatric gastrointestinal endoscopy trainers. J Pediatr Gastroenterol Nutr 2017;64: 501–4.
59. Walsh CM, Waschke KA. Training the endoscopic trainer. In: Cohen J, editor. Successful training in gastrointestinal endoscopy. Hoboken, New Jersey: John Wiley & Sons, Ltd; 2022. p. 33–42.
60. Ravindran S, Haycock A, Woolf K, et al. Development and impact of an endoscopic non-technical skills (ENTS) behavioural marker system. BMJ Simul Technol Enhanc Learn 2021;7:17–25.
61. Walsh CM, Scaffidi MA, Khan R, et al. Non-technical skills curriculum incorporating simulation-based training improves performance in colonoscopy among novice endoscopists: Randomized controlled trial. Dig Endosc 2020;32:940–8.
62. Chatur S, Islam S, Moore LE, et al. Incidence of syncope during pregnancy: Temporal trends and outcomes. J Am Heart Assoc 2019;8(10):e011608.
63. Meems M, Truijens SEM, Spek V, et al. Prevalence, course and determinants of carpal tunnel syndrome symptoms during pregnancy: a prospective study. BJOG An Int J Obstet Gynaecol 2015;122:1112–8.
64. Yarlagadda S, Poma P, Green L, et al. Syncope during pregnancy. Obstet Gynecol 2010;115:377–80.
65. Casagrande DM, Gugala Z, MD P, et al. Low back pain and pelvic girdle pain in pregnancy. J Am Acad Orthop Surg 2015;23:539–49.
66. Borg-Stein J, Dugan S. Musculoskeletal disorders of pregnancy, delivery and postpartum. Phys Med Rehabil Clin N Am 2007;18:459–76.
67. Ireland M, Lloyd M. The effects of pregnancy on the musculoskeletal system. Clin Orthop Relat Res 2000;372:169–79.
68. Szlachter B, Quagliarello J, Jewelewicz R, et al. Relaxin in normal and pathogenic pregnancies. Obs Gynecol 1982;59:167–70.
69. Schned E. DeQuervain tenosynovitis in pregnant and postpartum women. Obstet Gynecol 1986;68:411–4.

70. Austin K, Schoenberger H, Saha S. Special situations: performance of endoscopy while pregnant. Tech Gastrointest Endosc 2019;21:150–4.
71. Jackson R, Birsner ML, Terman S, et al. Employment considerations during pregnancy and the postpartum period. Obstet Gynecol 2018;131:E115–23.
72. Morrissey SJ. Work place design recommendations for the pregnant worker. Int J Ind Ergon 1998;21:383–95.
73. Shaw P, Duncan A, Vouyouka A, et al. Radiation exposure and pregnancy. J Vasc Surg 2011;53:28S–34S.
74. Cappell MS. Accidental occupational injuries to endoscopy personnel in a high-volume endoscopy suite during the last decade: Mechanisms, workplace hazards, and proposed remediation. Dig Dis Sci 2011;56:479–87.
75. Churgay CA, Smith M, Cain J. A practical guide to physician disability insurance. Fam Pract Manag 2021;28:10–6.
76. Pearson S. Disability insurance 101. In: Garrett P, Yoon-Flannery K, editors. A pediatrician's path. Cham, Switzerland: Springer; 2021. p. 307–14.
77. Parekh NK, McQuaid K. The injured endoscopist: a roadmap for recovery. Tech Gastrointest Endosc 2019;21:155–8.

Upskilling Pediatric Ileocolonoscopy

Wenly Ruan, MD[a,b], Priya Narula, MD[c], Douglas S. Fishman, MD[a,b],*

KEYWORDS

- Colonoscopy • Ileocolonoscopy • Upskilling • Pediatrics
- Gastrointestinal endoscopy • Quality improvement

KEY POINTS

- Devices have been created to enhance the performance of pediatric ileocolonoscopy, including variable stiffness endoscopes, magnetic imagers, as well as tools to enhance endoscopy ergonomics and facilitate optical diagnosis.
- There are many techniques that can be applied to aid with navigation through a difficult ileocolonoscopy, including dynamic position change and water-assisted endoscopy, as well as mucosal exposure devices such as transparent caps and cuffs.
- Training is a critical aspect of upskilling pediatric endoscopy. Achieving competency, maintenance of competence, and reassessment of skills are all important aspects of training.

INTRODUCTION

There are many unique aspects of performing endoscopy in pediatric patients due to differences in patient size, anatomy, disease processes, and the need for size-appropriate equipment. The acquisition of skills necessary to perform pediatric endoscopy is important and requires pediatric-focused training and upskilling to ensure that procedures are performed safely and efficiently. Upskilling is the learning of additional skills through education and training to improve one's expertise. In the last several years, there have also been advances in "train-the-trainer" activities, such that the trainer becomes proficient at teaching these skills.

Given the differences in patient size and equipment, pediatric ileocolonoscopy can be more technically challenging. Upskilling enables pediatric endoscopists to maintain and continually improve their skills over their careers as new techniques and devices are developed. This chapter will highlight devices and techniques to enhance performance of ileocolonoscopy and highlight the importance of endoscopy training.

[a] Department of Pediatrics, Baylor College of Medicine, Houston, TX, USA; [b] Division of Pediatric Gastroenterology, Hepatology, and Nutrition, Texas Children's Hospital, Houston, TX, USA; [c] Department of Paediatric Gastroenterology, Sheffield Children's NHS Foundation, TrustWestern Bank, Sheffield S10 2TH, United Kingdom
* Corresponding author. 6701 Fannin Street, D1010, Houston, TX 77030.
E-mail address: Douglas.fishman@bcm.edu

Gastrointest Endoscopy Clin N Am 33 (2023) 253–265
https://doi.org/10.1016/j.giec.2022.11.006
1052-5157/23/© 2022 Elsevier Inc. All rights reserved.

DEVICES TO ENHANCE PERFORMANCE OF ILEOCOLONOSCOPY

There are many devices that have been introduced to aid in the performance of endoscopy. These tools aim to improve the diagnostic and therapeutic outcomes for pediatric endoscopy as well as ergonomics during endoscopy. In this section, we explore some devices that can be used to enhance the performance of pediatric ileocolonoscopy, including variable stiffness endoscopes, magnetic endoscopic imagers, as well as tools to enhance endoscopy ergonomics and facilitate optical diagnosis.

Variable Stiffness Endoscopes

Loop formation in a mobile colon is a common issue that may create difficulty in procedural performance and completion. Excessive looping leads to transfer of force to the colonic wall and its mesenteric attachment (instead of forward advancement) which can increase patient discomfort and risk of perforation.[1] Increasing scope rigidity may help to prevent loop formation; however, this can also make it difficult to pass through tightly angulated sections of the colon. Colonoscopes that incorporate a variable-stiffness function have a rotatable dial on the control head that can be manually turned to adjust the stiffness of the endoscope via an adjustable tensioning coil. This enables the endoscopist to alter the stiffness of the endoscope depending on what is necessary to navigate through the colon. The insertion tube is stiffened beyond 30 cm from the endoscope tip, so that the distal portion remains easily deflectable.

Studies have shown that the use of a variable stiffness colonoscope may help to reduce cecal intubation time and patient discomfort.[2] A meta-analysis of eight randomized trials also supports that variable stiffness colonoscopes can improve cecal intubation rates and reduce the need for additional maneuvers during an ileocolonoscopy.[3] Additional endoscope design features that may facilitate procedure performance include slimmer designs, which are particularly useful in younger children and for fixed and tightly angulated colons (eg, postsurgical adhesions), as well as RetroView endoscopes with retroflexed tips that allow for a full view of the rectum and proximal aspects of interhaustral folds on withdrawal.

Magnetic Endoscopic Imagers

Another tool that can enhance endoscopic performance is magnetic endoscopic imaging (MEI). This technology allows for visualization of the colonoscope shaft in real time to facilitate navigation through the colon. MEI also enables visualization of loops to aid in loop reduction. This in theory can lead to more efficient ileocolonoscopies, less patient pain, and improved procedure safety.

In the past, understanding the colonoscope configuration within the patient required fluoroscopy. This innovation provides endoscopists with a three-dimensional display of the colonoscope positioning without exposure to radiation.[4] In one meta-analysis of twenty-one randomized controlled trials (RCTs) involving 7060 patients, MEI helped improve procedure completion rates for less experienced endoscopists and in the subgroup of patients who had technically difficult colonoscopies.[5] Use of the device was also associated with quicker loop resolution, shorter duration of abdominal pressure, and better lesion localization; however, there were no significant differences noted in the overall rate of procedure completion, cecal intubation time, the number of loops formed during a procedure or patient pain scores.[5] This likely is the result of the heterogeneity of the data, although it is generally thought that the true value of MEI is in facilitating loop resolution and training endoscopists.[6]

In one study, MEI improved colonoscopy performance when used by trainees.[7] In addition, a large RCT of 810 patients showed improved cecal intubation rates among less experienced endoscopists when they used MEI compared with standard colonoscopy.[8] The unpublished experience from the Canadian skills enhancement in endoscopy (SEE) Program has been that the use of MEI is extremely beneficial in fostering the conscious competence of trainees as it enables them to link what they are "feeling" to the image on the screen to develop a better understanding of the procedure. In addition, it enables endoscopy trainers to deconstruct ileocolonoscopy, thus facilitating the provision of real-time performance-enhancing instruction.

Devices to Improve Endoscopy Ergonomics

Often understated is the role of ergonomics in both the performance and safety of an endoscopy. Many gastroenterologists develop endoscopy-related injury during their career due to the repetitive nature of gastrointestinal endoscopy, with more women reporting upper extremity injuries.[9,10] The goal of ergonomics in endoscopy is to minimize the risk of injury while optimizing endoscopic performance. Modifications can be made to the endoscopy suite and to patient and endoscopist positioning to improve ergonomics.[11] In addition to these strategies, many tools have been introduced that further enhance endoscopy ergonomics. One such device is an "extender knob" that makes the dials on the endoscope control section.[12] This can facilitate access to the dials, improve maneuverability and decrease fatigue, particularly for endoscopists with smaller hands, which are more often female.[13,14]

Cologrip (Meditech Endoscopy) is another tool that aims to enhance the endoscopists' grip on the colonoscope to potentially decrease hand strain related to advancing and torquing the scope. It has not been systematically evaluated. Another device designed to improve ergonomics during ileocolonoscopy is the ColoWrap (ColoWrap LLC), an abdominal compression device that is applied as an alternative to abdominal pressure to decrease the risk of looping. One RCT found that the wrap did not decrease the need for manual pressure and patient repositioning; however, in adult patients with a higher body mass index (30–40 kg/m^2) it did improve cecal intubation time.[15] Other devices have also been developed to decrease strain related to the application of abdominal pressure and patient repositioning such as a positioning wedge that can be placed under the abdomen to decrease the need for external abdominal pressure, particularly for obese patients.[16] The applicability of these devices to pediatric endoscopy has not been systematically evaluated. As awareness of ergonomics in endoscopy is increasing, more devices will likely be developed to help decrease the risk of endoscopy-related injury.

Tools to Enhance Optical Diagnosis

Accurate diagnosis is another key aspect of endoscopy. To aid in this process, many technologies have been developed with the goal of improving visualization of pathology during endoscopies. One such device is confocal laser endomicroscopy (CLE) which allows for the mucosa to be visualized under microscopic analysis to aid in disease diagnosis in a rapid manner.[17] CLE can be built into the endoscope, or a probe-based system can be used. This technology is currently being used to diagnose neoplasms, celiac disease, inflammatory diseases, and even biliary diseases.[18–20] Adult studies evaluating confocal microscopy utilization for the diagnosis of these diseases have found CLE to have a high sensitivity and specificity.[21] Few studies have examined the utility of CLE in pediatric patients, however, case series have described its use in gastroesophageal reflux disease, Barrett's esophagus, peptic ulcer disease, celiac disease, inflammatory bowel disease, diarrhea, hematochezia, concern for familial adenomatous polyposis with APC mutation and graft versus host disease.[17,22,23]

Training for this device can typically be achieved via continuing medical education courses, training at expert centers, and online courses.[21]

As technology improves, other devices that use artificial intelligence are being developed to help in the detection and diagnosis of several gastrointestinal diseases, including polyps, dysplasia in Barrett's esophagus, and *Helicobacter pylori* infection, and neoplasms.[24–26] This is currently a rapidly evolving field in gastroenterology.

TECHNIQUES FOR ACHIEVING SUCCESSFUL ILEOCOLONOSCOPY

Difficult ileocolonoscopies can occur for a multitude of reasons. Patients may have redundant or long colons, prior surgeries, hernias, and other anatomic factors that can affect the ease of insertion. In pediatrics, ileocolonoscopies are challenging due to differences in pathology, sedation, tolerance of bowel preparation, patient size, and equipment limitations. Various techniques can be used to facilitate navigation and to help with diagnostic and therapeutic yields, including dynamic position change, water-assisted ileocolonoscopy, and use of mucosal exposure devices.

Dynamic Position Change

During ileocolonoscopy insertion and withdrawal, a patient's position can be changed dynamically to optimize the configuration of the colonic anatomy to aid with both navigation and visualization (**Fig. 1**). When evaluating starting positions for ileocolonoscopy, one meta-analysis and systematic review did not show any significant difference between starting in the left lateral or supine position.[27] However, during ileocolonoscopy insertion and withdrawal, strategic use of patient position change has been shown to improve cecal intubation rates, luminal distention, mucosal visualization, and adenoma detection.[28–30]

During ileocolonoscopy, visualization can be obscured due to patient positioning based on where the dependent area of the colon lies. Rotating the patient so that the segment of bowel being intubated and/or examined is superior allows gas to rise and distend or "open up" that segment of bowel. This improves visualization, decreases the amount of gas required for insufflation, and moves fluid and stool away from the colonic segment of interest, further facilitating navigation and visualization. For example, if the patient is in the left lateral position, the cecum and terminal ileum may be difficult to visualize as these are typically in the dependent position and collapsed. By changing the patient's position to the supine or even the right lateral position it often opens up the whole cecum and terminal ileum region, thereby enhancing visualization and facilitating ileal intubation.[31] Position changes can also help control loops and aid with navigation around sharp angles by opening up segments of the bowel.

Water-Assisted Ileocolonoscopy

Water-aided techniques are another tool in the endoscopists' toolbox for tackling difficult ileocolonoscopies. These include water immersion as well as water-exchange techniques. With water immersion, water is infused during insertion to expand the lumen and suctioning of the water primarily occurs on withdrawal. Water exchange, which involves infusion and near-simultaneous suctioning of water as one progresses during ileocolonoscopy, is particularly helpful when there is luminal residue as it maximizes cleanliness during insertion. In practice, a hybrid of water immersion and water exchange is often performed. Water-assisted ileocolonoscopy can be performed during the entire insertion or limited to the left colon. To increase efficiency and facilitate clearing of luminal debris when using water-assisted techniques it is essential to use a

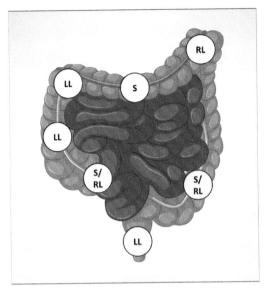

Fig. 1. Position change during ileocolonoscopy to facilitate advancement and visualization (image developed using image designed by Brgfx - Freepik.com).

water pump that is controlled via a foot pedal (using the non-dominant foot) and propels water through the water-jet channel or working channel of the endoscope. In pediatrics, it is also important to consider using warm water that approximates body temperature to reduce the risk of hypothermia.[32]

Water-assisted ileocolonoscopy can aid in the passage of the endoscope through difficult flexures, decrease loop formation, decrease colonic spasms, and decrease patient pain and discomfort. One RCT showed that the water exchange method is less painful than air insufflation and reduced the use of on-demand sedation during the procedure.[33] It has also been shown to improve adenoma detection rates, although it did prolong the procedure slightly (average 2 min).[33] Water-assisted colonoscopy is further supported by additional trials which have shown that water exchange, but not water immersion, achieves higher adenoma detection rates in adults compared with air insufflation.[34,35]

Mucosal Exposure Devices: Caps and Cuffs

More recently, devices have been developed to enhance the exposure of the mucosa during ileocolonoscopy which can aid with both insertion and withdrawal. Cap-assisted ileocolonoscopy employs a small transparent cap attached to the tip of the colonoscope (**Fig. 2**) which maintains a small space between the endoscope and the mucosal wall. This helps to prevent "red out," stabilizes the tip, and aids in navigation beyond angulations and folds to help minimize blind turns.[32] Cap-assisted ileocolonoscopy has been reported to increase cecal intubation rates and shorten the time for cecal intubation among endoscopy trainees.[36] In addition to helping with procedure completion, cap-assisted colonoscopy can improve polyp and adenoma detection rates while reducing procedure times.[37,38]

Newer cuff devices have been introduced to assist with visualization during ileocolonoscopy. These devices, which attach to the distal end of a colonoscope, can be used to increase scope stability and manipulate the colonic folds to enhance

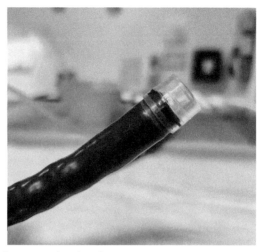

Fig. 2. Image showing cap-assisted endoscopy.

visualization. Studies have found that this device decreases insertion times and improves adenoma detection rates, although it may cause patient discomfort in some, requiring cuff removal.[39] These devices are contraindicated in active colitis.

TRAINING IN PEDIATRIC ILEOCOLONOSCOPY

Over the last decade, there has been growing recognition of the importance of high-quality endoscopic training, particularly the need for trainers who are aware of best practices in procedural skills education, use of a structured approach to training, and the strategic use of assessment to support learning. In addition, complementary endoscopy teaching methods are increasingly being used to enhance apprenticeship approaches, including magnetic endoscopic imagers and simulators.

Assessment to Support Learning and Quality Improvement

Variability in pediatric endoscopy training and in key performance indicators (eg, terminal ileum intubation rate) achieved at the completion of training, highlight the need to use competency assessment tools with strong validity evidence and defined competency milestones.[40] Formative assessments under direct observation can be used in a sequential manner throughout training to monitor and support competency development of the requisite cognitive, technical, and nontechnical skills, aid in the development of learning objectives, and eventually indicate readiness for a summative assessment and independent practice.[41,42]

There are several assessment tools that have been developed for colonoscopy; however, the Gastrointestinal Endoscopy Competency Assessment tool for pediatric colonoscopy ($GIECAT_{kids}$)[43,44] and the pediatric colonoscopy DOPS (direct observation of procedural skills)[45] have strong validity evidence for use in the pediatric context as compared with other assessments.[46] Both tools are well suited to formative assessment as they assess the full breadth of cognitive, technical, and nontechnical skills required to perform ileocolonoscopy, a factor that facilitates learning.[42]

The pediatric colonoscopy DOPS is implemented within the pediatric colonoscopy certification model in the United Kingdom.[47] The JAG, which represents all professional stakeholders involved in endoscopy services, oversees standards in endoscopy training and provides quality assurance for endoscopy services. The UK pediatric colonoscopy certification model requires trainees to record all colonoscopy procedures on the JAG endoscopy training system electronic portfolio along with their formative pediatric colonoscopy DOPS. Trainees are eligible to apply for certification when they achieve the pediatric colonoscopy criteria[48] and are then required to submit four summative DOPS assessments, followed by local trainer sign-off. Although a robust certification model for pediatric colonoscopy trainees exists in the United Kingdom, there is no formalized system for tracking assessment data in North America. Widespread implementation may be limited due to the lack of time, resources, and technological infrastructure for data tracking.[46]

Assessment is also important in practice to ensure endoscopists remain up to date and competent and to guide quality improvement efforts. Currently, however, there are no well-established recredentialing or recertification practices for independent pediatric endoscopists in the United Kingdom or elsewhere.[49] Web-based self-assessment quality improvement tools such as the pediatric endoscopy global rating scale (P-GRS)[50,51] developed in the United Kingdom and North American Society of Pediatric Gastroenterology, Hepatology and Nutrition (NASPGHAN) sponsored maintenance of certification modules have been developed as a means to promote quality improvement.[52] These tools encourage pediatric endoscopists to regularly review their procedural key performance indicators, capture procedural and performance data to identify gaps, and track their quality improvement efforts.[49]

A critical component of ensuring ongoing competence in endoscopy is monitoring of quality indicators. An international working group of the Pediatric Endoscopy Quality Improvement Network (PEnQuIN) recently identified quality indicators for high-quality pediatric ileocolonoscopy and set minimum targets for two key indicators: an unadjusted cecal intubation rate or $\geq$ 90% and an unadjusted terminal ileum intubation rate $\geq$ 85%.[53] These indicators can be continuously measured at an individual provider level to ensure endoscopists are achieving minimum recommended targets and promote continuous quality improvement throughout an endoscopists career.

Training Pediatric Endoscopy Trainers

Increasingly, it has been recognized that there is a need for pediatric endoscopy trainers to not only be competent in performing ileocolonoscopy but also in the ability to teach the procedure. A recent European Society of Pediatric Gastroenterology, Hepatology, and Nutrition (ESPGHAN) position paper encouraged the uptake of "train-the-trainer" or "train the colonoscopy trainer" workshops and courses to ensure a uniform approach.[54] "Conscious competence," a key concept at these courses, is the ability to effectively deconstruct colonoscopy technique and explain it to a trainee in an understandable manner.[55,56] Many trainers who perform ileocolonoscopy proficiently no longer need to think about the steps required to perform the procedure (ie, automaticity). To teach effectively, they must work on becoming consciously competent to be able to provide performance-enhancing instructions using clear, concise, and common language. "Train the colonoscopy trainer" courses emphasize the importance of a structured approach to teaching endoscopy—the "preparation-training-wrap-up" framework first developed by John Anderson in the United Kingdom.[57,58] This framework (**Fig. 3**) highlights the importance of establishing a clear educational contract, including setting specific, measurable, achievable, realistic, and timely objectives, providing performance-enhancing instruction during the procedure, and effectively wrapping up the teaching session with a feedback conversation that

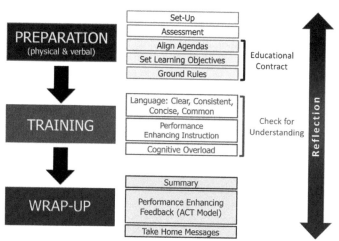

Fig. 3. Framework for endoscopy skills training. (*Adapted from* Walsh CM, Anderson JT, Fishman DS. Evidence-based Approach to Training Pediatric Gastrointestinal Endoscopy Trainers. J Pediatr Gastroenterol Nutr. 2017;64(4):501-504.)

can be used to review and reflect on the encounter and generate learning objectives for future training sessions.[49]

An adult observational study comparing quality indicators between centers participating in train-the-colonoscopy-trainer courses versus those who did not showed an improvement in colonoscopy quality indicators.[59] Although there are no similar pediatric studies, over the last decade there has been an increasing uptake of pediatric train-the-trainer courses in the United Kingdom (through JAG),[60] Canada (through the Canadian Association of Gastroenterology),[61] as well as Europe[62] and North America (through NASPGHAN), with self-reported improvements in knowledge and skills related to training pediatric endoscopy.[63] In addition, in the United Kingdom, the trainer skills outlined within the training domain of the P-GRS[50] encourage all pediatric endoscopy trainers to have undertaken a train-the-trainer course. This has helped to foster quality assurance related to training by standardizing the language, techniques, assessments, and performance-enhancing feedback used across centers.

Technologies to Support Endoscopy Training: Magnetic Endoscopic Imaging and Simulation

With recent advances in technology, there have been several instructional aids that have been developed to support endoscopy training. Use of MEI enables the trainer and trainee to visualize loop formation while performing ileocolonoscopy which can be particularly useful in teaching loop recognition and loop reduction techniques. Research indicates that use of an imager may enhance learners' understanding of loop formation and loop reduction maneuvers.[64] This may be particularly relevant in pediatrics as a recent pediatric prospective observational study looking at ileocolonoscopies performed using MEI showed that loops formed and re-formed very frequently.[65] Visual representation of the colonoscope configuration in three dimensions can also help endoscopy trainers to more easily pinpoint the problem when trainees encounter an area of difficulty, help trainers to deconstruct the procedure, and facilitate provision of performance-enhancing instruction without taking over the colonoscope.

Simulation is another technology that is increasingly being integrated into endoscopy training as it provides a learner-centered teaching environment where trainees can rehearse key aspects of procedures at their own pace and a simulated environment enables learners to make mistakes without placing patients at risks.[66] The extant literature supports simulation-based endoscopy training as an effective teaching modality, particularly for more novice endoscopists in helping them to developing the requisite skills in a safe and controlled environment, before clinical practice.[67] To enhance learning, however, the integration of simulation into training must be informed by evidence-based educational strategies, including incorporation of feedback, deliberate practice, mastery learning, interactivity, and range of difficulty.[68–73]

SUMMARY

High-quality training and continued upskilling in pediatric ileocolonoscopy are essential to ensure development and maintenance of competence and provision of high-quality endoscopic care. There are many devices and techniques that pediatric endoscopists can employ to improve the ease with which they perform procedures, enhance ergonomics and impact outcomes including procedure duration, patient comfort and lesion detection. Thoughtful integration of assessment during training and practice is essential support learning, document readiness for independent practice, and ensure ongoing maintenance of competence. In addition, measurement of quality indicators is critical to guide quality improvement efforts designed to enhance patient outcomes, maximize patient safety, and optimize efficiency. Structured, evidence-based endoscopic training and provision of training for endoscopy trainers are also an important as high-quality training is a key component to provision of safe, efficient, and effective endoscopic care for children.

CLINICS CARE POINTS

- Variable stiffness colonoscopes can reduce cecal intubation time and improve patient comfort.
- Magnetic endoscopic imagers aid with training in ileocolonoscopy and can improve procedural completion rates.
- Endoscopists encountering difficulties during pediatric ileocolonoscopies can try dynamic position changes, water-assisted ileocolonoscopy, and/or mucosal exposure devices to aid with navigation.
- Assessment of competence and recertification is important for ensuring quality assurance in pediatric ileocolonoscopy.
- "Train-the-trainer" courses can help endoscopists develop conscious competence and provide trainers with a uniform approach to training pediatric ileocolonoscopy.

DISCLOSURE

The authors do not have any commercial or financial conflicts of interest to disclose.

REFERENCES

1. Ginsberg GG. Colonoscopy with the variable stiffness colonoscope. Gastrointest Endosc 2003;58(4):579–84.

2. Brooker J, Saunders B, Shah S, et al. A new variable stiffness colonoscope makes colonoscopy easier: a randomized controlled trial. Gut 2000;46:801–5.

3. Xie Q, Chen B, Liu L, et al. Does the variable-stiffness colonoscope makes colonoscopy easier? A meta-analysis of the efficacy of the variable stiffness colonoscope compared with the standard adult colonoscope. BMC Gastroenterol 2012; 12(151):1–11.

4. Cirocco W, Rusin L. Surgical endoscopy. Surg Endosc 1996;10:1080--4.

5. Tan X, Yang W, Wichmann D, et al. Magnetic endoscopic imaging as a rational investment for specific colonoscopies: a systematic review and meta-analysis. Expert Rev Gastroenterol Hepatol 2021;15(4):447–58.

6. Rahman I, Pelitari S, Boger P, et al. magnetic endoscopic imaging: a useful ally in colonoscopy. J Gastrointest Dig Syst 2015;5(5):1–3.

7. Shah SG, Brooker JC, Williams CB, et al. Effect of magnetic endoscope imaging on colonoscopy performance: A randomised controlled trial. Lancet 2000;356: 1718–22.

8. Holme Ö, Höie O, Matre J, et al. Magnetic endoscopic imaging versus standard colonoscopy in a routine colonoscopy setting: A randomized, controlled trial. Gastrointest Endosc 2011;73(6):1215–22.

9. Pawa S, Banerjee P, Kothari S, et al. Are all endoscopy-related musculoskeletal injuries created equal? results of a national gender-based survey. Am J Gastroenterol 2021;116(March):530–8.

10. Ruan W, Walsh CM, Pawa S, et al. Musculoskeletal injury and ergonomics in pediatric gastrointestinal endoscopic practice. Surg Endosc 2023;37(1):248–54.

11. Walsh CM. Integrating ergonomics into pediatric endoscopy training and practice. Gastrointest Endosc Clin N Am 2023;33(2):235–51.

12. Parekh NK, McQuaid K. The injured endoscopist: A roadmap for recovery. Tech Gastrointest Endosc 2019;21(3):155–8.

13. Cappell MS, Co M. Endoscopes for endoscopists with small hands: A call to meet an unmet demand. Gastrointest Endosc 2013;78(4):670–2.

14. Akerkar GA, McQuaid KR, Terdiman JP, et al. An angulation dial adapter to facilitate endoscopy. Gastrointest Endosc 1999;49:AB120.

15. Crockett SD, Cirri HO, Kelapure R, et al. An abdominal compression device reduces cecal intubation time for some obese patients undergoing colonoscopy. Clin Gastroenterol Hepatol 2016;14(6):850–7.

16. Fetzer SJ. application of a positioning wedge during colonoscopy of obese patients to mitigate nurse pain. Work Heal Saf 2020;68(7):320–4.

17. Lerner DG, Mencin A, Novak I, et al. Advances in pediatric diagnostic endoscopy: a state-of-the-art review. JPGN Rep 2022;3(3):e224.

18. Pilonis ND, Januszewicz W, di Pietro M. Confocal laser endomicroscopy in gastro-intestinal endoscopy: Technical aspects and clinical applications. Transl Gastroenterol Hepatol 2022;7(7):1–20.

19. Jeong J, Hong ST, Ullah I, et al. Classification of the confocal microscopy images of colorectal tumor and inflammatory colitis mucosa tissue using deep learning. Diagnostics 2022;12(288):1–10.

20. Mi J, Han X, Wang R, et al. Diagnostic accuracy of probe-based confocal laser endomicroscopy and tissue sampling by endoscopic retrograde cholangiopancreatography in indeterminate biliary strictures: a meta-analysis. Sci Rep 2022; 12(7257):1–12.

21. Chauhan SS, Abu Dayyeh BK, Bhat YM, et al. Confocal laser endomicroscopy. Gastrointest Endosc 2014;80(6):928–38.

22. Venkatesh K, Cohen M, Evans C, et al. Feasibility of confocal endomicroscopy in the diagnosis of pediatric gastrointestinal disorders. World J Gastroenterol 2009; 15(18):2214–9.

23. Shavrov A, Kharitonova AY, Davis EM, et al. pilot study of confocal laser endomicroscopy to predict barrier dysfunction and relapse in pediatric inflammatory bowel disease. J Pediatr Gastroenterol Nutr 2016;62:873–8.

24. Pannala R, Krishnan K, Melson J, et al. Artificial intelligence in gastrointestinal endoscopy. VideoGIE 2020;5(12):598–613.

25. Dhaliwal J, Walsh CM. Artificial intelligence in pediatric enadoscopy. In: Gastrointest Endosc Clin N Am 2023;33(2):305–22.

26. Kröner PT, Engels MML, Glicksberg BS, et al. Artificial intelligence in gastroenterology: a state-of-the-art review. World J gastroenterol 2021;27(40):6794–824.

27. Lin SY, Yaow CYL, Ng CH, et al. Different position from traditional left lateral for colonoscopy? A meta-analysis and systematic review of randomized control trials. Chronic Dis Transl Med 2021;7:27–34.

28. Arya V, Singh S, Agarwal S, et al. Position change during colonoscopy improves caecal intubation rate, mucosal visibility, and adenoma detection in patients with suboptimal caecal preparation. Gastroenterol Rev 2017;12(4):296–302.

29. East JE, Bassett P, Arebi N, et al. Dynamic patient position changes during colonoscope withdrawal increase adenoma detection: a randomized, crossover trial. Gastrointest Endosc 2011;73(3):456–63.

30. East JE, Suzuki N, Arebi N, et al. Position changes improve visibility during colonoscope withdrawal: a randomized, blinded, crossover trial{A figure is presented. Gastrointest Endosc 2007;65(2):263–9.

31. Walsh CM, Qayed E, Aihara H, et al. Core curriculum for ergonomics in endoscopy. Gastrointest Endosc 2021;93(6):1222–7.

32. Trindade AJ, Lichtenstein DR, Aslanian HR, et al. Devices and methods to improve colonoscopy completion (with videos). Gastrointest Endosc 2018; 87(3):625–34.

33. Cadoni S, Gallittu P, Sanna S, et al. A two-center randomized controlled trial of water-aided colonoscopy versus air insufflation colonoscopy. Endoscopy 2014; 46(3):212–8.

34. Cadoni S, Falt P, Rondonotti E, et al. Water exchange for screening colonoscopy increases adenoma detection rate: A multicenter, double-blinded, randomized controlled trial. Endoscopy 2017;49(5):456–67.

35. Hsieh YH, Tseng CW, Hu CT, et al. Prospective multicenter randomized controlled trial comparing adenoma detection rate in colonoscopy using water exchange, water immersion, and air insufflation. Gastrointest Endosc 2017;86(1):192–201.

36. Park SM, Lee SH, Shin KY, et al. The cap-assisted technique enhances colonoscopy training: Prospective randomized study of six trainees. Surg Endosc 2012; 26:2939–43.

37. Nutalapati V, Kanakadandi V, Desai M, et al. Cap-assisted colonoscopy : a meta-analysis of high-quality randomized controlled trials. Endosc Int Open 2018;6: E1214–23.

38. Mir FA, Boumitri C, Ashraf I, et al. Cap-assisted colonoscopy versus standard colonoscopy: Is the cap beneficial? a meta-analysis of randomized controlled trials. Ann Gastroenterol 2017;30:640–8.

39. Rameshshanker R, Tsiamoulos Z, Wilson A, et al. Endoscopic cuff–assisted colonoscopy versus cap-assisted colonoscopy in adenoma detection: randomized tandem study—DEtection in Tandem Endocuff Cap Trial (DETECT). Gastrointest Endosc 2020;91(4):894–904, e1.

40. Broekaert IJ, Jahnel J, Moes N, et al. Evaluation of a European-wide survey on paediatric endoscopy training. Frontline Gastroenterol 2019;10(2):188–93.

41. Siau K, Hawkes ND, Dunckley P. Training in endoscopy. Curr Treat Options Gastroenterol 2018;16:345–61.

42. Walsh CM. In-training gastrointestinal endoscopy competency assessment tools: Types of tools, validation and impact. Best Pract Res Clin Gastroenterol 2016;30: 357–74.

43. Walsh CM, Ling SC, Mamula P, et al. The gastrointestinal endoscopy competency assessment tool for pediatric colonoscopy. J Pediatr Gastroenterol Nutr 2015;60: 474–80.

44. Walsh CM, Ling SC, Walters TD, et al. Development of the gastrointestinal endoscopy competency assessment tool for pediatric colonoscopy (GiECATKIDS). J Pediatr Gastroenterol Nutr 2014;59(4):480–6.

45. Siau K, Levi R, Iacucci M, et al. Paediatric colonoscopy direct observation of procedural skills: evidence of validity and competency development. J Pediatr Gastroenterol Nutr 2019;69:18–23.

46. Khan R, Zheng E, Wani SB, et al. Colonoscopy competence assessment tools: A systematic review of validity evidence. Endoscopy 2021;53(12):1235–45.

47. Royal College of Physicians, Joint Advisory Group on GI Endoscopy. JAG certification criteria and application process. Available at: https://www.thejag.org.uk/AboutUs/DownloadCentre.aspx. Accessed February 15, 2023.

48. Royal College of Physicians, Joint Advisory Group on GI Endoscopy. New DOPS and DOPyS forms and certification criteria. 2017. Available at: https://www.thejag.org.uk/AboutUs/DownloadCentre.aspx. Accessed February 15, 2023.

49. Narula P, Thomson M. Recertification and revalidation as concepts in pediatric endoscopy. In: Gershman G, Thomson M, editors. Practical Pediatric Gastrointestinal Endoscopy. 3rd Edition. Hoboken, New Jersey: Wiley Blackwell; 2022. p. 31–2.

50. Royal College of Physicians, Joint Advisory Group on GI Endoscopy. JAG Paediatric Global Rating Scale (P-GRS). Available at: https://www.thejag.org.uk/AboutUs/DownloadCentre.aspx. Accessed February 15, 2023.

51. Narula P, Broughton R, Howarth L, et al. Paediatric endoscopy global rating scale: development of a quality improvement tool and results of a national pilot. J Pediatr Gastroenterol Nutr 2019;69:171–5.

52. Sheu J, Chun S, O'Day E, et al. Outcomes from pediatric gastroenterology maintenance of certification using web-based modules. J Pediatr Gastroenterol Nutr 2017;64(5):671–8.

53. Walsh CM, Lightdale JR, Leibowitz IH, et al. pediatric endoscopy quality improvement network quality standards and indicators for pediatric endoscopists and endoscopists in training: a joint NASPGHAN/ESPGHAN guideline. J Pediatr Gastroenterol Nutr 2022;74:S44–52.

54. Broekaert I, Tzivinikos C, Narula P, et al. European society for paediatric gastroenterology, hepatology and nutrition position paper on training in paediatric endoscopy. J Pediatr Gastroenterol Nutr 2020;70:127–40.

55. Waschke KA, Anderson J, Macintosh D, et al. Training the gastrointestinal endoscopy trainer. Best Pract Res Clin Gastroenterol 2016;30:409–19.

56. Walsh CM, Anderson JT, Fishman DS. Evidence-based approach to training pediatric gastrointestinal endoscopy trainers. J Pediatr Gastroenterol Nutr 2017; 64(4):501–4.

57. Anderson J. The future of gastroenterology training: the trainee's perspective. Frontline Gastroenterol 2012;3(Suppl 1):i9–12.

58. Anderson J. Teaching colonoscopy. In: Waye J, Rex D, Williams C, editors. Colonoscopy: principles and practice. 2nd edition. Malden MA: Wiley Blackwell; 2009. p. 141–53.
59. Hoff G, Botteri E, Huppertz-Hauss G, et al. The effect of train-the-colonoscopy-trainer course on colonoscopy quality indicators. Endoscopy 2021;53(12): 1229–34.
60. Joint Advisory Group on GI Endoscopy. Course finder. Available at: https:// jetsapp.thejag.org.uk/courses/JAG_CRP2(P). Accessed February 15, 2023.
61. Canadian Association of Gastroenterology. Skills Enhancement for Endoscopy (SEE™) Program. Available at: https://www.cag-acg.org/education/see-program. Accessed February 15, 2023.
62. ESPGHAN. Endoscopy training the trainers. Available at: https://www.espghan. org/knowledge-center. Accessed February 15, 2023.
63. Kaul I, Queliza K, Waschke KA, et al. Sa2054 colonoscopy skills and "train the trainer" courses for pediatric endoscopy: north american experience. Gastrointest Endosc 2019;89(6):AB287–8.
64. Shah SG, Thomas-Gibson S, Lockett M, et al. Effect of real-time magnetic endoscope imaging on the teaching and acquisition of colonoscopy skills: Results from a single trainee. Endoscopy 2003;35(5):421–5.
65. Thomson M, Belsha D, Nedelkopoulou N, et al. colonoscope "looping" during ileo-colonoscopy in children is significantly different to that observed in adult practice. J Pediatr Gastroenterol Nutr 2022;74:651–6.
66. Walsh CM, Cohen J, editors. Endoscopic simulators. In: Clinical gastrointestinal endoscopy. 3rd edition. philadelphia, PA: Elsevier; 2018. p. 141–51.
67. Khan R, Plahouras J, Johnston BC, et al. Virtual reality simulation training for health professions trainees in gastrointestinal endoscopy. Cochrane Database Syst Rev 2018;8(8):CD008237.
68. Khan R, Scaffidi MA, Grover SC, et al. Simulation in endoscopy: Practical educational strategies to improve learning. World J Gastrointest Endosc 2019;11(3): 209–18.
69. Cook DA, Hamstra SJ, Brydges R, et al. Comparative effectiveness of instructional design features in simulation-based education: Systematic review and meta-analysis. Med Teach 2013;35(1):e867–98.
70. Walsh CM, Ling SC, Wang CS, et al. Concurrent versus terminal feedback: It may be better to wait. Acad Med 2009;84(10):54–7.
71. Grover SC, Scaffidi MA, Khan R, et al. Progressive learning in endoscopy simulation training improves clinical performance: a blinded randomized trial. Gastrointest Endosc 2017;86(5):881–9.
72. Walsh CM, Scaffidi MA, Khan R, et al. Non-technical skills curriculum incorporating simulation-based training improves performance in colonoscopy among novice endoscopists: Randomized controlled trial. Dig Endosc 2020;32(6):940–8.
73. Yen AW, Leung JW, Leung FW. A novel method with significant impact on adenoma detection: Combined water-exchange and cap-assisted colonoscopy. Gastrointest Endosc 2013;77(6):944–8.

Electronic Medical Records
Use as Tools for Improving Quality in Pediatric Endoscopy

Jeannie S. Huang, MD, MPH, F-NASPGHAN[a,b,*], Catharine M. Walsh, MD, MEd, PhD[c,d]

KEYWORDS

- Pediatric endoscopy • Quality improvement • Metrics • Gastrointestinal endoscopy
- Electronic health record • Electronic medical record • Key performance indicators
- Quality standards

KEY POINTS

- The international Pediatric Endoscopy Quality Improvement Network (PEnQuIN) has identified pediatric endoscopy quality standards and indicators that define best practice.
- Data collection of quality indicators is essential to quality improvement (QI) efforts in pediatric endoscopy.
- Increasing functionality of electronic medical record (EMR) systems in pediatric care can enable point of care collection and monitoring of quality indicators in real-time.
- Setting up EMR protocols and frameworks for active collection and monitoring of pediatric endoscopy quality indicators can also enable "big data" analyses and sharing across endoscopy services that can be used to inform and support QI efforts.

INTRODUCTION

Gastrointestinal endoscopic procedures are fundamental to pediatric gastrointestinal clinical care. However, unwarranted variation in clinical endoscopic services limits the assurance of high-quality pediatric endoscopic care, as well as engagement in continuous quality improvement (QI) activities by multiple stakeholders. Quality metrics in pediatric endoscopy, recently identified through the international Pediatric Endoscopy Quality Improvement Network (PEnQuIN),[1,2] are now available for regular monitoring in

[a] Department of Pediatrics, University of California San Diego, 9500 Gilman Drive, MC 0984, La Jolla, CA 92093, USA; [b] Division of Pediatric Gastroenterology, Rady Children's Hospital San Diego, 3020 Children's Way, San Diego, CA, USA; [c] Division of Gastroenterology, Hepatology, and Nutrition, and the SickKids Research and Learning Institutes, The Hospital for Sick Children, Toronto, ON, Canada; [d] Department of Paediatrics and The Wilson Centre, University of Toronto, Temerty Faculty of Medicine, University of Toronto, Toronto, ON, Canada
* Corresponding author.
E-mail address: jshuang@ucsd.edu

Gastrointest Endoscopy Clin N Am 33 (2023) 267–290
https://doi.org/10.1016/j.giec.2022.11.004
1052-5157/23/© 2022 Elsevier Inc. All rights reserved.

a scheduled fashion. Ideally, such monitoring will enable real-time identification of gaps in care so that QI interventions and protocols can be implemented, and an ideal standard of endoscopic performance and periprocedural care can be assured.

During the past few decades, there have been several efforts promoting quality in pediatric endoscopy. These have included single institution projects, multicenter data registries and collaborations, as well as the convening of expert panels to identify standards of care and quality metrics.[1,3–5] Common components of these efforts have included identification and measurement of outcome metrics and identification of processes needing improvement. There have also been iterative and evolving actions to address identified processes in need of improvement that can ideally enhance patient outcomes. Prior work, however, has been limited to date by a lack of consensus on key pediatric-specific quality indicators that can accurately measure quality in a standardized way within endoscopy services, provider groups and individual endoscopists, and thereby promote QI through data capture, feedback, and intervention. The recent PEnQuIN guidelines from the North American and European Societies of Pediatric Gastroenterology, Hepatology and Nutrition[1,2] have helped to address this gap.

The advent and adoption of electronic medical record (EMR) systems during the past several decades also provides a means to standardize care and care measurement. EMR systems also contribute to the electronic health record (EHR), defined as a comprehensive integration of many EMRs that can enable sharing of health information across institutions. According to HealthIT.gov, identified care gaps that local EMRs and the EHR can address that are relevant to endoscopy include legible complete documentation, accurate streamlined coding and billing, improved patient and provider interaction and communication, and a reduction in health-care costs through reduced paperwork and duplication of testing.[6] The following state-of-the art review aims both to outline the potential role EMRs can play in QI, and to provide practical tips for harnessing functionalities available in the EMR at a local level that can facilitate data acquisition and visualization. In the process, we will discuss how use of the EMR can support continuous QI within and across pediatric endoscopy services.

Quality Improvement

According to the United States Health Resources and Services Administration, QI consists of "systematic and continuous actions that lead to measurable improvement in health care services and the health status of targeted patient groups."[7] This definition acknowledges several key features of QI, namely that it is ongoing and involves system interventions (beyond the individual) and measurement. The Associates in Process Improvement has developed The Model for Improvement[8] that incorporates a Plan-Do-Study-Act (PDSA) cycle (**Fig. 1**), which encompasses baseline data collection to identify the gap or need to be addressed, the goal aspired to, and the intervention to be performed, followed by intervention performance and repeat data collection (inclusive of outcome, process, and balancing measures) to determine what improvements (and the costs of such improvements), if any, resulted from the intervention. Subsequent cycle performance is determined based on ongoing need or suboptimal performance until a stipulated goal is achieved. This model provides a useful framework for developing, testing, and implementing changes leading to improvement.

Measurement and Reporting

A major requirement of QI is data collection, which must be scheduled and occur on a regular basis. Data collection is required to initially determine where one is starting

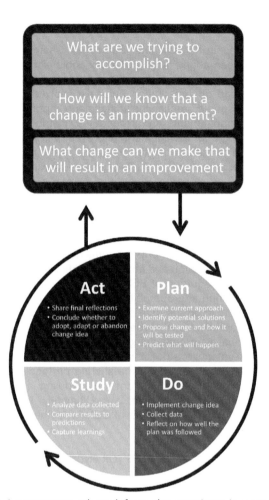

Fig. 1. Model for improvement adapted from the associates in process improvement. (*Adapted from* Langley G, Moen R, Nolan K, Nolan T, Norman C, Provost L. The Improvement Guide: A Practical Approach to Enhancing Organizational Performance. 2nd ed. San Francisco, CA: Jossey-Bass Publishers; 2009.)

(baseline) and then, in subsequent, iterative PDSA cycles, the effects of interventions. Scheduled intervals between data collections must be of sufficient length to allow for the collection of enough meaningful data resulting from QI interventions, while also being short enough to provide prompt feedback on whether the tested intervention has succeeded in improving care, to determine whether additional intervention is needed to effect the desired change. Ideally, this should be monthly, at minimum, to keep the interest of involved parties (eg, if it takes a year to receive feedback on an intervention performed daily, it is unlikely that persons involved will continue that intervention on a regular basis). In general, outcomes measured at a given regular interval should be reported at the next highest consolidated schedule level (ie, if an intervention is expected to be performed every hour, one should report it daily or per worker shift; if an intervention is performed daily, one should report it weekly; and if an intervention is reported a few times a week, one should report it monthly).

ENDOSCOPIC ELECTRONIC MEDICAL RECORD SYSTEMS

As expertly summarized in an American Society of Gastrointestinal Endoscopy guideline,[9] there has been a long history of endoscopic electronic medical record (EEMR) systems. Initially created in the 1980s, these systems were created for endoscopy reporting and documentation but have evolved over time to include other elements of endoscopic practice including image capture, automated coding, scheduling of future appointments and procedures, distribution of patient hand-outs, instrument tracking and management, and even the beginnings of pathology report integration.[9,10] The data generated from such systems can service various aspects of an endoscopic practice, including quality assurance, risk management, practice management, and research. Related to QI, many EEMRs permit tracking of quality indicators for self-assessment and quality benchmarking within an endoscopy practice and enabled reporting of select metrics to endoscopy out-comes registries for broader comparison and multicenter endoscopy QI initiatives.[3,4]

Unfortunately, the development of EMR systems during recent decades to docu-ment and store patient information and facilitate workflow across services have not routinely accounted for integration of EEMR capabilities. As a result, there have been challenges to ensuring interoperability or communication between systems, and rarely simple ways to integrate data collected in stand-alone EEMRs into cur-rent EMR systems. In addition, such endeavors have been found to be expensive, and to require additional time-consuming programming efforts for ultimate suc-cess. Recently, EMR systems are beginning to enter the EEMR space themselves by designing their own templates and data-sharing protocols in ways that allow data integration across all clinical platforms (scheduling, reporting, pathologic condition) necessary to influence clinical care. Ultimately, these maneuvers and developments may reduce the relevance of EEMRs in the current digital health arena.

UTILITY OF ELECTRONIC MEDICAL RECORDS FOR ENDOSCOPY QUALITY DATA ACQUISITION

Two prerequisites for beginning any improvement in care or quality in care project are (1) delineation of clinical workflows involved in delivery of care and (2) identifica-tion of outcome metrics that define quality of care in a given clinical scenario. Clin-ical workflows involved in endoscopy involve 3 phases of endoscopic care encompassing *preprocedure* scheduling and procedural preparation, *intraprocedure* performance and documentation, and *postprocedure* communication. Endoscopy quality outcome indicators, defined as measurable and auditable key performance metrics, have already been identified by a rigorous consensus process and pub-lished in the PEnQuIN guidelines.[1,2,11–15] Additional indicators are presented below for consideration.

In each section below, we outline the phase of endoscopic care, specific PEnQuIN indicators, and EMR programming considerations around each mentioned quality in-dicator as needed for appropriate data capture. It is expected that indicators can be measured, at minimum monthly, which satisfies the criteria for interval data collection, as stated above. Further, it is recommended that indicators be displayed in an ongoing fashion for ready access, with multiple indicators displayed and organized by phase of care for ease of access and interpretation. Construction of the related PEnQuIN indi-cators is included in the tables below. For justification of a specified quality indicator, please refer to the reference articles.[1,2,11–15]

Preprocedure: Scheduling and Preparation

In the phase before performing pediatric endoscopy, planning is required to ensure patients and caregivers are adequately prepared to undergo procedures in a safe and timely manner. At a minimum, this phase includes considerations related to efficient procedure scheduling and high-quality bowel preparation.

Procedure scheduling

Scheduling issues directly affect the flow of patients receiving endoscopic care and thus significantly affect both clinical outcomes and financial viability of endoscopy services. For example, a delay in scheduling a procedure may lead to a delay in diagnosis, which in certain conditions can increase morbidity (ie, delay in scheduling a procedure to confirm a diagnosis of Crohn disease may risk worsening of anemia, higher likelihood of abdominal pain, weight loss). Alternatively, expediently scheduling a procedure before obtaining prior authorization for insurance coverage in the United States can risk denial of payment to providers and facilities.

At a basic level, fundamental processes in scheduling an endoscopic procedure involve the procedure order and communication with the patient and/or caregiver to schedule a date and time. Additional considerations include the time required to complete the insurance authorization process for financial coverage of the procedure (where applicable), procedure duration and room turnover time, and unique considerations in pediatrics related to the need for anesthesia and desire to coordinate multiple procedures at the same time for convenience and to mitigate anesthetic-related risk.[16,17]

Monitoring procedure scheduling metrics can be a helpful way to identify problematic or bottleneck processes that can reduce endoscopy service capacity. Proposed quality metrics are listed in **Table 1**.

Bowel preparation

Preparation of the gastrointestinal tract is crucial to successful performance of endoscopy, in particular lower endoscopy or ileocolonoscopy. However, inadequate bowel preparations still occur commonly, with more than 25% of pediatric lower endoscopies affected.[18] Poor bowel preparation is associated with lower ileal intubation rates, longer procedure times, higher costs, and increased need to repeat procedures to obtain the required clinical data to inform management.[19,20] There remains great variation in pediatric bowel preparation, with no ideal regimen identified.[4,19–22] Additionally, although standardized tools to assess bowel preparation have been developed, their application to pediatrics has not been examined systematically. Overall, bowel preparation remains an inadequately addressed arena where a supporting and sustaining framework is required to support much needed QI efforts. Quality indicators related to bowel preparation are outlined in **Table 2**. Use of the EMR to track and visualize rates of bowel preparation adequacy at the facility and/or individual endoscopist level may help identify opportunities for QI and assess efficacy of QI activities to improve bowel preparations in pediatric patients undergoing lower endoscopic procedures.

Intraprocedure: Procedural Performance and Documentation

Procedural outcome metrics are important to assess whether pediatric endoscopic procedures are performed ideally, to monitor adverse event rates, and to identify gaps in providing high-quality endoscopic care. Relevant quality indicators and considerations related to the intraprocedural phase of care are listed in **Table 3**.

High-quality procedural documentation, defined by the inclusion of all key reporting elements with an endoscopy report, is also essential to ensure clear communication of

Table 1
Quality indicators related to procedure scheduling

Indicator Construct	PEnQuIN Quality Indicators[1]	Dashboard Monthly Indicator	EMR Specifics, Modifiers, and Considerations
Time from placement of order to scheduling of the procedure	n/a	• *Construct:* Median time from order placement to procedure date. This should be calculated by procedure type (eg, upper endoscopy, ileocolonoscopy) • *Calculation:* Median (range) time in days	• Ideally measured in business and not calendar days
Rate with which endoscopies are performed within a timeframe as specified in guidelines	Rate with which endoscopies are performed within a timeframe as specified in guidelines, when available (eg, button battery removal, endoscopy for suspected inflammatory bowel disease) (I1)	• *Numerator:* Number of pediatric endoscopies occurring in an endoscopy facility that are performed within a guideline-specified timeframe • *Denominator:* All pediatric endoscopies occurring in an endoscopy facility that are subject to a guideline-specified timeframe • *Calculation:* Proportion (%)	• Ideally measured in business and not calendar days
Time for completion of insurance authorization (time from authorization request to approval)	n/a	• *Numerator:* Number of pediatric endoscopies receiving authorization from a specific insurance carrier within a specified timeframe (eg, 48 h) • *Denominator:* All pediatric endoscopies requiring authorization from a given insurance carrier • *Calculation:* Proportion (%)	• Should be evaluated by insurance carrier to identify potential need for discussion with payors to improve workflows
Rate of scheduling cancellations and no-shows	n/a	• *Numerator:* Number of pediatric endoscopies canceled within a specified timeframe, precluding filling of the endoscopy schedule (eg, 24 or 48 h)	• Since the ability to quickly fill an endoscopy unit schedule depends on the need for bowel preparation, calculations may be performed by procedure type (ie, those requiring bowel preparation vs not)

		• *Denominator:* All pediatric endoscopies • *Calculation:* Proportion (%)	• Similarly, reasons for cancellations should be recorded (discrete categories might include provider cancellation, patient illness, lack of transportation, loss of insurance, unknown)
Procedure time	Procedure time (I27)	• *Construct:* Median procedure time from first insertion until final removal of endoscope. This should be calculated by procedure type (eg, upper endoscopy, ileocolonoscopy) • *Calculation:* Median (range) time in minutes	• Time needed to perform a procedure must be adequately incorporated into the endoscopy schedule • Although there are standard procedure times for different procedure types, practical awareness of how long a given endoscopist takes can be very valuable for scheduling and for running an efficient endoscopy unit. Accordingly, procedure times should be calculated by procedure type and proceduralist • Although controversial, the need to determine endoscopic competence across the provider continuum has been recently highlighted.[34,35] Although competency assessment standards have yet to be agreed upon, the EMR enables continual monitoring of procedure performance to ensure continuous quality and patient safety • Confounder to consider: One may want to filter both the numerator and denominator to include only lower endoscopies where there was an adequate bowel preparation when assessing procedure time for a given endoscopist

Abbreviations: EMR, electronic medical record; PEnQuIN: Pediatric Endoscopy Quality Improvement Network.

Table 2
Quality indicators related to procedure preparation

Indicator Construct	PEnQuIN Quality Indicators[1]	Dashboard Monthly Indicator	EMR Specifics, Modifiers, and Considerations

Delivery of bowel preparation instructions	Rate with which patients receive adequate instructions on bowel preparation (I13)	• *Numerator:* Number of pediatric endoscopies occurring in an endoscopy facility where adequate instructions on bowel preparation were communicated to patients, and this is documented
		• *Denominator:* All pediatric endoscopies occurring in an endoscopy facility where bowel preparation is required
		• *Calculation:* Proportion (%)
			• Documentation should reflect:
			  ○ To whom (patient and/or caregiver)
			  ○ When (relative to scheduled procedure)
			  ○ Communication modality (in-person, telemedicine, telephone)
			  ○ Format (written, written with oral review, oral, app)
			  ○ Which bowel preparation instructions were given

Adequacy of bowel preparation	Rate of adequate bowel preparation (I28)	• *Numerator:* Number of pediatric endoscopies with adequate bowel preparation. This should be assessed formally, using a tool with strong validity evidence (eg, Ottawa Bowel Preparation Scale,[36,37] Boston Bowel Preparation Scale[38,39]) or, at a minimum, using standardized language with clear definitions (eg, excellent, good, or fair) • *Denominator:* All pediatric endoscopies for which bowel preparation is required • *Calculation:* Proportion (%) • *Minimum target:* ≥80% (unadjusted)	• A uniform score should be used per group/facility • Consider capturing whether suboptimal bowel preparation results require a repeat procedure

Abbreviations: EMR, electronic medical record; PEnQuIN: Pediatric Endoscopy Quality Improvement Network.

Table 3
Relevant intraprocedure quality indicators

Indicator Construct	PEnQuIN Quality Indicators[1]	Dashboard Monthly Indicator	EMR Specifics, Modifiers, and Considerations
Indication for the procedure	Rate with which the endoscopy report documents the indication for the procedure (117)	• *Numerator:* Number of procedure reports for pediatric endoscopies that clearly document the indication for the procedure • *Denominator:* All pediatric endoscopies performed • *Calculation:* Proportion (%)	• Specific data collection items to be incorporated into the endoscopy report include indication and type of procedure • PEnQuIN Indicator #18 (Rate with which endoscopy is performed for an indication that is in accordance with current evidence-based guidelines and/or published standards, when available) is related to this indicator • Determination of PEnQuIN indicator 18 will likely require post hoc analysis of data. Discrete entry of indication and procedure type would facilitate post hoc analysis
Informed consent	Rate with which informed consent/assent is obtained (119)	• *Numerator:* Number of pediatric endoscopies for which informed consent/assent is obtained and this process is documented • *Denominator:* All pediatric patients undergoing endoscopies • *Calculation:* Proportion (%)	• Specific data collection items to be incorporated into the endoscopy report include whether informed consent/assent was obtained (yes/no) and from whom (parent, guardian, patient) • Depending on jurisdiction, assent is often not required for procedural performance; however, it is ideal to also document assent whenever possible

(continued on next page)

Table 3
(continued)

Indicator Construct	PEnQuIN Quality Indicators[1]	Dashboard Monthly Indicator	EMR Specifics, Modifiers, and Considerations
Whether a preprocedural team pause was conducted	Rate with which a preprocedural team pause is conducted (I4)	• *Numerator:* Number of pediatric endoscopies for which a preprocedural team pause (time-out) is conducted and this is documented • *Denominator:* All pediatric endoscopies occurring at an endoscopy facility/group/provider level • *Calculation:* Proportion (%)	• Simple yes/no metric • Usually documented by nurses/endoscopy team and this documentation can be used for the dashboard indicator (if not documented in the endoscopy report). • If a preprocedure team pause is documented by both the nurse/team and endoscopist, the metrics should match for the indicator to be marked as performed
Anesthesia documentation	Rate with which the sedation/anesthetic plan is documented (I20)	• *Numerator:* Number of pediatric endoscopies that document the sedation/anesthetic plan • *Denominator:* All pediatric endoscopies performed that involve sedation/anesthetic • *Calculation:* Proportion (%)	• It is recommended to document the sedation/anesthesia plan in the endoscopy report. The type and level of sedation administered should also be documented within the endoscopy report • NOTE: This section also refers to PEnQuIN indicators #23 (rate of documentation of all medications and associated details during the procedure), #24 (rate of documentation of patient comfort during the procedure), #25 (rate with which reversal agents are used), and #26 (rate with which procedure interrupted or prematurely terminated due to sedation/anesthesia-related issue) • These indicators may use related anesthesiologist and nonanesthesiologist sedation documentation

Rate with which ASA status is documented (I21)	• *Numerator:* Number of pediatric endoscopies that document ASA status • *Denominator:* All pediatric endoscopies performed that involve sedation/anesthetic • *Calculation:* Proportion (%)	
Rate with which patient monitoring during sedation/anesthesia is performed (I22)	• *Numerator:* Number of pediatric endoscopies in which patient monitoring during sedation/anesthetic is performed and this is documented • *Denominator:* All pediatric endoscopies performed that involve sedation/anesthetic • *Calculation:* Proportion (%)	
Prophylactic antibiotic administration Rate of appropriate prophylactic antibiotic administration in accordance with accepted guidelines (I3)	• *Numerator:* Number of pediatric endoscopies where prophylactic antibiotics are *administered* in accordance with currently accepted guidelines • *Denominator:* All pediatric endoscopies occurring at an endoscopy facility/group/provider level where prophylactic antibiotics are *indicated* in accordance currently accepted guidelines • *Calculation:* Proportion (%)	• Additional data capture items to be considered include which antibiotics were administered, indications for the procedure, and procedure(s) or intervention(s) performed • Post hoc analysis will be necessary to determine whether antibiotic administration was performed in accordance with guidelines
Quality of visualization Rate of adequate bowel preparation (I28)	• *Numerator:* Number of pediatric endoscopies with adequate bowel preparation. This should be assessed formally, using a tool with strong validity evidence (eg, Ottawa Bowel Preparation Scale,[36,37] Boston Bowel Preparation Scale[38,39]) or, at a minimum, using standardized language with clear definitions (eg, excellent, good, or fair)	• Standardization of bowel prep documentation is best performed using tools which use standardized definitions with accompanying picture examples for validity • Although tool references can be posted in endoscopy suites for reference by endoscopists, it is best if such references are incorporated into the EMR documentation itself

(continued on next page)

Table 3
(continued)

Indicator Construct	PEnQuIN Quality Indicators[1]	Dashboard Monthly Indicator	EMR Specifics, Modifiers, and Considerations
		• *Denominator*: All pediatric endoscopies for which bowel preparation is required • *Calculation*: Proportion (%) • *Minimum target*: ≥80% (unadjusted)	• Standardized documentation of relevant findings (and thus inspection) using discrete data capture (not free text), quality of visualization, whether biopsies are performed by location, and whether the procedure was completed per standard should ideally be incorporated into an endoscopy reporting template
Procedure completeness (documentation of inspection of all areas, acquisition of appropriate biopsies and procedure completion of per standards)	Rate of procedure completeness as defined by inspection of all relevant areas, acquisition of appropriate biopsies and successful completion of interventions (I30)	• *Numerator*: Number of cases in which completeness of the procedure (inspection of all relevant areas, acquisition of appropriate biopsies and successful completion of interventions) is documented • *Denominator*: All pediatric endoscopies performed • *Calculation*: Proportion (%)	• Use of free text is common but is not amenable to subsequent data analysis. Although natural language processing may be a solution in the future to extract data from free text in clinical documentation,[40,41] such capabilities are not universally available
	Rate with which biopsies are obtained or eschewed, appropriately (I33)	• *Numerator*: Number of pediatric endoscopies in which biopsies are obtained appropriately, in accordance with currently accepted guidelines (eg, number of duodenal biopsies in a patient with suspected celiac) *plus* the number of pediatric endoscopies in which biopsies are not obtained for appropriate reasons that are documented • *Denominator*: All pediatric endoscopies performed • *Calculation*: Proportion (%)	• EMR endoscopy report templates can incorporate many procedure types and account for all these indicators. Ideally, one should use one EMR template from which the various procedures can be selected for complete documentation By standardizing a common workflow, one can more easily incorporate required changes in documentation when necessary
	Rate with which the endoscopy report documents findings (I34)	• *Numerator*: Number of procedure reports for pediatric endoscopies that document findings. Both written and photo documentation is preferable. If no findings, this should be documented	

	Rate with which the endoscopy report documentation is complete (I35)	• *Denominator:* All pediatric endoscopies performed • *Calculation:* Proportion (%) • *Numerator:* Number of procedure reports for pediatric endoscopies for which documentation is complete (all recommended reporting elements included) • *Denominator:* All pediatric endoscopies performed • *Calculation:* Proportion (%)	
Standardized reporting of endoscopy findings by disease	Pediatric endoscopic procedures should be reported using standardized disease-related terminology and/or scales, when available (Standard 38)	• *Numerator:* Number of procedure reports for pediatric endoscopies which use standardized disease-related terminology or scales (when available) to document findings for a given disease • *Denominator:* All pediatric endoscopies performed for a given disease • *Calculation:* Proportion (%)	• Endoscopy findings are increasingly being used to define clinical status (eg, remission and disease severity in inflammatory bowel disease and eosinophilic esophagitis). Accordingly, to better communicate how a given patient is doing, common standards will have to be utilized • It is recommended to use validated standardized disease-related terminology and/or scales, when available, to document endoscopy findings • Similar to bowel preparation quality rating scales, when incorporating such terminology and/or scales into endoscopy report templates, it is best to provide clear definitions and examples within the documentation template itself to facilitate accurate completion

(continued on next page)

Table 3
(continued)

Indicator Construct	PenQuIN Quality Indicators[1]	Dashboard Monthly Indicator	EMR Specifics, Modifiers, and Considerations
Endoscopic interventions performed	Rate with which endoscopic interventions are performed or eschewed, appropriately (I31)	• *Numerator:* Number of pediatric endoscopies in which interventions are performed appropriately (in accordance with the indication and findings) and documented *plus* the number of pediatric endoscopies in which interventions are not performed for appropriate reasons that are documented • *Denominator:* All pediatric endoscopies performed • *Calculation:* Proportion (%)	• Elements to be incorporated into the endoscopy report include procedure indication(s), endoscopic intervention(s) performed, the results of the intervention(s), and whether they were performed to completion
	Rate of endoscopic intervention completion (I32)	• *Numerator:* Number of pediatric endoscopies in which interventions (eg, polypectomy) are performed to completion • *Denominator:* All pediatric endoscopies in which interventions are performed • *Calculation:* Proportion (%)	
Adverse events	Rate of *documented* intraprocedural adverse events (I7)	• *Numerator:* Number of intraprocedural adverse events that are *documented* for a procedure/facility/group/provider • *Denominator:* All intraprocedural adverse events occurring at a procedure/facility/group/provider level • *Calculation:* Proportion (%)	• Additional considerations here are to have documentation specify not only yes/no (whether an intraprocedural adverse event occurred) but what type of adverse event occurred (eg, intestinal perforation, uncontrolled or significant bleeding requiring intervention, hemodynamic instability)

Procedure time	Procedure time (I27)	• *Construct:* Median procedure time from first insertion until final removal of endoscope. This should be calculated by procedure type (eg, upper endoscopy, ileocolonoscopy) • *Calculation:* Median (range) time in minutes	• It is also helpful to document resulting interventions (eg, surgical repair, hospitalization, intensive care unit stay) • As always, discrete data collection should be preferred over free text • Additional time-based data indicators to consider include time to cecum and time to terminal ileum. In general, endoscopy skill is related to ability to reach these sites within stipulated time frames, and thus these indicators can be used as surrogate measures of endoscopist competence
Endoscopy report finalization	Rate with which the endoscopy report documentation is finalized (I36) Rate with which endoscopy report documentation is finalized in a timely manner (I37)	• *Numerator:* Number of procedure reports for pediatric endoscopies for which documentation is finalized (ie, signed and entered into the medical record) • *Denominator:* All pediatric endoscopies performed • *Calculation:* Proportion (%) • *Numerator:* Number of procedure reports for pediatric endoscopies for which documentation is finalized (ie, signed and entered into the medical record) within a specified timeframe, per institutional/regulatory policies • *Denominator:* All pediatric endoscopies performed • *Calculation:* Proportion (%)	• These indicators are important not only for patient safety considerations but also for financial reimbursement • Documentation should ideally be available immediately after the procedure as documentation is crucial for subsequent evaluation should a procedure-related adverse event occur

Abbreviations: EMR, electronic medical record; PEnQuIN: Pediatric Endoscopy Quality Improvement Network.

procedural events and outcomes, guide patient care, and facilitate QI. Standardized endoscopy reporting elements for pediatric endoscopy procedure reports have been identified by PEnQuIN,[11] which will help to serve as a basis for QI activities.

Postprocedure: Communications

Considerations related to endoscopy quality do not end on completion of the procedure. Instead, it is also important to measure quality to ensure maintenance of patient safety and procedural effectiveness during postprocedure care and follow-up, as outlined in **Table 4**. Postprocedure quality indicators relate to safety monitoring after the procedure and ensuring timely follow-up of the procedure results, including tissue sampling, with patients and caregivers.

Special Considerations: Monitoring Quality During Training

Procedural education is a key aspect of all pediatric gastroenterology training programs, and "competence thresholds" (target numbers of supervised procedures to be performed before competence should be assessed), have been identified primarily based on expert opinion due to limited data.[23] Although adequate volume is necessary to achieve competence, the number of procedures performed does not directly correlate with competence in performing endoscopy when measured using standardized assessment tools with strong validity evidence.[24,25] Furthermore, for rare procedures, such as gastrointestinal bleeding control, the infrequent and erratic nature of clinical cases with such issues can result in trainees having a restricted range of procedural experience. In practice, continued exposure is also required to ensure maintenance of competence. Considered together, it is essential for training programs to monitor the types and numbers of procedures, as well as PEnQuIN quality indicators, for endoscopies performed by trainees to facilitate assessment of competence and help identify trainees who may require additional support.[12]

Quality metrics complement detailed feedback provided by direct observation assessment tools by helping to assess trainees at the "does" level of Miller's pyramid (ie, performance in practice).[26] Additionally, incorporation of collection and regular review of quality metrics as a standard component of an educational curriculum helps trainees to understand the importance of quality metrics, to cultivate self-reflection, and to foster a culture of quality assessment and improvement, which endoscopists will carry forward into their future careers. The key features of a system for assessing procedural competence, which incorporates quality metrics include (1) a clear definition of all quality metrics coupled with a transparent assessment process; (2) systematic collection and analysis of quality metrics; and (3) feedback that integrates quality metrics with other assessment data, including direct observational assessment tools.[27] Future research is required to delineate how quality metrics, such as terminal ileal intubation rate, change over the course of pediatric endoscopic training.

Special Considerations: Monitoring Quality in Practice

Monitoring the types and numbers of procedures performed by a given endoscopist over specified time periods (generally a year) also represent ongoing metrics that should be followed by endoscopy services.[12] Typically speaking, the number of procedures performed annually is often queried during the process of obtaining continued privileging at institutions supporting endoscopy services. For the same reasons as listed above for trainees, endoscopy quality indicators should be measured continually for active endoscopists to document maintenance of competence.[25] They also may be useful in helping to determine whether a proceduralist is safe to resume endoscopic practice after a prolonged absence or whether they require supports to

Table 4
Relevant postprocedure quality indicators

Indicator Construct	PEnQuIN Quality Indicators[1]	Dashboard Monthly Indicator	EMR Specifics, Modifiers, and Considerations
Patient/caregiver receipt of postprocedure instructions, including when pathology follow-up will occur	Rate with which patients/caregivers receive written postprocedure instructions on discharge (138)	• *Numerator:* Number of patients/caregivers who receive written postprocedure instructions on discharge and communication of these instructions is documented. Instructions should include potential symptoms that may indicate a procedure-related adverse event, along with instructions on what to do should these symptoms develop • *Denominator:* All pediatric patients undergoing endoscopies • *Calculation:* Proportion (%)	• As with all patient communications, the modality and format of communication will affect patient understanding • As with all forms of communication, documentation should include to whom (patient and/or caregiver), when (relative to performed procedure), the communication modality (in person, telemedicine, telephone) and format (written, written with oral review, oral) by which postprocedure instructions were delivered
	Rate with which the plan for pathology follow-up is communicated to patients/caregivers (139)	• *Numerator:* Number of patients/caregivers who receive a plan for pathology follow-up after a pediatric endoscopy, and this plan is documented • *Denominator:* All pediatric patients undergoing endoscopies • *Calculation:* Proportion (%)	
Pathology findings review with patient/caregiver	Rate with which pathology findings are reviewed with the patient and/or caregiver (140)	• *Numerator:* Number of patients/caregivers who receive communication about pathology findings after a pediatric endoscopy and this communication is documented • *Denominator:* All pediatric patients undergoing endoscopies where pathology is expected • *Calculation:* Proportion (%)	• As with all patient communications, the modality and format of communication affects patient understanding • As with all forms of communication, documentation should include to whom (patient and/or caregiver), when (relative to performed procedure—ideally in business days), the communication modality (in person, telemedicine, telephone, patient portal) and format (written, written with oral review, oral) by which pathology follow-up was performed

(continued on next page)

Table 4
(continued)

Indicator Construct	PEnQuIN Quality Indicators[1]	Dashboard Monthly Indicator	EMR Specifics, Modifiers, and Considerations
Adverse event rate	Rate of *documented* immediate postprocedural adverse events (I8)	• *Numerator:* Number of immediate postprocedural adverse events that are documented for a procedure/facility/group/provider • *Denominator:* All immediate postprocedural adverse events occurring at a procedure/facility/group/provider level • *Calculation:* Proportion (%)	• Although PEnQuIN Indicator #7, intraprocedural adverse events (**Table 3**), can be easily extracted from a templated endoscopy report that documents intraprocedural adverse events, postprocedural adverse events are difficult to identify without proactive intervention • Methods that have been utilized to identify potential postprocedural adverse events include identifying whether patients undergoing endoscopy have been evaluated at the emergency department or admitted to the hospital within a specific timeframe from the procedure. However, such methods still often require extensive chart review to determine whether the reason for emergency department evaluation or hospital admission was related to the preceding endoscopic procedure • Some facilities use a more proactive approach to identify adverse events by reaching out to patients/families within 72 h of the endoscopy to evaluate the patient's status
	Rate of *documented* late adverse events (I9)	• *Numerator:* Number of late adverse events, defined as procedure-related adverse events identified after an endoscopy is complete, that are *documented* for a procedure/facility/group/provider • *Denominator:* All late adverse events occurring at a procedure/facility/group/provider level • *Calculation:* Proportion (%)	

Abbreviations: EMR, electronic medical record; PEnQuIN: Pediatric Endoscopy Quality Improvement Network.

enhance their skills. Active monitoring of endoscopic performance, through the documentation of procedural numbers and PEnQuIN indicators in the EMR, may also represent opportunities to identify needs for clinical retraining, upskilling, or refresher courses.[28]

UTILITY OF ELECTRONIC MEDICAL RECORDS FOR ENDOSCOPY QUALITY DATA VISUALIZATION

Appropriate visualization of data is paramount to conveying important trends to a wide range of users in an easy-to-comprehend manner. In QI, a fundamental method for displaying QI data collection over time is a run chart.[29] Key elements in run charts that facilitate a user's understanding of the data are displayed in **Fig. 2** and include the following:

- Measured data over time with a connecting line (so the user can understand directionality),
- The current data mean and/or median,
- The project goal (so the user can understand the threshold above or below which datapoints should fall and/or the range from minimally acceptable to ideal), and
- Intervention timelines (so the user can decipher which interventions have and have not been effective).

Definitions of the metrics being measured should be clearly displayed to facilitate interpretation as well as the time mark when such measurements occurred.

Although run charts are not currently commonly found in available EMR displays, data tables of endoscopy quality indicators by scheduled frequencies can be made available, along with corresponding graphs, in some EMRs, and can be used to track performance over time. Display considerations should include determining whether there may be utility in the grouping of data output by facility, division, and/or endoscopist. This will vary by indicator. Grouping of data at various levels can help supervisors determine optimal interventions to promote improvement and where QI interventions should be targeted (ie, at the individual, divisional, or facility level).

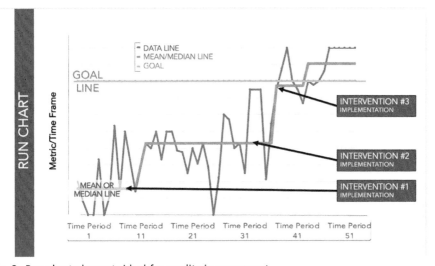

Fig. 2. Run chart elements ideal for quality improvement.

Access to and sharing of data can be a sensitive topic during initial implementation of QI activities. However, being transparent about the purposes of QI monitoring and the importance of data sharing to guide improvement and facilitate benchmarking can help reduce users' dismay at seeing their data relative to others. The goals of QI should be reviewed to highlight that data sharing is not meant to identify outliers but rather to foster performance improvement of the group. Data sharing can also help endoscopists conform to standards by showing them how they compare to their peers and provides a means for identifying areas for intervention that may enhance the quality of patient-centered and family-centered care, as well as patient safety. Assurance and reassurance of provision of support must be repeatedly offered to endoscopists engaged in QI activities to keep the focus on group performance and meeting standards of care.

Ensuring complete and standardized endoscopy reports is central to continuous QI activities because they can facilitate longitudinal monitoring for auditing and benchmarking purposes. In the surgical context, operative note templates have been shown to improve the quality, comprehensiveness, and timely production of electronic surgical notes following procedures.[30,31] Related to endoscopy, there is limited evidence that documentation rates of quality metrics can be enhanced if they are incorporated into a standardized endoscopy report template.[32]

Recently, Choi and colleagues[32,33] developed an endoscopy documentation template incorporating PEnQuIN indicators (**Fig. 3**) and extracted select PEnQuIN endoscopy indicators from endoscopy documentation and endoscopy workflows in the 3 identified phases of endoscopic care for display in data dashboards (**Fig. 4**).[33] Capitalizing on ongoing endoscopy documentation workflows by replacing a preexisting endoscopy reporting template with a new template incorporating PEnQuIN indicators enabled an almost immediately successful implementation of the template and related data visualization. Further, data displayed on the dashboard in the scheduling phase enabled improvements in scheduling protocols that reduced wait times for patients.

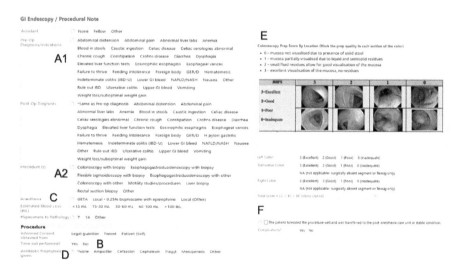

Fig. 3. Sample endoscopy electronic medical record note template demonstrating relevant data capture elements for select PEnQuIN indicators: (A) Indicator #17–Indications for Procedure, (B) Indicator #4–Preprocedural Pause Performance, (C) Indicator #20–Anesthesia Plan, (D) Indicator #3–Antibiotic Prophylaxis, (E) Indicator #28–Bowel Preparation Adequacy, and (F) Indicator #7–Intraprocedural Adverse Event Documentation.

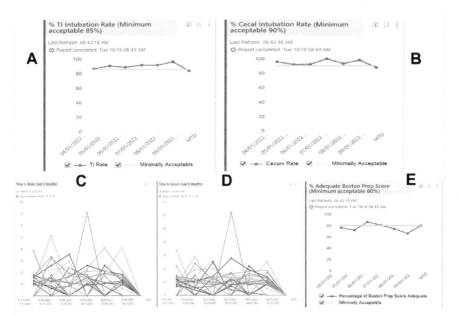

Fig. 4. Sample data dashboard elements demonstrating visualization of PEnQuIN indicators over time, including: (*A*) Terminal Ileum Intubation Rate (group summary), (*B*) Cecal Intubation Rate (group summary), (*C*) Time to Ileum (by proceduralist), (*D*) Time to Cecum (by proceduralist), and (*E*) Adequacy of Bowel Prep (group summary).

Lessons learned included the need to reprogram recorded endoscopy procedure times (including total procedure times, as well as time to cecum and time to ileum) to account for training (times assigned to trainees, whenever present, as opposed to the staff proceduralist), the need to organize displayed indicators and metrics according to phase of care for ease of user access and interpretation, and the need to display adverse events at a group level to preserve endoscopists' privacy around sensitive events.

FUTURE OPPORTUNITIES

The concepts introduced in this review are intended to lay out a framework by which EMR functionalities can be harnessed to enable active monitoring of pediatric endoscopy quality indicators, including the standards identified by PEnQuIN. Although this article provides advice for individual endoscopy services seeking to set up their EMR to optimize data collection and visualization, the hope is that using this functionality of the EMR could occur not only at the local level but also at national and even international levels. In short, implementing multicenter EMR protocols where quality indicators are measured in standard ways across pediatric endoscopy services will enable EHR interoperability (convenient sharing of data). In turn, such data can be shared across systems and transmitted in real-time to multicenter registries to enable the validation of quality indicators and standards and inform QI efforts. To accomplish this, a standardized data structure to ensure transferability across EMR systems is critical.

Currently, many of the PEnQuIN indicators and standards are "conditional" recommendations (ie, suggested vs recommended) owing to need for additional and broader data collection than has been available to date to determine whether and to what degree such indicators and standards affect patient outcomes in pediatric gastrointestinal, hepatic, pancreatic, and nutritional disease.[1,2] Only by setting up common EMR data collection frameworks can we contribute to this much needed multisite data collection to evaluate and test the meaningful relevance of these indicators and standards to patient outcomes. Only then can we answer whether active and ongoing measurement of PEnQuIN quality indicators to meet identified standards should be implemented as standards of care.

CLINICS CARE POINTS

- Pediatric endoscopy services are encouraged to implement the PEnQuIN quality standards and indicators to inform their local QI efforts.
- Measurement of endoscopy quality indicators helps to identify clinical care gaps, potential interventions, and related improvements, and can enhance quality by motivating endoscopy services and providers to institute changes.
- Setting up EMR protocols and frameworks for active quality indicator monitoring facilitates ongoing QI efforts and helps to ensure maintenance of achieved QI goals.
- Standardizing data capture and reporting of quality indicators across pediatric endoscopy services will help to expand the evidence basis for endoscopic practice in children, while also helping to validate the PEnQuIN standards and indicators as predictors of patient outcomes.

FUNDING/SUPPORT

C.M. Walsh holds an Early Researcher Award from the Ontario Ministry of Research and Innovation. The funders had no role in the design and conduct of the review, decision to publish and preparation, review, or approval of the article.

DISCLOSURE

The authors have nothing to disclose.

REFERENCES

1. Walsh CM, Lightdale JR, Mack DR, et al. Overview of the pediatric endoscopy quality improvement network quality standards and indicators for pediatric endoscopy: a joint NASPGHAN/ESPGHAN guideline. J Pediatr Gastroenterol Nutr 2022;74:S3–15.
2. Walsh CM, Lightdale JR. Pediatric Endoscopy Quality Improvement Network (PEnQuIN) quality standards and indicators for pediatric endoscopy: an ASGE-endorsed guideline. Gastrointest Endosc 2022;96(4):593–602.
3. Gilger M a, Gold BD. Pediatric endoscopy: new information from the PEDS-CORI project. Curr Gastroenterol Rep 2005;7(3):234–9.
4. Thakkar K, Holub JL, Gilger MA, et al. Quality indicators for pediatric colonoscopy: results from a multicenter consortium. Gastrointest Endosc 2016;83(3):533–41.
5. Alaifan M, Barker C. Colonoscopy quality assurance and maintenance of competency among pediatric gastroenterology staff members: a Canadian center experience. Cureus 2022;14(6):e26126.

6. HealthIT.gov. Frequently asked questions: advantages of electronic health records. 2022. Available at. https://www.healthit.gov/topic/health-it-and-health-information-exchange-basics/frequently-asked-questions. Accessed November 15, 2022.
7. U. S. Department Of Health And Human Services Health Resources And Services Administration. QUALITY Improvement. 2011. Available at. https://www.hrsa.gov/sites/default/files/quality/toolbox/508pdfs/qualityimprovement.pdf.   Accessed November 15, 2022.
8. Langley G, Moen R, Nolan K, et al. The improvement guide: a practical approach to enhancing organizational performance. 2nd ed. San Francisco, CA: Jossey-Bass Publishers; 2009.
9. Manfredi MA, Chauhan SS, Enestvedt BK, et al. Endoscopic electronic medical record systems Prepared by. Gastrointest Endosc 2016;83(1):29–36.
10. Enns RA, Barkun AN, Gerdes H. Electronic endoscopic information systems: what is out there? Gastrointest Endosc Clin N Am 2004;14(4 SPEC. ISS):745–54.
11. Walsh CM, Lightdale JR, Fishman DS, et al. Pediatric endoscopy quality improvement network pediatric endoscopy reporting elements: a joint NASPGHAN/ESPGHAN guideline. J Pediatr Gastroenterol Nutr 2022;74(S1 Suppl 1):S53–62.
12. Walsh CM, Lightdale JR, Leibowitz IH, et al. Pediatric endoscopy quality improvement network quality standards and indicators for pediatric endoscopists and endoscopists in training: a joint NASPGHAN/ESPGHAN guideline. J Pediatr Gastroenterol Nutr 2022;74(S1 Suppl 1):S44–52.
13. Lightdale JR, Thomson MA, Walsh CM. The pediatric endoscopy quality improvement network joint NASPGHAN/ESPGHAN guidelines: a global path to quality for pediatric endoscopy. J Pediatr Gastroenterol Nutr 2022;74(S1 Suppl 1):S1–2.
14. Lightdale JR, Walsh CM, Oliva S, et al. Pediatric Endoscopy Quality Improvement Network quality standards and indicators for pediatric endoscopic procedures: a joint NASPGHAN/ESPGHAN guideline. J Pediatr Gastroenterol Nutr 2022;74(S1 Suppl 1):S30–43.
15. Lightdale JR, Walsh CM, Narula P, et al. Pediatric endoscopy quality improvement network quality standards and indicators for pediatric endoscopy facilities: a joint NASPGHAN/ESPGHAN GUIDELINE. J Pediatr Gastroenterol Nutr 2022;74(S1 Suppl 1):S16–29.
16. McCann ME, Soriano SG. Does general anesthesia affect neurodevelopment in infants and children? BMJ 2019;367:l6459.
17. Davidson AJ, Disma N, De Graaff JC, et al. Neurodevelopmental outcome at 2 years of age after general anaesthesia and awake-regional anaesthesia in infancy (GAS): an international multicentre, randomised controlled trial. Lancet 2016;387(10015):239–50.
18. Mamula P, Nema N. Bowel preparation for pediatric colonoscopy. Front Pediatr 2021;9:705624.
19. Rex DK, Imperiale T, Latinovich D, et al. Impact of bowel preparation on efficiency and cost of colonoscopy. Am J Gastroenterol 2002;97(7):1696–700.
20. Pall H, Zacur GM, Kramer RE, et al. Bowel preparation for pediatric colonoscopy: report of the NASPGHAN Endoscopy and Procedures Committee. J Pediatr Gastroenterol Nutr 2014;59(3):409–16.
21. Singh HK, Withers GD, Ee LC. Quality indicators in pediatric colonoscopy: an Australian tertiary center experience. Scand J Gastroenterol 2017;52(12):1453–6.
22. Parmar R, Martel M, Rostom A, et al. Validated scales for colon cleansing: a systematic review. Am J Gastroenterol 2016;111(2):197–204.

23. Leichtner AM, Gillis LA, Gupta S, et al. NASPGHAN guidelines for training in pediatric gastroenterology. J Pediatr Gastroenterol Nutr 2013;56(Suppl. 1):1–38.
24. Walsh CM. Training and assessment in pediatric endoscopy. Gastrointest Endosc Clin N Am 2016;26(1):13–33.
25. Walsh CM. In-training gastrointestinal endoscopy competency assessment tools: types of tools, validation and impact. Best Pract Res Clin Gastroenterol 2016; 30(3):357–74.
26. Miller GE. The assessment of clinical skills/competence/performance. Acad Med 1990;65(9):S63–7.
27. Rizk MK, Vargo JJ. Incorporating quality metrics into training. Tech Gastrointest Endosc 2012;14(1):3–7.e1.
28. Walsh CM, Anderson JT, Fishman DS. Evidence-based approach to training pediatric gastrointestinal endoscopy trainers. J Pediatr Gastroenterol Nutr 2017;64(4).
29. Perla RJ, Provost LP, Murray SK. The run chart: a simple analytical tool for learning from variation in healthcare processes. BMJ Qual Saf 2011;20(1):46–51.
30. Theivendran K, Hassan S, I Clark D. Improving the quality of operative notes by implementing a new electronic template for upper limb surgery at the Royal Derby Hospital. BMJ Qual Improv Rep 2016;5(1). u208727.w3498.
31. Laflamme MR, Dexter PR, Graham MF, et al. Efficiency, comprehensiveness and cost-effectiveness when comparing dictation and electronic templates for operative reports. AMIA Annu Symp Proc 2005;2005:425–9.
32. Sawh M, Hemperly A, Gorsky G, et al. Improving adherence to quality metrics using the electronic medical record in the endoscopy suite. J Pediatr Gastroenterol Nutr 2019;69(2S):S167–8.
33. Choi L, Richardson A, Smith N, et al. Standardization of reporting and capturing quality metrics in pediatric endoscopy. J Pediatr Gastroenterol Nutr 2022;75(S1): S156–7.
34. Frazer A, Tanzer M. Hanging up the surgical cap: assessing the competence of aging surgeons. World J Orthop 2021;12(4):234–45.
35. Council on Medical Education. Guiding principles and appropriate criteria for assessing the competency of physicians across the professional continuum (CME Report 01-N-21). 2021. Available at: https://www.ama-assn.org/system/files/ n21-cme-01.pdf. Accessed November 15, 2022.
36. Rostom A, Jolicoeur E. Validation of a new scale for the assessment of bowel preparation quality. Gastrointest Endosc 2004;59(4):482–6.
37. Gofton WT, Dudek NL, Wood TJ, et al. The ottawa surgical competency operating room evaluation (O-SCORE): a tool to assess surgical competence. Acad Med 2012;87(10):1401–7.
38. Calderwood AH, Jacobson BC. Comprehensive validation of the boston bowel preparation scale. Gastrointest Endosc 2010;72(4):686.
39. Lai EJ, Calderwood AH, Doros G, et al. The Boston bowel preparation scale: a valid and reliable instrument for colonoscopy-oriented research. Gastrointest Endosc 2009;69(3 Pt 2):620–5.
40. Sheikhalishahi S, Miotto R, Dudley JT, et al. Natural language processing of clinical notes on chronic diseases: Systematic review. JMIR Med Inform 2019; 7(2):1–18.
41. Li I, Pan J, Goldwasser J, et al. Neural Natural Language Processing for unstructured data in electronic health records: A review. Computer Sci Rev 2022;46: 100511.

Artificial Intelligence in Pediatric Endoscopy
Current Status and Future Applications

Jasbir Dhaliwal, MBBS, MSc[a],*, Catharine M. Walsh, MD, MEd, PhD[b,c]

KEYWORDS

- Artificial intelligence • Pediatric gastrointestinal endoscopy
- Computer-aided diagnosis • CADe • CADx • Convolutional neural network
- Artificial neural networks • Deep learning

KEY POINTS

- Artificial intelligence (AI) is a powerful and increasingly prevalent technology that has great potential to improve the quality of patient-centered and family-centered endoscopic care for children.
- An important consideration in the development of an AI algorithm is being aware of the potential limitations of the training data set. The data may be inherently biased, and as such, the algorithm may potentially amplify the societal biases and discriminate disproportionately.
- The majority of preclinical endoscopy studies using AI have been undertaken in adults, and, at present, only three computer-aided diagnostic systems for the detection of colorectal polyps have received regulatory approval. These systems are yet to be fully integrated into colorectal cancer screening and surveillance practices.
- The potential applications of AI to endoscopy training are continually expanding, including the delivery of real-time instruction during procedures, feedback provision, competency assessment, and quality metric tracking.

INTRODUCTION

Artificial intelligence (AI) is a powerful and increasingly prevalent technology that will likely transform pediatric endoscopic practice. Endoscopy, which lends itself to imaging data, is well suited for the application of AI.[1] Preclinical studies, the majority of which have been undertaken in adults, have focused on the identification of colonic, gastric, and esophageal findings; distinguishing dysplastic from benign lesions; and

[a] Division of Pediatric Gastroenterology, Hepatology and Nutrition, Cincinnati Children's Hospital Medical Center, University of Cincinnati, OH, USA; [b] Division of Gastroenterology, Hepatology, and Nutrition, and the SickKids Research and Learning Institutes, The Hospital for Sick Children, Toronto, ON, Canada; [c] Department of Paediatrics and The Wilson Centre, University of Toronto, Temerty Faculty of Medicine, University of Toronto, Toronto, ON, Canada
* Corresponding author. University of Cincinnati, 3333 Burnet Avenue, Cincinnati, OH, 45229.
E-mail address: jasbir.dhaliwal@cchmc.org

Gastrointest Endoscopy Clin N Am 33 (2023) 291–308
https://doi.org/10.1016/j.giec.2022.12.001   **giendo.theclinics.com**

grading mucosal damage from endoscopic images. There is great promise for the application of these models in pediatric care, with the caveat that adaptation (eg, transfer learning) and fine-tuning will most likely be required. Although AI has tremendous capabilities, high-quality pediatric endoscopic care will remain heavily reliant on the technical, cognitive, and non-technical skills of endoscopists, as AI cannot interpret what is not captured and visualized during a procedure. Endoscopists must also remain clinically vigilant when using this emerging technology, as AI tools are not without diagnostic error.

In this state-of-the-art review, we outline key terminology and concepts related to AI, summarize the literature on AI in gastrointestinal endoscopy, and describe its potential application to pediatric endoscopy, particularly pertaining to lesion detection and diagnosis. Additionally, we discuss AI as it relates to endoscopy education.

KEY TERMINOLOGY AND CONCEPTS

AI is an umbrella term and should be perceived more as a goal than a methodological approach (**Fig. 1**). It refers to machines that can mimic human cognitive function.[2] *Machine learning*, which is an application of AI, refers to the ability of a computer to identify and learn from patterns in data without explicit programming. It then generates predictions based on mathematical computations from the provided data, which can take many forms, including numeric, image, and video data, depending on the AI application. The overall goal of machine learning is to build an algorithm (a collection of specific mathematical formulas that form the basis of a computational learning method), based on inputted data, with the power to make data-driven predictions or decisions. In this review, we use the terms algorithm and model interchangeably.

Machine learning can be *supervised*, which requires both the input (predictors) and outcome data to be labeled (**Fig. 2**). For example, if an algorithm being developed to detect small bowel gastrointestinal bleeding is fed capsule endoscopy images that are labeled "blood content" or "no blood," supervised learning models predict the labels of new data based on what they learn from the labeled examples. A drawback of supervised learning is that labels should be assigned by domain experts, which can be a time-consuming and costly task. Alternatively, *unsupervised* machine learning uses unlabeled data to identify patterns, commonly for clustering, representation learning, and density estimation tasks.[3] Data characteristics that help distinguish them as unique (eg, ulceration size and shape) are termed features.

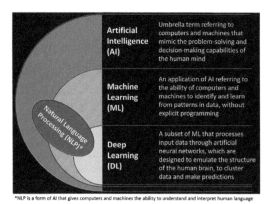

*NLP is a form of AI that gives computers and machines the ability to understand and interpret human language

Fig. 1. Key terminology related to artificial intelligence.

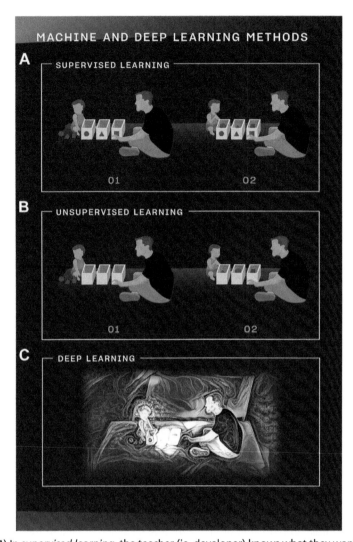

Fig. 2. (*A*) In *supervised learning*, the teacher (ie, developer) knows what they want to teach the child (ie, artificial intelligence), they define the expected answer, and the child learns to excel at the task. (*B*) In *unsupervised learning*, the teacher does not influence how the child learns the task but observes the conclusions the child can draw from solving it. (*C*) In *deep learning*, it is possible to analyze vastly more complex data sets from images and videos through multi-layered systems, that mimic how neural networks in the brain work, to process complex information and make predictions. *Adapted from* Meskó B, Görög M. A short guide for medical professionals in the era of artificial intelligence. NPJ Digit Med. 2020 Sep 24;3:126.

Deep learning, a subset of machine learning, processes input data through artificial neural networks that are designed to emulate the structure of the human brain. The data are processed through neural layers that contain millions of parameters and hundreds of layers, and the final layer compiles the weighted inputs to a given output.[3] These models automatically discover, learn, and extract the hierarchical data representations required for a detection or classification task.[4] The internal logic of these complex models is hidden, the "black box." Most recent AI systems have been based on deep learning given the depth and complexity achievable by deep learning–based algorithms.

Computer vision refers to computer systems processing images or videos (eg, endoscopy videos, radiological imaging) and using artificial neural networks called convolutional neural network (CNN) models. CNN models are data-hungry and typically trained using large data sets, for example, banks of images annotated by endoscopists (ie, ground truth) for the presence or location of specific endoscopic features (eg, polyps). These models are trained to imitate expert performance. To evaluate a model's performance, the algorithm should be tested on a new set of unseen images.

MODEL DEVELOPMENT, VALIDATION, AND TESTING

Data are used in the development, validation, and implementation of AI algorithms. Training data sets are the input data that are initially fed into the algorithm to "teach" it to recognize patterns in the data set to inform model development. Validation data sets are then used to evaluate and optimize the model's performance. Finally, test data sets are independent data that are used to fully evaluate the accuracy and efficiency of the algorithm and ensure generalizability.[5] The generalizability of an AI algorithm refers to how well the model adapts to new and unseen data.[6]

It is essential to ensure that the data sets used in model development and evaluation in the preclinical setting involve imaging data representative of the population for the intended use and that technical differences between sites (eg, different endoscopes used to capture images) and variations in local clinical and administrative practices (eg, different health care systems or local infrastructure) are considered during testing. A limitation to widespread application is the lack of standardization of imaging characteristics (eg, resolution, color, field of view) across vendors, resulting in poor performance of models when using equipment that is different from that used in model development.[7] It is also important to ensure that data sets are large and heterogenous, from across multiple sites. Another important consideration is algorithmic bias.[8] Algorithms are typically trained on historical data, and various biases may be implicitly encoded, which have the potential to amplify societal biases and racial discrimination.[9] Such discriminatory models will perform disproportionately worse in underrepresented populations.[10] To minimize possible discrimination and ensure equitable care delivery, evaluation in these subpopulations before implementation is imperative. Finally, when training data sets are labeled, it is essential to ensure the labels were assigned in a systematic and rigorous manner, ideally using multiple experts to label each image and multiple iterations of review, if required, to ensure adequate interrater reliability.

The success of an AI system does not solely depend on statistical validity (ie, accuracy, area under the receiver operator curve, sensitivity, specificity, and so forth) but also on pragmatic and ecological validity, which involves evaluating the usability and impact of the AI system in the real-world health care setting.[11] The widely publicized Google DeepMind's diabetic retinopathy algorithm[12] was integrated for the first time for point-of-care, real-time use in Thailand's national diabetic retinopathy screening program. The deep learning system was deployed across 11 primary care clinics and had performance comparable to that of human readers. Despite the observed robustness of the computer-aided diagnostic system, the study investigators highlighted the challenges of the system in real-time clinical workflow. They noted the absence of universal electronic health records, slow internet connectivity, and ungradable images due to poor image quality as a result of operator- and camera-dependent technical issues.[12] Measuring the compliance of a system within clinical practice and evaluating the financial impact are crucial for sustainability. Designing such a system should be interdisciplinary to ensure that the complexity of the health care system is considered in the development process. We echo the sentiments of Schmitz and colleagues[13] that the endoscopy community should make a concerted effort to be involved in the development and testing phases of computer-aided diagnostic systems on a continuous basis and at an early stage. This type of user-centered design will require both institutional support and dedicated funding.

APPLICATIONS IN ENDOSCOPY

Related to gastrointestinal endoscopy, AI is being applied to fulfill many functions. However, broadly speaking, AI has focused largely on computer-aided detection (CADe) and computer-aided characterization or diagnosis (CADx). Algorithms focused on CADe are developed primarily to detect a pathology such as polyps. Alternatively, algorithms focused on CADx are developed for optical diagnosis and lesion characterization, such as polyp histology. Other potential applications of AI in endoscopic practice include offering technical assistance to improve endoscopy performance (eg, guiding scope insertion or mucosal visualization) and therapeutic assistance (eg, lesion delineation). This section provides an overview of some of the most promising applications of AI in endoscopy that have the potential to impact pediatric endoscopic practice.

Polyps: Lesion Detection

The greatest advancement in endoscopy AI so far has been the development of CADe systems automating polyp detection that has occurred over the last 10 years, from early systems using still endoscopic images to current state-of-the-art systems that use real-time videos. These systems have largely been used in the context of colorectal cancer screening and surveillance, and the applications in pediatric gastroenterology are limited. However, the lessons learned from their developmental history carry high relevance to implementing AI in pediatric endoscopy.

Before any development of an AI algorithm, evaluating its suitability and potential clinical utility is important. In clinical practice, the pooled missed rates of adenomas are as high as 26% overall, 9% for advanced adenomas, and 27% for serrated polyps.[14] Thus, a CADe system that can draw attention to polyps in real time which may otherwise be overlooked would certainly be of value. Earlier models were supervised and developed using shallow "handcrafted" features, such as color and shape, that were extracted from polyps in still endoscopic images. Their accuracy was reported to range from 48% to 90%.[15] The variable performance was attributed to the initial data source used for training, an open-access polyp database (CVC-ColonDB and ASUMayo) with fewer than 20 different polyps.[16] An algorithm trained on such a limited data set that does not encompass the full spectrum of the disease will lack generalizability. Furthermore, the use of "handcrafted" features may not be able to discriminate the distinct variations in polyps, and the algorithm could potentially learn false positives such as vessels, fecal matter, and folds.

It was only with the advent of deep learning CNN models, which can learn and incorporate the complexity of imaging data, that the prospect of implementing these algorithms into clinical practice became conceivable. The reported accuracy of CNN models using video data has increased to greater than 90%.[17-19] The improvement in accuracy is not only attributed to advances in computational approaches, but also to the use of data sets with several images and a variety of polypoid lesions.

These models typically require large data sets with the high data variability reflective of clinical practice, and to facilitate their development, it would be of value to establish large, publicly available, high-quality labeled data sets.[20] Such efforts were undertaken by Misawa and colleagues[21] to develop a publicly accessible, large-scale colonoscopy video "polyp" database that contains 56,668 annotated images. Developing such databases is labor-intensive and cost-intensive and involves hospital partnerships, robust information system infrastructure, and multi-institutional funding. The vast number of coronavirus disease AI models, which were developed using publicly available imaging data that lacked both reproducibility and demonstrated high bias, serve as a cautionary tale for using poor-quality data.[22]

Nonetheless, huge strides have been made in recent years. Between 2019 and 2020, six prospective randomized controlled trials (5 Chinese, 1 Italian) using in vivo CADe real-time systems have been evaluated, with favorable findings.[23–28] In a meta-analysis of these studies, the pooled adenoma detection rate (ADR) with the use of CADe endoscopy was greater than that with standard colonoscopy (rate ratio = 1.5 [95% confidence interval {CI} 1.3–1.72], $P < .0001$, $I^2 = 56\%$).[29] These findings did not translate to an increase in advanced ADR or sessile serrated ADR, with pooled rate ratios of 1.0 (95% CI 0.74–1.36) and 1.29 (95% CI 0.89–1.89), respectively.[29] These equivocal findings may be attributed to CADe systems unable to identify blind spots which may occur because of poor visualization or slipping of the scope. Gong and colleagues[25] developed a CADe system focused on improving the quality of endoscopy that can recognize cecal intubation, endoscope slippage, and withdrawal speed. It was the only system that reported significantly higher detection rates for large (>10 mm) colorectal polyps among users.[25] Furthermore, five of the studies were single-center studies undertaken in one region, which limits the generalizability of the findings globally.

Most recently, a randomized trial undertaken in five academic and community centers in the United States (US) tested the SKOUT CADe system (Cambridge, MA, USA).[30] Similar to the GI-Genius Medtronic,[27] the system analyzes colonoscopy video feeds in real time to identify polyps and produce a visual indicator via a bounding box. The system was implemented into practice, and the clinical benefit of the device was assessed in a US-based screening and surveillance population. Interestingly, among experienced endoscopists, the CADe device statistically improved overall adenoma detection per colonoscopy (standard vs CADe: 0.83 vs 1.05, $P = .002$) without a concomitant rise in resection of nonneoplastic lesions or a statistically significant increase in ADR (43.9% vs 47.8%, $P = .065$). The authors attributed the nonsignificant increase in ADR of 3.9% to the lower risk population and the considerable experience of the participating endoscopists in high-volume centers. Randomized controlled trials using CADe systems for adenoma detection are outlined in **Table 1**. There have been few tandem studies undertaken, perhaps due to difficulties recruiting patients to undergo two colonoscopies. Brown and colleagues[31] carried out a US multicenter randomized tandem colonoscopy study (CADe T-CS Trial) which found a lower adenoma miss rate in the CADe first group than that in the high-definition white light colonoscopy first group (20.1% vs 31.1%, $P = .0007$). The study was among the few that specifically showed the potential benefit of reducing the miss rate of sessile serrated lesions.

Another consideration to improve the detection of polyps is to improve colonoscopy quality, namely the field of view to ensure the entire colonic surface is evaluated. Endoscopic mucosal visibility is impaired by several factors, including a poor endoscopy technique (eg. improper camera orientation), poor bowel preparation, inadequate positioning, occlusion by colonic structures (eg, folds), and endoscopist limitations in recognizing missed areas. Ma and colleagues[32] developed a deep-learning 3D-reconstruction, localization, and mapping system of the colon. The system

Randomized controlled trials using computer-aided detection systems for adenoma detection

Author Year	Type	Population CADe	Population Control	Intervention CADe System	Control (CON)	ADR CADe	ADR Control	OR/RR (95% CI)
Wang et al,[23] 2019	Single center	522	536	CADe (Shanghai Wision AI Co. Ltd)	Standard colonoscopy	29.1%	20.3%	OR 1.61 CI 1.21–2.14
Wang et al,[26] 2020	Single center	484	478	CADe (EndoScreener; Wision AI, Shanghai, China)	White-light colonoscopy + sham system	34%	28%	OR 1.36 CI 1.03–1.79
Gong et al,[25] 2020	Single center	355	349	CADe (ENDOANGEL)	Standard colonoscopy	Intention to treat 16% Per protocol analysis 17%	8% 8%	OR 2.3 1.40–3.77 OR 2.18 CI 1.31–3.62
Su et al,[24] 2020	Single center	308	315	CADe (automatic quality control system AQCS, DCNN model)	Standard colonoscopy	28.9%	16.5%	OR 2.06 CI 1.40–3.02
Liu et al,[28] 2020	Single center	508	518	CADe (Henan Xuanweitang Medical Information Technology Co, LTD., Zhengzhou, China)	Standard colonoscopy	39.1%	23.8%	OR 1.64 CI 1.20–2.22
Repici et al,[27] 2020	Multicenter	341	344	CADe (Convolutional Neural Network (GI-Genius; Medtronic)	Standard colonoscopy	54.8%	40.4%	RR 1.30 CI 1.14–1.45
Repici et al,[93] 2022	Multicenter	330	330	CADe (GI Genius Medtronic)	High-definition colonoscopy	53.3%	44.5%	RR 1.22 CI 1.04–1.40
Shaukat et al,[30] 2022	Multicenter	682	677	CADe (SKOUT CADe system)	Standard colonoscopy	Screening 38.4% Surveillance 59.4%	41.3% 55.2%	Difference 2.9; CI-3.7–9.5 Difference 4.2; CI-5.5–13.2

Abbreviations: ADR, adenoma detection rate; AQCS, Automatic quality control system; CADe, Computer aided detection; CI, confidence interval; DCNN, Deep convolutional neural network; OR, odds ratio; RR, risk ratio.

reconstructs the endoscopic video into a 3D surface in real time and leaves poorly visualized regions blank, thereby alerting the endoscopist to survey previously unseen regions.[32] If such 3D-reconstruction systems are developed and implemented, they could not only aid in polyp detection (CADe) but could also be used to concurrently characterize pathology (CADx) in real time. Other AI applications related to endoscopy quality include systems that provide real-time evaluation of bowel preparation quality,[25,33] as well as systems that monitor withdrawal time to ensure the endoscopist takes enough time to examine each segment adequately.[25,33]

At present, three CADe systems for polyp detection have regulatory (Food and Drug Administration) approval in the US, GI Genius (Medtronic), Endoscreener (Wision AI), and, as of September 2022, SKOUT (Iterative Scopes).[34] Although the existing literature base points to the potential for AI to improve quality through improvements in ADR and consequent reductions in interval malignancy, the majority of missed adenomas in studies to date have been small (<9 mm), and current systems do not necessarily increase the rate of detection of advanced neoplasia.[35] Additionally, the long-term impact on colorectal carcinoma rates remains unknown. There is also limited literature evaluating the impact of CADe systems in authentic health care settings. Furthermore, although there has been an exponential growth of research examining AI focused on improving automated detection of polyps in adults, its application in pediatrics, and hereditary cancer predisposing syndromes in particular, has not been explored.

Polyps: Lesion Characterization

Although polyp detection is key, AI also has the potential to facilitate polyp characterization. Preclinical studies are promising. For example, Ozawa and colleagues[36] were able to develop a CNN model to detect and characterize a polyp simultaneously using stored still images during colonoscopy, with 83% accuracy. The system, trained on 16,418 images from 4752 polyps and 4013 images of normal colorectum, could predict five histopathological categories.[36]

Endoscopic societies such as the American Society for Gastrointestinal Endoscopy (ASGE) have introduced a "resect and discard" strategy (ie, no histopathological examination) for small (≤5 mm) polyps and a "diagnose and leave" strategy for hyperplastic polyps in the rectosigmoid colon when an optical diagnosis is completed with high certainty during endoscopy. CADx systems that can accurately differentiate between hyperplastic and neoplastic polyps in vivo may, therefore, have great potential to reduce workload, costs, and adverse events when integrated appropriately into clinical workflow. Recent research has corroborated this potential. Mori and colleagues[37] found that a CADx system designed to enable the "diagnose and leave" strategy for nonneoplastic diminutive polyps resulted in substantial cost reductions. Although this area of investigation is still in its infancy, future CADx algorithms will hopefully be developed which can be applied to children with hereditary cancer-predisposing syndromes who have high polyp burdens to help identify potentially dysplastic lesions that should be prioritized for removal.

Inflammatory Bowel Disease

The progress made in developing and implementing polyp CADe and CADx systems is exciting, but crucially, it tells a development story that occurred over a decade, moving from still images to video and preclinical, proof-of-concept studies to the clinical setting, while receiving regulatory approval in parallel. In comparison, the CADx systems in inflammatory bowel disease (IBD) are very much in their infancy.

The treatment target in IBD is to achieve endoscopic remission.[38] There are numerous endoscopic indices[39,40] to assess the severity of disease activity, but the complexity of some of these indices makes them a challenge to use in routine clinical practice. Furthermore, the interobserver and intraobserver variability can be high.[41] A CADx system could standardize scoring in real time to aid in therapeutic decision-making.

There are two distinct phenotypes of IBD, ulcerative colitis and Crohn disease. Ulcerative colitis is typically characterized by diffuse inflammation of the colonic mucosa, extending proximally from the rectum, whereas Crohn disease is patchy and discontinuous. The morphologic variation in Crohn disease may explain why studies to date have focused on developing CADx systems in ulcerative colitis. The majority of deep learning models have focused on predicting the Mayo Endoscopic Score (MES)[42–44] and Ulcerative Colitis Endoscopic Index of Severity Score (UCEIS).[45,46] Stidham and colleagues[42] developed a still image MES classifier that could accurately predict the Mayo score, with a sensitivity of 83%, specificity of 96%, and area under the curve of 0.97. In a preliminary study, the classifier was incorporated into an automated whole-video workflow, as a first step to real-time assessment, and performed well with an accuracy of 83%.[47] Gottlieb and colleagues[45] developed a deep learning algorithm from clinical trial data to predict levels of ulcerative colitis severity from full-length endoscopy videos. The CADx system was able to select informative frames and remove unsatisfactory frames (eg, due to poor bowel preparation) in an automated fashion. The agreement between the algorithm score and a human central reader score was found to be excellent, with a quadratic weighted kappa of 0.84 (95% CI 0.79–0.90) for MES and 0.86 (95% CI 0.80–0.91) for UCEIS.[45] There have also been efforts to develop deep learning systems that can predict endoscopic inflammation and histologic remission in ulcerative colitis from a single endoscopic image; however, these have not yet been applied in clinical care.[46]

The majority of IBD CADx systems have centered around replicating disease severity indices, which are still subject to human interpretation. Indices may also evolve over time, and perhaps efforts are better directed toward annotating endoscopic features such as ulcers and erosions. Building robust well-annotated data sets will be expensive and time-consuming, but the long-term utility of such data sets, in our opinion, will be of a greater value. Such work has been undertaken using video capsule endoscopy data to identify mucosal ulcerations and abnormalities in Crohn disease.[48,49] This may help to better delineate endoscopic features of IBD, assist in the identification of associations between variables, and even evaluate diseases in new ways (eg, as more of a spectrum as opposed to one of fixed categories).

Upper Gastrointestinal Pathology

In contrast to colonoscopy, the use of AI in upper endoscopy is at present limited, and there are currently no commercially available AI-based products. Nonetheless, promising data have been reported, which have potential application to pediatric endoscopic practice. The applications of AI for nonmalignant upper gastrointestinal pathology that are most applicable to pediatrics relate to *Helicobacter pylori* (*H. pylori*) and celiac disease. Several preclinical studies have evaluated the use of AI for *H. pylori* infection prediction based on endoscopic images.[50–55] As the accuracy of these models improves, they may help determine whether biopsies are required, potentially reducing the cost and burden of endoscopic procedures. Additionally, AI may eventually permit real-time diagnosis, thus enabling treatment to be initiated immediately after the procedure. Similarly, for celiac disease, while few studies have been conducted to date,[56–62] AI models may eventually be able to determine whether biopsies are required and identify the location for a biopsy, given the patchy nature of the disease.

Similar to colonoscopy, measurement of key performance indicators for upper endoscopy is a future potential target for AI.[63,64] For example, documented examination of certain anatomic landmarks is a marker of procedural quality, and AI has the potential to detect landmark visualization and to assist the endoscopist in ensuring adequate visualization.[65]

Capsule Endoscopy

While capsule endoscopy has revolutionized investigation of the small bowel, analysis is time-consuming. Capsule endoscopy is a prime candidate for early adoption of AI, as diagnostic assistance could help to improve reading efficiency, cost, and accuracy. To date, most research has focused on CADe algorithms to assist in the detection of active gastrointestinal bleeding or angioectasia. Recent research has demonstrated that AI-guided detection of blood is close to 100% accurate,[66] and a deep learning model developed by Tsuboi and colleagues[67] based on the CNN for angioectasia achieved an area under the curve of 0.998 with a sensitivity and specificity of 98.8% and 98.4%, respectively. CADe systems focused on the detection of small-intestinal ulcerations have also been developed. For example, Klang and colleagues[48,49] developed a deep learning model based on the CNN that used over 17,000 capsule endoscopy images to identify small bowel ulcers in Crohn disease, achieving an area under the curve of 0.99. Celiac disease has been another area of investigation, with developed models reporting high accuracies.[56,68–70] Additional studies have evaluated algorithms for the detection of small intestinal polyps[71,72] and even intestinal hookworm infections.[73]

There have also been efforts to develop models capable of differentiating normal from abnormal frames and, therefore, able to detect several different types of lesions. Ding and colleagues[74] developed and validated a CNN-based algorithm to identify and categorize a large array of small bowel abnormalities on capsule endoscopy images, including ulcers, polyps, bleeding lymphangiectasia, follicular hyperplasia, protruding lesions, diverticula, and inflammation. The model, which was developed using over 110 million images, was able to identify abnormalities with higher levels of sensitivity (99.90% vs 74.57%) and specificity (99.88% vs 76.89%) in the per-lesion analysis compared with conventional screening by gastroenterologists and had significantly shorter reading times (5.9 vs 96.6 minutes). It also had an error rate of only 3%.

Application of AI to capsule endoscopy may also help to address current issues with this technology, such as poor localization of anatomic landmarks and findings in the small bowel, measuring lesions, and evaluating bowel preparation quality. Proof of concept of capsule localization has been established using an AI system that could discriminate between the esophagus, stomach, small intestine, and colon based on the automated recognition of the respective tissues and anatomic landmarks, using color and texture handcrafted image features.[75] Combining such approaches with AI-enabled methods for estimating capsule motion may enable more accurate localization of pathology within the small bowel itself.[76] With regard to examination quality, Leenhardt and colleagues[77] and Noorda and colleagues[78] have developed CNN models to assess the quality of bowel preparation during capsule endoscopy, both achieving an accuracy rate of over 95%.

Overall, studies pertaining to capsule endoscopy have shown promising results; however, current research is based on retrospective studies with a high risk of bias, and video-level evaluations are limited. Prospective studies are needed before endoscopists can fully rely on such solutions. Additionally, a next step will be to categorize findings in terms of diagnosis and clinical relevance. Based on the time-consuming nature of reading capsule endoscopies and recent research in this area, it can be expected that AI will soon start to be integrated into clinical practice, and much of the work to date may have potential applicability in pediatric endoscopic practice.

TRAINING AND ARTIFICIAL INTELLIGENCE

With the introduction of any new technology, it is critical to reflect on how best to integrate it into training to optimize learning and assessment practices and carefully consider potential pitfalls associated with its widespread application. The endoscopic cognitive skill of pattern recognition takes time to master, and whether and how AI impacts the acquisition of these skills remain unknown. CADe systems may help to draw trainees' eyes toward frequently missed lesions, helping them to recognize subtle signs and adding to their mental repository of images for future pattern recognition.[79] Alternatively, trainees may become dependent on AI technology.

Studies from the educational literature have highlighted that when feedback is provided too frequently during procedures, trainees can become reliant on it, and their performance falters when it is not available.[80,81] In the same way, trainees may potentially become dependent on AI technology and fail to construct and automate cognitive schemas in their long-term memory that are required for expertise development.[82] One recent study, which examined the eye-tracking patterns of endoscopists viewing colonoscopy videos with and without AI support, found that eye travel distance was significantly reduced, and the gaze was more focused when endoscopists viewed videos with AI support.[83] These results suggest that AI may predispose endoscopists to missing polyps not captured by the system. Furthermore, the authors found differential visual gaze patterns between novice and experienced endoscopists, with the novice gaze pattern bearing similarity to that of endoscopists with low polyp-detection rates.[83–85] This raises the possibility that AI may impact trainees' learning by preventing them from developing the gaze pattern of high-performing endoscopists. Additionally, false positives detected by AI systems may reinforce faulty pattern recognition. Furthermore, AI systems may act to distract trainees during procedures and impose extraneous cognitive overload, which can interfere with learning, especially early in training.[82]

As AI evolves so likely will its potential applications in training, including the delivery of real-time instruction during procedures (eg, ensuring proper orientation during polyp resection), feedback provision, and competency assessment. Additionally, AI has great potential to automate the collection of trainee quality metrics (eg, terminal ileal intubation rates, mucosal visualization) to better track their progress during training and, if standardized across programs, to generate data to establish training benchmarks for pediatric endoscopy. Integration of AI into training may also help to improve endoscopy quality. In line with experienced endoscopists, AI may help to improve adenoma miss rates among trainees, but this requires further study.[86] Similarly, tools aimed at enhancing mucosal visualization or those that provide guidance regarding endoscopic lesion characterization may improve trainees' diagnostic accuracy. This concept has shown promise in a recent study that used an AI system to improve the accuracy of trainees in the analysis of hyperplastic versus adenomatous polyps, enabling trainees to reach near-expert levels of performance.[87]

How best to integrate AI into training remains unknown. Rodrigues and Keswani[79] have suggested a staged approach, starting with didactic content focused on understanding how data are processed in AI, the strengths and limitations of AI models, model validation, and clinical implications, with the aim of improving trainees' understanding of how AI systems produce specific output. Subsequently, the application of AI could focus on feedback, assessment of competence, and quality metric tracking with the aim to facilitate skills acquisition. Finally, once trainees have mastered the fundamentals of endoscopy, the diagnostic and therapeutic features of AI could be introduced to augment the skills they have acquired. This type of staged integration would help to ensure AI is thoughtfully incorporated to augment traditional endoscopy education, as opposed to relying solely on AI for endoscopic training.

Not only it is important to consider the impact of AI on trainee education, but it is also essential to consider practicing endoscopists. The implementation of AI is often encountered with trepidation from health care providers, which arises largely from feelings of unpreparedness, a lack of willingness to "trust" algorithms, worry about the potential increased administrative burden, and the fear of role replacement.[88,89] As the health care community prepares for this shift, education will be essential. As highlighted in the ASGE Summit on AI in Endoscopy, it is important that endoscopists are educated regarding current applications and the basics of AI in a comprehensible way to ensure broad understandability.[90] Literature on implementing health information systems indicates that education has a favorable impact on health care professionals' views of the technology and their ongoing use of the system.[91,92] Moving forward, it will be essential to develop evidence-informed educational programs to build clinicians' knowledge, skills, and abilities to translate the potential power of AI into effective clinical practice. By educating and empowering faculty, it will also help to ensure that trainees have mentors to help them contextualize AI and benefit maximally from its implementation.

SUMMARY

AI-assisted endoscopy has the potential to standardize and improve the quality of pediatric endoscopic practice and potentially reduce workload. The spectrum of possible clinical applications is vast, including improved detection and differentiation of lesions, risk stratification, and evaluation of endoscopy key performance metrics. However, there are challenges and possible shortcomings that must be considered before full implementation can be realized.

The greatest advances in the use of this technology have been in polyp detection in screening colonoscopies, and it remains to be seen what impact AI systems will have across the disease spectrum and in pediatrics. Moving forward, advances in deep learning may permit improved characterization of gastrointestinal disorders and ultimately lead to enhanced treatment selection and improved patient outcomes. To date, AI has not been tested for large-scale clinical applications related to endoscopy, and the long-term impact and efficacy of AI systems in clinical practice remain unknown. Randomized controlled trials are considered the gold standard in evaluating efficacy, but in the case of CAD systems, where evaluation goes beyond accuracy measurements and the system itself relies on integration into the daily clinical workflow, pragmatic trials would be more appropriate to determine how AI serves to benefit clinicians and patients in meaningful ways. These systems are typically built at one time point, but the clinical environment is not stationary; with evolution in clinical and operational practices, model performance may decline over time. Ethical design thinking is essential at every stage of development and application to ensure AI systems provide ethical, user-friendly, and cost-effective solutions.[90] Additionally, research is required to determine how best to integrate AI into trainee education as well as the potential impact of this technology on endoscopy skills acquisition.

Given its inherent reliance on imaging, endoscopy is emerging as one of the first areas in medicine in which AI is being integrated into clinical practice. It is important for us as a pediatric gastroenterology community to play a lead role in deciding how best to integrate this technology into endoscopic care to support decision-making, enhance efficiency, improve workflow, and augment performance. Ongoing collaboration among pediatric endoscopists, patient advocates, data scientists, industry experts, and regulatory agencies will be important to ensure progress is clinically meaningful, with the ultimate goal of improving the quality of patient-centered and family-centered endoscopic care for children.

CLINICS CARE POINTS

- The application of AI systems to pediatric endoscopy is very much in its infancy, which provides a unique opportunity for the pediatric gastroenterology community to work collectively with data scientists to design clinically meaningful systems that will have the greatest benefit for pediatric patients and their families.

- At present, no endoscopic computer-aided diagnostic system has been fully evaluated in the clinical setting. It is critical to understand and measure how AI will benefit both pediatric endoscopists and patients.

- Trainees and practicing endoscopists should be educated on the effective, appropriate, safe, and compassionate use of AI to ensure they are equipped with the knowledge, skills, and abilities to help shape AI practices and accelerate the appropriate adoption of data-driven and AI-enhanced care.

- Research is required to examine the potential impact of AI on endoscopy training and skills acquisition to inform thoughtful integration of AI-enabled technologies into training.

FUNDING/SUPPORT

J. Dhaliwal holds a Career Development Award from Crohn's & Colitis Foundation. C.M. Walsh. holds an Early Researcher Award from the Ontario Ministry of Research and Innovation. The funders had no role in the design and conduct of the review, decision to publish and preparation, review, or approval of the manuscript.

DISCLOSURE

The authors have nothing to disclose.

REFERENCES

1. Le Berre C, Sandborn WJ, Aridhi S, et al. Application of artificial intelligence to gastroenterology and hepatology. Gastroenterology 2020;158(1):76–94.e2.
2. Russell SJ. Artificial intelligence: a modern approach. 3rd edition. Upper Saddle River, NJ: Prentice Hall; 2010.
3. Schmidhuber J. Deep learning in neural networks: an overview. Neural Netw 2015;61:85–117.
4. Linardatos P, Papastefanopoulos V, Kotsiantis S. Explainable AI: a review of machine learning interpretability methods. Entropy (Basel) 2020;23(1):18.
5. Chahal D, Byrne MF. A primer on artificial intelligence and its application to endoscopy. Gastrointest Endosc 2020;92(4):813–20.e4.
6. Kelly CJ, Karthikesalingam A, Suleyman M, et al. Key challenges for delivering clinical impact with artificial intelligence. BMC Med 2019;17(1):195.
7. Sohn JH, Chillakuru YR, Lee S, et al. An open-source, vender agnostic hardware and software pipeline for integration of artificial intelligence in radiology workflow. J Digit Imaging 2020;33(4):1041–6.
8. Wiens J, Price WN, Sjoding MW. Diagnosing bias in data-driven algorithms for healthcare. Nat Med 2020;26(1):25–6.
9. Yuan A, Lee AY. Artificial intelligence deployment in diabetic retinopathy: the last step of the translation continuum. Lancet Digit Health 2022;4(4):e208–9.

10. Seyyed-Kalantari L, Zhang H, McDermott MBA, et al. Underdiagnosis bias of artificial intelligence algorithms applied to chest radiographs in under-served patient populations. Nat Med 2021;27(12):2176–82.

11. Cabitza F, Zeitoun J-D. The proof of the pudding: in praise of a culture of real-world validation for medical artificial intelligence. Ann translational Med 2019;7(7):161.

12. Ruamviboonsuk P, Tiwari R, Sayres R, et al. Real-time diabetic retinopathy screening by deep learning in a multisite national screening programme: a prospective interventional cohort study. Lancet Digital Health 2022;4(4):e235–44.

13. Schmitz R, Werner R, Repici A, et al. Artificial intelligence in GI endoscopy: stumbling blocks, gold standards and the role of endoscopy societies. Gut 2022; 71(3):451–4.

14. Zhao S, Wang S, Pan P, et al. Magnitude, Risk Factors, and Factors Associated With Adenoma Miss Rate of Tandem Colonoscopy: A Systematic Review and Meta-analysis. Gastroenterology 2019;156(5):1661–74.e11.

15. Misawa M, Kudo SE, Mori Y, et al. Current status and future perspective on artificial intelligence for lower endoscopy. Dig Endosc 2021;33(2):273–84.

16. Tajbakhsh N, Gurudu SR, Liang J. Automated polyp detection in colonoscopy videos using shape and context information. IEEE Trans Med Imaging 2016; 35(2):630–44.

17. Misawa M, Kudo SE, Mori Y, et al. Artificial intelligence-assisted polyp detection for colonoscopy: initial experience. Gastroenterology 2018;154(8):2027–9.e3.

18. Wang P, Xiao X, Glissen Brown JR, et al. Development and validation of a deep-learning algorithm for the detection of polyps during colonoscopy. Nat Biomed Eng 2018;2(10):741–8.

19. Yamada M, Saito Y, Imaoka H, et al. Development of a real-time endoscopic image diagnosis support system using deep learning technology in colonoscopy. Sci Rep 2019;9(1):14465.

20. Houwen BBSL, Nass KJ, Vleugels JLA, et al. Comprehensive review of publicly available colonoscopic imaging databases for artificial intelligence research: availability, accessibility and usability. Gastrointest Endosc 2023;97(2):184–99.e16.

21. Misawa M, Kudo S-e, Mori Y, et al. Development of a computer-aided detection system for colonoscopy and a publicly accessible large colonoscopy video database (with video). Gastrointest Endosc 2021;93(4):960–7.e3.

22. Roberts M, Driggs D, Thorpe M, et al. Common pitfalls and recommendations for using machine learning to detect and prognosticate for COVID-19 using chest radiographs and CT scans. Nat Machine Intelligence 2021;3:199–217.

23. Wang P, Berzin TM, Glissen Brown JR, et al. Real-time automatic detection system increases colonoscopic polyp and adenoma detection rates: a prospective randomised controlled study. Gut 2019;68(10):1813–9.

24. Su JR, Li Z, Shao XJ, et al. Impact of a real-time automatic quality control system on colorectal polyp and adenoma detection: a prospective randomized controlled study (with videos). Gastrointest Endosc 2020;91(2):415–24.e4.

25. Gong D, Wu L, Zhang J, et al. Detection of colorectal adenomas with a real-time computer-aided system (ENDOANGEL): a randomised controlled study. Lancet Gastroenterol Hepatol 2020;5(4):352–61.

26. Wang P, Liu X, Berzin TM, et al. Effect of a deep-learning computer-aided detection system on adenoma detection during colonoscopy (CADe-DB trial): a double-blind randomised study. Lancet Gastroenterol Hepatol 2020;5(4):343–51.

27. Repici A, Badalamenti M, Maselli R, et al. Efficacy of real-time computer-aided detection of colorectal neoplasia in a randomized trial. Gastroenterology 2020; 159(2):512–20.e7.
28. Liu W-N, Zhang Y-Y, Bian X-Q, et al. Study on detection rate of polyps and adenomas in artificial-intelligence-aided colonoscopy. Saudi J Gastroenterol 2020; 26(1):13–9.
29. Mohan BP, Facciorusso A, Khan SR, et al. Real-time computer aided colonoscopy versus standard colonoscopy for improving adenoma detection rate: A meta-analysis of randomized-controlled trials. EClinicalMedicine 2020;29-30:100622.
30. Shaukat A, Lichtenstein DR, Somers SC, et al. Computer-aided detection improves adenomas per colonoscopy for screening and surveillance colonoscopy: a randomized trial. Gastroenterology 2022;163(3):732–41.
31. Glissen Brown JR, Mansour NM, Wang P, et al. Deep learning computer-aided polyp detection reduces adenoma miss rate: a United States multi-center randomized tndem colonoscopy study (CADeT-CS Trial). Clin Gastroenterol Hepatol 2022;20(7):1499–507.e4.
32. Ma R, Wang R, Zhang Y, et al. RNNSLAM: Reconstructing the 3D colon to visualize missing regions during a colonoscopy. Med Image Anal 2021;72:102100.
33. Zhou J, Wu L, Wan X, et al. A novel artificial intelligence system for the assessment of bowel preparation (with video). Gastrointest Endosc 2020;91(2): 428–35, e2.
34. US Food and Drug Administration. Artificial Intelligence and Machine Learning (AI/ML) - Enabled Medical Devices. 2022. Available at: https://www.fda.gov/medical-devices/software-medical-device-samd/artificial-intelligence-and-machine-learning-aiml-enabled-medical-devices. Accessed January 1, 2023.
35. Barua I, Vinsard DG, Jodal HC, et al. Artificial intelligence for polyp detection during colonoscopy: a systematic review and meta-analysis. Endoscopy 2021;53(3): 277–84.
36. Ozawa T, Ishihara S, Fujishiro M, et al. Automated endoscopic detection and classification of colorectal polyps using convolutional neural networks. Therap Adv Gastroenterol 2020;13. 1756284820910659.
37. Mori Y, Kudo SE, East JE, et al. Cost savings in colonoscopy with artificial intelligence-aided polyp diagnosis: an add-on analysis of a clinical trial (with video). Gastrointest Endosc 2020;92(4):905–11.e1.
38. Turner D, Ricciuto A, Lewis A, et al. STRIDE-II: an update on the Selecting Therapeutic Targets in Inflammatory Bowel Disease (STRIDE) initiative of the International Organization for the Study of IBD (IOIBD): Determining therapeutic goals for treat-to-target strategies in IBD. Gastroenterology 2021;160(5):1570–83.
39. Khanna R, Nelson SA, Feagan BG, et al. Endoscopic scoring indices for evaluation of disease activity in Crohn's disease. Cochrane Database Syst Rev 2016; 2016(8):Cd010642.
40. Mohammed Vashist N, Samaan M, Mosli MH, et al. Endoscopic scoring indices for evaluation of disease activity in ulcerative colitis. Cochrane Database Syst Rev 2018;1(1):CD011450.
41. Osada T, Ohkusa T, Yokoyama T, et al. Comparison of several activity indices for the evaluation of endoscopic activity in UC: inter- and intraobserver consistency. Inflamm Bowel Dis 2010;16(2):192–7.
42. Stidham RW, Liu W, Bishu S, et al. Performance of a deep learning model vs human reviewers in grading endoscopic disease severity of patients with ulcerative colitis. JAMA Netw Open 2019;2(5):e193963.

43. Ozawa T, Ishihara S, Fujishiro M, et al. Novel computer-assisted diagnosis system for endoscopic disease activity in patients with ulcerative colitis. Gastrointest Endosc 2019;89(2):416–21.e1.

44. Gutierrez Becker B, Arcadu F, Thalhammer A, et al. Training and deploying a deep learning model for endoscopic severity grading in ulcerative colitis using multicenter clinical trial data. Ther Adv Gastrointest Endosc 2021;14. 2631774521990623.

45. Gottlieb K, Requa J, Karnes W, et al. Central reading of ulcerative colitis clinical trial videos using neural networks. Gastroenterology 2021;160(3):710–9.e2.

46. Takenaka K, Ohtsuka K, Fujii T, et al. Development and validation of a deep neural network for accurate evaluation of endoscopic images from patients with ulcerative colitis. Gastroenterology 2020;158(8):2150–7.

47. Yao H, Najarian K, Gryak J, et al. Fully automated endoscopic disease activity assessment in ulcerative colitis. Gastrointest Endosc 2021;93(3):728–36.e1.

48. Klang E, Barash Y, Margalit RY, et al. Deep learning algorithms for automated detection of Crohn's disease ulcers by video capsule endoscopy. Gastrointest Endosc 2020;91(3):606–13.e2.

49. Klang E, Grinman A, Soffer S, et al. Automated eetection of crohn's disease intestinal strictures on capsule endoscopy images using deep neural networks. J Crohns Colitis 2021;15(5):749–56.

50. Wang CC, Chiu YC, Chen WL, et al. A deep learning model for classification of endoscopic gastroesophageal reflux disease. Int J Environ Res Public Health 2021;18(5):2428.

51. Shichijo S, Endo Y, Aoyama K, et al. Application of convolutional neural networks for evaluating Helicobacter pylori infection status on the basis of endoscopic images. Scand J Gastroenterol 2019;54(2):158–63.

52. Shichijo S, Nomura S, Aoyama K, et al. Application of convolutional neural networks in the diagnosis of Helicobacter pylori infection based on endoscopic images. EBioMedicine 2017;25:106–11.

53. Nakashima H, Kawahira H, Kawachi H, et al. Artificial intelligence diagnosis of Helicobacter pylori infection using blue laser imaging-bright and linked color imaging: a single-center prospective study. Ann Gastroenterol 2018;31(4):462–8.

54. Nakashima H, Kawahira H, Kawachi H, et al. Endoscopic three-categorical diagnosis of Helicobacter pylori infection using linked color imaging and deep learning: a single-center prospective study (with video). Gastric Cancer 2020; 23(6):1033–40.

55. Zheng W, Zhang X, Kim JJ, et al. High accuracy of convolutional neural network for evaluation of Helicobacter pylori infection based on endoscopic images: preliminary experience. Clin Transl Gastroenterol 2019;10(12):e00109.

56. Wimmer G, Vécsei A, Uhl A. CNN transfer learning for the automated diagnosis of celiac disease. IEEE 2016;1–6.

57. Hegenbart S, Uhl A, Vécsei A, et al. Scale invariant texture descriptors for classifying celiac disease. Med Image Anal 2013;17(4):458–74.

58. Hegenbart S, Uhl A, Vécsei A. Systematic assessment of performance prediction techniques in medical image classification: a case study on celiac disease. Inf Process Med Imaging 2011;22:498–509.

59. Kwitt R, Hegenbart S, Rasiwasia N, et al. Do we need annotation experts? A case study in celiac disease classification. Med Image Comput Comput Assist Interv 2014;17(Pt 2):454–61.

60. Gadermayr M, Kogler H, Karla M, et al. Computer-aided texture analysis combined with experts' knowledge: Improving endoscopic celiac disease diagnosis. World J Gastroenterol 2016;22(31):7124–34.
61. Vécsei A, Amann G, Hegenbart S, et al. Automated Marsh-like classification of celiac disease in children using local texture operators. Comput Biol Med 2011;41(6):313–25.
62. Ojala T, Pietikäinen M, Harwood D. A comparative study of texture measures with classification based on featured distributions. Pattern Recognition 1996;29(1):51–9.
63. Walsh CM, Lightdale JR. Pediatric Endoscopy Quality Improvement Network (PEnQuIN) quality standards and indicators for pediatric endoscopy: an ASGE-endorsed guideline. Gastrointest Endosc 2022;96(4):593–602.
64. Walsh CM, Lightdale JR, Mack DR, et al. Overview of the Pediatric Endoscopy Quality Improvement Network Quality Standards and Indicators for Pediatric Endoscopy: a Joint NASPGHAN/ESPGHAN Guideline. J Pediatr Gastroenterol Nutr 2022;74(S1):S3–15.
65. Wu L, Zhang J, Zhou W, et al. Randomised controlled trial of WISENSE, a real-time quality improving system for monitoring blind spots during esophagogastroduodenoscopy. Gut 2019;68(12):2161–9.
66. Aoki T, Yamada A, Kato Y, et al. Automatic detection of blood content in capsule endoscopy images based on a deep convolutional neural network. J Gastroenterol Hepatol 2020;35(7):1196–200.
67. Tsuboi A, Oka S, Aoyama K, et al. Artificial intelligence using a convolutional neural network for automatic detection of small-bowel angioectasia in capsule endoscopy images. Dig Endosc 2020;32(3):382–90.
68. Tenório JM, Hummel AD, Cohrs FM, et al. Artificial intelligence techniques applied to the development of a decision-support system for diagnosing celiac disease. Int J Med Inform 2011;80(11):793–802.
69. Zhou T, Han G, Li BN, et al. Quantitative analysis of patients with celiac disease by video capsule endoscopy: A deep learning method. Comput Biol Med 2017;85:1–6.
70. Wang X, Qian H, Ciaccio EJ, et al. Celiac disease diagnosis from videocapsule endoscopy images with residual learning and deep feature extraction. Comput Methods Programs Biomed 2020;187:105236.
71. Saito H, Aoki T, Aoyama K, et al. Automatic detection and classification of protruding lesions in wireless capsule endoscopy images based on a deep convolutional neural network. Gastrointest Endosc 2020;92(1):144–51.e1.
72. Yuan Y, Meng MQ. Deep learning for polyp recognition in wireless capsule endoscopy images. Med Phys 2017;44(4):1379–89.
73. He JY, Wu X, Jiang YG, et al. Hookworm detection in wireless capsule endoscopy images with deep learning. IEEE Trans Image Process 2018;27:2379–92.
74. Ding Z, Shi H, Zhang H, et al. Gastroenterologist-level identification of small-bowel diseases and normal variants by capsule endoscopy using a deep-learning model. Gastroenterology 2019;157(4):1044–54.e5.
75. Zou Y, Li L, Wang Y, et al. Classifying digestive organs in wireless capsule endoscopy images based on deep convolutional neural network. IEEE Int Conf Digital Signal Process (Dsp) 2015;1274–8.
76. Dray X, Iakovidis D, Houdeville C, et al. Artificial intelligence in small bowel capsule endoscopy - current status, challenges and future promise. J Gastroenterol Hepatol 2021;36(1):12–9.
77. Leenhardt R, Souchaud M, Houist G, et al. A neural network-based algorithm for assessing the cleanliness of small bowel during capsule endoscopy. Endoscopy 2021;53(9):932–6.

78. Noorda R, Nevárez A, Colomer A, et al. Automatic evaluation of degree of cleanliness in capsule endoscopy based on a novel CNN architecture. Sci Rep 2020; 10(1):17706.
79. Rodrigues T, Keswani R. Endoscopy training in the age of artificial intelligence: deep learning or artificial competence? Clin Gastroenterol Hepatol 2023; 21(1):8–10.
80. Walsh CM, Ling SC, Wang CS, et al. Concurrent versus terminal feedback: it may be better to wait. Acad Med, 84(10 Suppl) 2009;S54–S57..
81. Salmoni AW, Schmidt RA, Walter CB. Knowledge of results and motor learning: a review and critical reappraisal. Psychol Bull 1984;95(3):355–86.
82. Young JQ, Van Merrienboer J, Durning S, et al. Cognitive load theory: implications for medical education: AMEE Guide No. 86, Med Teach 2014;36(5):371–84.
83. Troya J, Fitting D, Brand M, et al. The influence of computer-aided polyp detection systems on reaction time for polyp detection and eye gaze. Endoscopy 2022; 54(10):1009–14.
84. Lami M, Singh H, Dilley JH, et al. Gaze patterns hold key to unlocking successful search strategies and increasing polyp detection rate in colonoscopy. Endoscopy 2018;50(7):701–7.
85. Almansa C, Shahid MW, Heckman MG, et al. Association between visual gaze patterns and adenoma detection rate during colonoscopy: a preliminary investigation. Am J Gastroenterol 2011;106(6):1070–4.
86. Wallace MB, Sharma P, Bhandari P, et al. Impact of artificial intelligence on miss rate of colorectal neoplasia. Gastroenterology 2022;163(1):295–304.e5.
87. Jin EH, Lee D, Bae JH, et al. Improved accuracy in optical diagnosis of colorectal polyps using convolutional neural networks with visual explanations. Gastroenterology 2020;158(8):2169–79.e8.
88. Briganti G, Le Moine O. Artificial intelligence in medicine: today and tomorrow. Front Med (Lausanne) 2020;7:27.
89. Paranjape K, Schinkel M, Nanayakkara P. Short keynote paper: Mainstreaming personalized healthcare-transforming healthcare through new era of artificial intelligence. IEEE J Biomed Health Inform 2020;24(7):1860–3.
90. Parasa S, Wallace M, Bagci U, et al. Proceedings from the First Global Artificial Intelligence in Gastroenterology and Endoscopy Summit. Gastrointest Endosc 2020;92(4):938–45.e1.
91. Kraus S, Barber TR, Briggs B, et al. Implementing computerized physician order management at a community hospital. Jt Comm J Qual Patient Saf 2008;34(2):74–84.
92. Bredfeldt CE, Awad EB, Joseph K, et al. Training providers: beyond the basics of electronic health records. BMC Health Serv Res 2013;13:503.
93. Repici A, Spadaccini M, Antonelli G, et al. Artificial intelligence and colonoscopy experience: lessons from two randomised trials. Gut 2022;71(4):757–65.

Pediatric Unsedated Transnasal Endoscopy

Rajitha D. Venkatesh, MD[a,b,*], Kristina Leinwand, DO[c,d], Nathalie Nguyen, MD[e]

KEYWORDS

- Unsedated transnasal endoscopy • Esophagoscopy • Pediatrics
- Ultrathin endoscope

KEY POINTS

- Unsedated transnasal endoscopy (TNE) provides direct visualization of the esophagus and enables acquisition of biopsy samples while eliminating the risks associated with sedation and anesthesia.
- Unsedated TNE is feasible, safe, and cost-effective in pediatric populations. It is well accepted and tolerated, provides time-saving to patients and families, enables caregivers to be present during the procedure, and has the potential to improve access to endoscopy.
- Unsedated TNE should be considered in the evaluation and monitoring of disorders of the upper gastrointestinal tract, particularly in diseases such as eosinophilic esophagitis that often require repeated endoscopy.

INTRODUCTION

Pediatric unsedated transnasal endoscopy (TNE) is a promising alternative to esophagogastroduodenoscopy (EGD) which, during the last 2 decades, has shifted toward using anesthesiologist-administered sedation in children and adolescents.[1,2]

Disclosure Statement: R.D. Venkatesh has nothing to disclose. K. Leinwand has received speaker honoraria from EvoEndo and participated in EvoEndo Physician Preference Testing. N. Nguyen has consulted for EvoEndo and Regeneron.
[a] Division of Pediatric Gastroenterology, Hepatology, and Nutrition, Nationwide Children's Hospital, 700 Childrens Drive, Columbus, OH 43205, USA; [b] Department of Pediatrics, The Ohio State University College of Medicine, Columbus, OH, USA; [c] Section of Pediatric Gastroenterology, Hepatology and Nutrition, Northwest Permanente, Portland, OR, USA; [d] Department of Pediatric Gastroenterology, Hepatology, and Nutrition, Doernbecher Children's Hospital at Oregon Health and Science University, Portland, OR, USA; [e] Gastrointestinal Eosinophilic Diseases Program, Section of Pediatric Gastroenterology, Hepatology and Nutrition, Children's Hospital of Colorado, Digestive Health Institute, Children's Hospital Colorado, University of Colorado School of Medicine
* Corresponding author. Division of Gastroenterology, Hepatology and Nutrition, Nationwide Children's Hospital, 700 Childrens Drive, Columbus, OH 43205.
E-mail address: Rajitha.venkatesh@nationwidechildrens.org

Gastrointest Endoscopy Clin N Am 33 (2023) 309–321
https://doi.org/10.1016/j.giec.2022.10.006
1052-5157/23/© 2022 Elsevier Inc. All rights reserved.

Unsedated TNE uses an ultrathin endoscope, defined as having a diameter ranging from 2.8 to 6 mm, inserted through the nasal cavity and advanced down the esophagus and stomach, to perform an upper endoscopic examination. TNE was first used by gastroenterologists as a cost-effective tool to screen for Barrett's esophagus and esophageal cancer in adults in the early 1990s.[3] Since then, there has been increasing use of unsedated TNE in both adults and children for various indications and several subsequent studies have shown that TNE is feasible, cost-effective, safe, and well tolerated.[4,5]

In comparison to local or topical anesthesia, which is used for TNE, sedation and general anesthesia are associated with increased adverse events, added monitoring and staffing requirements, higher costs, and a longer overall procedure and recovery time. Pediatric studies describe an overall adverse event rate for EGD of 2.3%, including a specific risk of respiratory issues in 1.5% of procedures.[6–10] Most cardiopulmonary adverse events associated with pediatric endoscopy relate to procedural sedation and anesthesia, and sedation-related complications may account for up to 60% of all adverse events during pediatric endoscopic procedures.[6,10] In 2017, the US Food and Drug Administration issued a "Drug Safety Communication" warning that repeated use of anesthetics may affect young children's neurodevelopment.[11] Therefore, concerns related to anesthesia are particularly relevant in pediatrics. Additionally, deep sedation and anesthesia are expensive, owing to direct costs related to anesthesia and indirect costs of taking time off from work or school for the procedure.[5] The purpose of this article is to provide an overview of unsedated TNE in pediatrics including indications, advantages and limitations, and implementation.

INDICATIONS FOR TRANSNASAL ENDOSCOPY

In pediatrics, TNE has been described largely for the evaluation and management of patients with eosinophilic esophagitis (EoE), who often require serial endoscopic assessments for disease monitoring.[5] In the largest study of TNE in pediatric patients, 190 children and young adults aged 3 to 22 years underwent the procedure with a 98% success rate (294 of 300 attempts successful).[5] In this cohort, 54 patients had multiple TNEs to evaluate response to management changes in EoE.[5] Visual findings, which are similar to traditional EGD (**Fig. 1**A–C), and histologic findings were adequate for diagnosis. There were no significant adverse events, and the cost of unsedated TNE was 53.4% less than the patient's previous endoscopy.

Unsedated TNE is particularly useful in disease that required repeated esophageal assessments. Other indications for TNE described in pediatrics include the evaluation

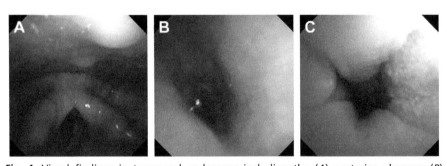

Fig. 1. Visual findings in transnasal endoscopy including the (A) posterior pharynx; (B) normal esophagus; and (C) edema, linear furrows, and exudate seen in patients with eosinophilic esophagitis.

of dysphagia, Barrett esophagus, candida esophagitis, monitoring of esophagitis in patients with tracheoesophageal fistula/esophageal atresia, abdominal pain, gastroesophageal reflux disease (GERD), and celiac disease.[5] In general, TNE allows for the evaluation of esophageal disorders by visually assessing the esophageal mucosa and obtaining mucosal biopsies of the esophagus. In adults, TNE has been used for a broader list of indications in the upper gastrointestinal tract, including dysphagia, globus pharyngeus, GERD or reflux symptoms, Barrett esophagus, eosinophilic esophagitis, esophageal varices, vomiting, gastric carcinoma, esophageal varices, gastroduodenal ulcers, esophagitis, gastritis, duodenitis, Helicobacter pylori infection, and celiac disease.[4] Use of TNE has even been described for therapeutic procedures in adults, including esophageal dilation, nasogastric and percutaneous endoscopic gastrostomy tube placement, and foreign body identification and removal.[4,12] Although there are no absolute contraindications for unsedated TNE, relative contraindications to consider include patients with abnormal nasal anatomy that would preclude passage of the endoscope, significant coagulopathy, or epistaxis.

PATIENT SELECTION, PREPARATION, AND DISTRACTION TECHNIQUES

Patient selection and preparation are important determinants of procedural completion because success largely depends on a cooperative patient. TNE has been performed in children aged as young as 3 years but most centers currently perform the procedure in children aged 8 years and older.[5] Some experienced centers routinely perform TNE in children aged 5 years and older. Outside of age, it is important to consider developmental readiness including the ability to follow instructions and cooperation. Importantly, anxiety is not necessarily a contraindication to performing unsedated TNE.

Precounseling and patient and family education are recommended ahead of the procedure to help alleviate anxiety and ensure the patient knows what to expect. This can be done in-person or over the phone and educational resources such as videos can be helpful. Child life specialists can play a critical role in orienting patients and families to the required steps of the procedure.[13,14] They can help prepare patients and families, either in advance or on the day of the procedure, by facilitating conversations about coping skills as well as expectations regarding comfort, pain, and other sensations before and during the procedure and help to alleviate anxiety related to the procedure.[13,14]

Distraction techniques can be helpful both in preparation for and during unsedated TNE. One widely used distraction technique for pediatric patients is the use of virtual reality (VR) headsets,[5,15–17] which may positively impact procedural success rate in children and adolescents.[18,19] VR consists of a fully immersive 3-dimensional environment displayed in surround stereoscopic vision on a head-mounted display. VR is an effective pain and anxiety management tool for pediatric patients during specific medical procedures.[19] Although there are no specific studies examining the use of VR in TNE as a distraction technique, its use has been well described in the preparation for outpatient surgical procedures and as distraction method during painful medical procedures (eg, intravenous line placements, burn care) where it has been shown to reduce pain and anxiety and improve patient satisfaction.[18,20–23]

VR is available in many different forms, from a stand-alone VR system to a set of VR goggles (disposable or reusable) that is paired with a cellular phone. There are many options for VR distraction systems, and important considerations when choosing a device or system for unsedated TNE are finding an acceptable and adjustable face/head fit for pediatric patients and using a system that enables unobstructed access to the nares rather than using a VR device where the nares are positioned inside the device. Typically for TNE, the VR headset is positioned after topical anesthesia is applied and the patient wears the headset for the duration of the procedure.[5,15] Other distraction techniques patients may opt for include music/headphones, light systems, projection systems, or a multisensory environment machine. Often a combination of distraction techniques can be helpful based on the patient's age and developmental stage.[24] Some pediatric patients choose not to use a distraction technique and prefer to watch the procedure on the endoscopy monitor.

Qualitative research examining the utility of preparation and distraction strategies in pediatric TNE highlighted the perceived value of online videos, clear preprocedural communication, physician coaching and comforting during the procedures, presence of a caregiver and use of distraction techniques, including VR headsets and stress balls.[17] Overall, the procedure is well tolerated and accepted by pediatric patients and their caregivers.[17] Studies in pediatric and adult patients have found that it is more comfortable than EGD and many patients who have undergone TNE, when given the choice, would select TNE over EGD for their subsequent procedure.[15,25,26]

PERFORMING TRANSNASAL ENDOSCOPY

TNE uses an ultrathin endoscope, which enables it to be passed through the nasal cavity. In preparation for unsedated TNE, patients are nil per os for 2 hours before the scheduled procedure. Although other patient positions can be used, pediatric TNE is traditionally performed with the patient sitting upright in an adjustable chair, where the adjustable arm and backrest will provide the patient comfort while optimizing their position during the TNE after informed consent (and assent as required) is obtained and a preprocedure "time out" is completed, topical anesthesia (4% lidocaine spray or gel) should be applied in the nose and mouth to minimize nasal pain and discomfort. A vasoconstrictor such as oxymetazoline may also be applied to facilitate nasal decongestion and improve ease of endoscope insertion via turbinate shrinkage. Nasal passage has been reported to be the most painful area during endoscope insertion, highlighting the importance of proper nasal preparation.[27,28] However, these medications can taste and feel unpleasant, so it is important to forewarn patients.[17] Distraction techniques, as mentioned, are incorporated after topical anesthesia is applied. For pediatric patients, a family member may often be present in the room to observe the procedure, which can help with facilitate procedural acceptance and tolerance, as parental presence is known to be one of the most comforting factors for children when in pain.[29] Parental presence may also be reassuring for caregivers and help to increase their understanding of the procedure and their child's illness.[17]

The ultrathin endoscope is lubricated and passed through the nasal passageway either below the inferior turbinate or between the middle and inferior turbinate (**Fig. 2**). It is important to apply gentle pressure on the shaft of the scope and avoid sudden movement as it enters the nose because this can cause intranasal pressure and patient discomfort. Nasopharyngeal closure, the tongue base, the hypopharynx, vocal fold motion, and pooling of oral secretions should all be evaluated during this portion of the procedure. The patient should then be asked to swallow as the endoscope is gently advanced midline through the upper esophageal sphincter similar to standard EGD. Once the endoscope is in the esophagus, image acquisition and mucosal biopsies can be performed in the standard fashion. The working channel of ultrathin endoscopes, which range from 1.2 to 2 mm, is smaller compared with a standard gastroscope (2.8 mm) and, therefore, requires use of smaller diameter biopsy forceps to obtain biopsies. However, previous studies have shown that specimens

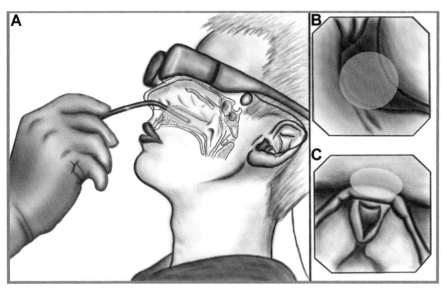

Fig. 2. Upright positioning for TNE with (*A*) the TNE insertion pathway below the inferior turbinate (*green*). After insertion, the transnasal endoscope should (*B*) be passed lateral and inferior to the inferior turbinate, and then (*C*) passed midline from the pharyngeal location to the esophagus (directly superior to the arytenoid cartilage). (*Courtesy of* Robert E. Kramer, MD, FASGE, Aurora, CO.)

obtained using smaller biopsy forceps are adequate for histologic examination and comparable in diagnostic yield to samples obtained using conventional EGD biopsy forceps.[5] The endoscope can be advanced into the stomach and duodenum and biopsies obtained. The ability to reach the stomach and duodenum while the patient is unsedated depends on the gastroenterologists' experience with unsedated TNE with a limited view and minimal insufflation, the length of the endoscope and patient cooperation.

During the removal of the endoscope, the tip should be kept in the middle of the lumen by hand control to prevent it from rubbing against the nasal septum and turbinates as it is withdrawn. After the procedure is finished, patients can eat and drink once the topical anesthetic has worn off, typically within 30 minutes of TNE completion, and can resume normal activities.

ADVANTAGES AND LIMITATIONS OF TRANSNASAL ENDOSCOPY

There are clear advantages to TNE, including a reduction in the risk and cost associated with anesthesia, decreased costs and time associated with postprocedure monitoring, and a reduction in time away from school and work. In the pediatric population, sedation or general anesthesia require additional staffing, including an anesthesiologist and a postanesthesia care unit to enable close monitoring. When costs for TNE and EGD were compared in a large retrospective pediatric study, there was a 53.4% reduction in charges for TNE, largely due to costs associated with anesthesia as well as decreased in-office time.[5] Similar prospective studies that have examined the economic impact associated with use of TNE in adult patients have shown comparable cost reductions.[30] Although the preparation time may be slightly longer for TNE and the time to complete the procedure is similar, research has shown that the recovery time and the overall procedural time is lower.[25,31–33] A large pediatric center reported an average procedure time of 8.6 minutes with a total office time of 60 to 90 minutes.[5,15]

Another positive aspect of TNE is that caregivers are often able to be in the room with their child during the procedure, which enables them to directly comfort their child and may help to alleviate both patient and parental anxiety. A qualitative study of pediatric patients' and parents' experiences with TNE found that the procedure is overall well accepted.[17] Perceived positive aspects of the procedure were the lack of intravenous anesthetic, the decreased cost, shorter procedure time, and the ability of parents to accompany the patient. Another important advantage of unsedated TNE includes low rate of reported adverse events, including brief emesis in 5.2% of patients, nasal irritation in 2.6%, self-limited episodes of epistaxis during 2% of cases, 0.9% with presyncopal events, 0.5% with reported anxiety, 0.4% with procedural nausea, and only one report of esophageal perforation to date.[5,34]

One must also be aware of the limitations of TNE, including the limited capabilities of current ultrathin endoscopes, lower reimbursement rates, and limited access because few pediatric centers currently perform TNE. Working channel size limits the choice of accessories currently available for use with ultrathin endoscopes. Although ultrathin endoscopes accommodate smaller biopsy forceps for diagnostic evaluation, many currently available accessories that are required for therapeutic procedures do not fit down in smaller working channel. Limited therapeutic devices including grasping forceps (eg, Olympus, Boston Scientific), argon plasma coagulation (APC) probes (ie, ERBE) and nets (ie, US Endoscopy) have been made to accommodate some ultrathin endoscope channels. There are case reports of therapeutic procedures such as esophageal dilation,[35] nasoenteric tube,[36–38] and percutaneous endoscopic gastrostomy placement[12] performed on adult patients; however, the use of TNE for therapeutic procedures has not been described in the pediatric literature. The endoscope size also limits the size of the suction channel and resultant flow rate when suctioning. Adequate visualization is important to appropriately evaluate many upper gastrointestinal tract lesions. Because patients are awake during TNE, minimal air insufflation is used for patient comfort; therefore, visibility may be limited compared with EGD where full insufflation of the esophagus and stomach can be achieved.

Other limitations of current ultrathin endoscopes, depending on model, may include lack of a standard water channel, shorter length, and lack of high-definition imaging. However, studies that have evaluated the quality of views obtained from TNE and conventional gastroscopes found no difference in video quality.[39] In addition, reimbursement rates are lower for TNE than EGD under sedation or general anesthesia, which may deter some physicians from performing TNE. Finally, although TNE has the potential to ultimately improve access to care because it requires fewer health-care resources, access to TNE in pediatrics is currently limited to a few centers across North America. Because the availability of TNE is currently limited, some patients and families may choose to travel to access TNE, which ultimately does not lower cost or decrease time away from school and work.

There are several reasons to consider using pediatric TNE; however, there are instances where it may not be as successful. Large adult studies suggest that reasons for failure of TNE include transnasal insertion failure, patient refusal, or nasal pain and factors that may predict failure include younger age (<35 years), female gender, and larger endoscope diameter.[4] In the largest pediatric study to date, 294 of 300 TNE attempts were performed completely.[5] The procedure was unsuccessful in 6 patients as a result of transnasal insertion failure secondary to movement of the child and patient refusal (ages 5–10 years).[5] Hence, the authors recommend offering TNE to children aged 5 years and older, who are cooperative and do not have a history of untreated anxiety.

STARTING A TRANSNASAL ENDOSCOPY PROGRAM

As interest in unsedated TNE continues to increase, many have considered offering this procedure at their center. Start-up funding is often the biggest barrier to establishing a TNE program; therefore, formulating a business proposal is a key strategy in getting an initial approval for a program. Potential options for funding may include foundational support, donations, and/or grants. Sharing resources between departments (eg, pulmonology and gastroenterology) should also be considered.

A business plan should include pro forma projections and financial statements for the number of patients eligible by diagnostic code/indication within the appropriate age range, with a focus on anticipated monthly and yearly procedure numbers, and anticipated revenue and/or anticipated cost savings based on the individual business practice model. The most common CPT codes for TNE, including transnasal esophagoscopy and transnasal EGD, are listed in **Table 1**. The business plan should also detail proposed expenses, including variable costs that depend on patient volume such as labor and materials, as well as fixed costs such as lease/rental payments, insurance. The overall goal of the business plan is to establish a value analysis, which is a systematic approach and decision-making process to evaluate a current technology such as TNE with the goal of highlighting value-based procurement of the equipment and resources needed by decreasing expenses and enhancing revenue, while balancing issues of quality and safety in patient care.[40]

Understanding the options for TNE products and endoscopes is helpful when formulating a business plan with the goal of decreasing expenses. The cost of endoscope(s) is often the largest portion of the start-up expenses in setting up a TNE program. Major manufacturers of ultrathin endoscopes that can be used to perform TNE include, but are not limited to, Fujinon (Wayne, NJ) Pentax (Montvale, NJ) and Olympus (Center Valley, PA) **(Table 2)**. There is also a dedicated transnasal esophagoscope available from Vision Sciences (see **Table 2**) but this option has an outer diameter that is at the larger end for ultrathin endoscopes (5.4–5.8 mm). Although all of these ultrathin endoscopes can be used for TNE, most centers performing pediatric TNE in the United States prefer scopes with the smallest outer diameter possible to ensure patient comfort and tolerability. Reflective of this, physician preference has been largely toward using a flexible bronchoscope to perform unsedated TNE in children and adolescents, as the outer diameter of the bronchoscope ranges from 2.8 to 4.2 mm. Although the flexible bronchoscopes are the most widely used instrument for unsedated TNE in pediatric patients, limitations include lack of a standard water channel, limited suctioning capabilities, and shorter length. However, these limitations have not impeded successful performance of unsedated pediatric TNE. Technological advancements in endoscope design have been occurring rapidly, and there are now several single-use (ie, disposable) endoscope and bronchoscope systems available through Ambu, Boston

Table 1	
Common CPT codes for transnasal endoscopy	
CPT Code	**Description**
43197	Esophagoscopy, flexible, transnasal; diagnostic
43198	Esophagoscopy, flexible, transnasal; with biopsy, single or multiple
0652T	Esophagogastroduodenoscopy, flexible, transnasal; diagnostic
0653T	Esophagogastroduodenoscopy, flexible, transnasal; with biopsy, single or multiple

Table 2
Common multiuse ultrathin transnasal endoscopes/bronchoscopes and their specifications

Model	Type	Angulation (deg)	Field of View (deg)	Outer Diameter (mm)	Accessory Channel Diameter (mm)	Working Length (mm)
Olympus (Center Valley, Pa)						
GIF-XP190 N	Gastroscope	210 up/90 down 100 left/100 right	140	5.4	2.2	1100
GIF-H190 N	Gastroscope	210 up/90 down 100 left/100 right	140	5.4	2.2	1100
GIF N180	Gastroscope	210 up/90 down	120	4.9	2	1100
PEF-V	Transnasal	180 up/130 down	120	5.3	2	650
BF-XP190/290	Bronchoscope	210 up/130 down 120 left/120 right	110	3.1	1.2	600
BF-P190/290	Bronchoscope	210 up/130 down 120 left/120 right	110	4.2	2	600
Fujinon (Wayne, NJ)						
EG-740N	Gastroscope	210 up/90 down 100 left/100 right	140	5.9	2.4	1100
EB-530P	Bronchoscope	180 up/130 down	120	3.8	1.2	600
EB-580s	Bronchoscope	210 up/130 down	120	5.3	2.2	600
EB-530H	Bronchoscope	180 up/130 down	140	5.4	2	600
EB-580T	Bronchoscope	180 up/130 down	120	5.9	2.8	600
Pentax (Montvale, NJ)						
EG 1690K	Gastroscope	210 up/120 down 120 left/120 right	120	5.4	2	1100
EB-1170K	Bronchoscope	210 up/130 down	120	3.8	1.2	600
EB15-J10	Bronchoscope	210 up/130 down	120	5.4	2	600

Scientific (Marlborough, MA), EvoEndo (Denver, CO), and Olympus (**Table 3**). These single-use scope systems may change the way unsedated TNE is performed in both pediatric and adult patients. Benefits of the single-use endoscopes to consider when establishing a TNE program include easy accessibility for the outpatient setting, and avoidance of time-consuming and costly sterilization procedures, maintenance, and repairs needed for multiuse systems. However, the cost, covered by either the program or patient, for a single-use system may preclude its use in some centers. Depending on the type of endoscope system chosen, there will be various compatible disposable and/or reusable biopsy forceps, which is also a consideration in total cost.

In addition to the wide variety of available endoscopes or bronchoscopes, there are many options regarding location to perform unsedated TNE. Many programs perform TNE in an outpatient clinic room. Benefits of this model include convenience for physician workflow and staffing and cost savings related to avoiding hospital or surgical center fees. Limitations with using an outpatient clinical setting may include the lack of onsite facilities for sterile instrument processing but this may be circumvented through single-use endoscope systems or by using a courier system to transport endoscopes to a sterile instrument-processing center. Other options for performing unsedated TNE include ambulatory surgical centers or within hospital operating rooms where sterile processing and equipment storage is onsite. However, these may be associated with higher costs and facility fees for the procedure.

Table 3
Ultrathin single-use gastroscopes and bronchoscopes and their specifications

Model	Type	Angulation (deg)	Field of View (deg)	Outer Diameter (mm)	Accessory Channel Diameter (mm)	Working Length (mm)
Ambu (Columbia, MD)						
aScope 4 Broncho Slim	Bronchoscope	180 up/180 down	85	3.8	1.2	600
aScope 4 Broncho Reg	Bronchoscope	180 up/180 down	85	5	2	600
aScope 4 Broncho Large	Bronchoscope	180 up/160 down	85	5.8	2.8	600
Boston Scientific (Marlborough, MA)						
EXALT Model B Slim	Bronchoscope	180 up/180 down	90	3.8	1	600
EXALT Model B Reg	Bronchoscope	180 up/180 down	90	5	2	600
EvoEndo (Denver, CO)						
Model LE	Gastroscope	210 up/90 down 100 left/100 right	120	3.5	2	1100
Olympus (Center Valley, PA)						
H-SteriScope Slim BCV1-C2	Bronchoscope	210 up/210 down 90 left/90 right	110	3.2	1.2	600
H-SteriScope Normal BCV1-M2	Bronchoscope	210 up/210 down 90 left/90 right	110	4.9	2.2	600
H-SteriScope Large BCV1-S2	Bronchoscope	210 up/210 down 90 left/90 right	110	5.8	2.8	600

Recommended staff for unsedated TNE include the endoscopists and a procedure assistant, who can be a trained medical assistant, registered nurse, or procedure center technician. One additional highly recommended staff consideration for pediatric TNE is using a Child Life specialist before and during the procedure.

TRAINING IN TRANSNASAL ENDOSCOPY

Currently, there are just over a dozen centers performing unsedated TNE in pediatrics in North America. As a first step in learning to perform TNE on pediatric patients, it is recommended to contact established pediatric TNE programs with experienced pediatric endoscopists who perform unsedated TNE regularly. Contacting multiple physicians experienced in unsedated TNE is highly recommended when establishing a TNE program due to the wide variation in practice types, distraction techniques, equipment/materials, and location options. A vital component of setting up a TNE program and learning to perform TNE is a site visit to an existing pediatric TNE program to observe pediatric TNE procedures as well as preprocedural and postprocedural aspects of TNE including patient preparation and consent, equipment set-up and, postprocedure communication, recovery, and endoscope reprocessing. It can also be helpful for the medical assistant or registered nurse who will be assisting with the unsedated TNE procedures to attend the site visit(s) as well. This facilitates the understanding of the technician role and the nuances with assisting in unsedated TNE.

After a site visit or discussion with experienced TNE program, learning the nasal anatomy and practicing endoscope navigation from the nare into the esophagus is key. This is often best achieved using a dual approach, including collaboration with other procedural colleagues and simulation-based practice. Options for collaboration include working with ear, nose, and throat surgeons to observe and assist with in-office flexible fiberoptic laryngoscopy and nasal endoscopy, and/or pulmonologist colleagues to pass bronchoscopes through the nare on sedated patients in the operating room. Hands-on practice with nasal endoscope intubation can be very helpful in the learning process but it is also vital to practice TNE with the endoscopes/bronchoscopes that will be used within the TNE program.

Simulation-based endoscopy training has been widely studied and has become an acceptable method for trainees to acquire basic skills for medical procedures.[41–43] Use of simulators allows for sustained deliberate practice of TNE without compromising patient safety and comfort. Endoscopy simulators, including inanimate models (mechanical simulators), VR simulators and ex vivo and live animal models, have been successfully used by health professionals to supplement procedural training in related techniques ranging from fiberoptic endoscopic evaluation of swallowing[44] to gastrointestinal endoscopy,[41,42] and skills have been shown to transfer to the clinical setting.[43] Furthermore, acquiring a TNE simulator is not necessarily a high-cost endeavor because many pediatric medical centers have access to patient simulators for pediatric advanced life support training or for medical code simulation training, which can be used for TNE practice.

SUMMARY

In conclusion, unsedated TNE is feasible, safe, effective, and well-tolerated procedure, which is acceptable to pediatric patients and their parents. Because it can be performed without sedation, it is cost-effective and reduces the risk and costs associated with sedation and anesthesia that are recommended for endoscopy in children. Given its benefits, TNE should be considered in the evaluation of disorders of the upper gastrointestinal tract in children and adolescents, particularly for diseases such as EoE that can require serial endoscopy. Although many centers across Asia, Europe, and North America[45] perform TNE on adult patients, further research and educational are needed to expand the indications, training opportunities, and available centers that perform unsedated TNE in pediatric patients.

CLINICS CARE POINTS

- The ability to perform unsedated TNE at a clinic office visit could allow for rapid assessment of common upper gastrointestinal symptoms.

- When considering TNE in a pediatric patient, selecting a candidate is not based solely on age but on developmental readiness as well as adequate preparation of the patient and family.

- Consider TNE in the evaluation and monitoring of patients with disorders of the upper gastrointestinal tract, which can require serial endoscopy, such as eosinophilic esophagitis. Avoid TNE in patients with nasal pain and transnasal insertion failure.

- Distraction techniques such as VR goggles and using child life specialists may improve tolerability of the procedure in children.

ACKNOWLEDGMENTS

The authors would like to acknowledge the contributions of Dr Joel Friedlander to transnasal endoscopy in pediatrics.

REFERENCES

1. Walsh CM, Lightdale JR, Mack DR, et al. Overview of the Pediatric Endoscopy Quality Improvement Network Quality Standards and Indicators for Pediatric Endoscopy: A Joint NASPGHAN/ESPGHAN Guideline. J Pediatr Gastroenterol Nutr 2022;74:S3–15.
2. Hartjes KT, Dafonte TM, Lee AF, et al. Variation in Pediatric Anesthesiologist Sedation Practices for Pediatric Gastrointestinal Endoscopy. Front Pediatr 2021;9:709433.
3. Leisser A, Delpre G, Kadish U. Through the nose with the gastroscope. Gastrointest Endosc 1990;36:77.
4. Dumortier J, Napoleon B, Hedelius F, et al. Unsedated transnasal EGD in daily practice: results with 1100 consecutive patients. Gastrointest Endosc 2003;57:198–204.
5. Nguyen N, Lavery WJ, Capocelli KE, et al. Transnasal Endoscopy in Unsedated Children With Eosinophilic Esophagitis Using Virtual Reality Video Goggles. Clin Gastroenterol Hepatol 2019;17:2455–62.
6. Thakkar K, El-Serag HB, Mattek N, et al. Complications of pediatric EGD: a 4-year experience in PEDS-CORI. Gastrointest Endosc 2007;65:213–21.
7. Lightdale JR, Liu QY, Sahn B, et al. Pediatric Endoscopy and High-risk Patients: A Clinical Report From the NASPGHAN Endoscopy Committee. J Pediatr Gastroenterol Nutr 2019;68:595–606.
8. Mark JA, Kramer RE. Impact of fellow training level on adverse events and operative time for common pediatric GI endoscopic procedures. Gastrointest Endosc 2018;88:787–94.
9. ASoP Committee, Lightdale JR, Acosta R, et al. Modifications in endoscopic practice for pediatric patients. Gastrointest Endosc 2014;79:699–710.
10. Gilger MA, Gold BD. Pediatric endoscopy: new information from the PEDS-CORI project. Curr Gastroenterol Rep 2005;7:234–9.

11. FDA Drug Safety Communication: FDA review results in new warnings about using general anesthetics and sedation drugs in young children and pregnant women. Volume 2022, 2016. Available at: https://www.fda.gov/drugs/drug-safety-and-availability/fda-drug-safety-communication-fda-review-results-new-warnings-about-using-general-anesthetics-and. Accessed February 14, 2023.

12. Dumortier J, Lapalus MG, Pereira A, et al. Unsedated transnasal PEG placement. Gastrointest Endosc 2004;59:54–7.

13. Brewer S, Gleditsch SL, Syblik D, et al. Pediatric anxiety: child life intervention in day surgery. J Pediatr Nurs 2006;21:13–22.

14. Romito B, Jewell J, Jackson M, et al. Child life services. Pediatrics 2021;147(1): e2020040261.

15. Friedlander JA, DeBoer EM, Soden JS, et al. Unsedated transnasal esophago-scopy for monitoring therapy in pediatric eosinophilic esophagitis. Gastrointest Endosc 2016;83:299–306.e1.

16. Friedlander JA, Fleischer DM, Black JO, et al. Unsedated transnasal esophago-scopy with virtual reality distraction enables earlier monitoring of dietary therapy in eosinophilic esophagitis. J Allergy Clin Immunol Pract 2021;9:3494–6.

17. Scherer C, Sosensky P, Schulman-Green D, et al. Pediatric Patients' and Parents' Per-spectives of Unsedated Transnasal Endoscopy in Eosinophilic Esophagitis: A Qual-itative Descriptive Study. J Pediatr Gastroenterol Nutr 2020;74:558–62.

18. Ali S, Rajagopal M, Stinson J, et al. Virtual reality-based distraction for intrave-nous insertion-related distress in children: a study protocol for a randomised controlled trial. BMJ Open 2022;12:e057892.

19. Bernaerts S, Bonroy B, Daems J, et al. Virtual Reality for Distraction and Relaxa-tion in a Pediatric Hospital Setting: An Interventional Study With a Mixed-Methods Design. Front Digit Health 2022;4:866119.

20. Eijlers R, Utens E, Staals LM, et al. Systematic Review and Meta-analysis of Vir-tual Reality in Pediatrics: Effects on Pain and Anxiety. Anesth Analg 2019;129: 1344–53.

21. Walther-Larsen S, Petersen T, Friis SM, et al. Immersive Virtual Reality for Pediat-ric Procedural Pain: A Randomized Clinical Trial. Hosp Pediatr 2019;9:501–7.

22. Chan E, Hovenden M, Ramage E, et al. Virtual Reality for Pediatric Needle Proce-dural Pain: Two Randomized Clinical Trials. J Pediatr 2019;209:160–7.e4.

23. Lambert V, Boylan P, Boran L, et al. Virtual reality distraction for acute pain in chil-dren. Cochrane Database Syst Rev 2020;10:CD010686.

24. Stunden C, Stratton K, Zakani S, et al. Comparing a Virtual Reality-Based Simu-lation App (VR-MRI) With a Standard Preparatory Manual and Child Life Program for Improving Success and Reducing Anxiety During Pediatric Medical Imaging: Randomized Clinical Trial. J Med Internet Res 2021;23:e22942.

25. Alexandridis E, Inglis S, McAvoy NC, et al. Randomised clinical study: compari-son of acceptability, patient tolerance, cardiac stress and endoscopic views in transnasal and transoral endoscopy under local anaesthetic. Aliment Pharmacol Ther 2014;40:467–76.

26. Sami SS, Subramanian V, Ortiz-Fernandez-Sordo J, et al. Performance character-istics of unsedated ultrathin video endoscopy in the assessment of the upper GI tract: systematic review and meta-analysis. Gastrointest Endosc 2015;82:782–92.

27. Thota PN, Zuccaro G Jr, Vargo JJ 2nd, et al. A randomized prospective trial comparing unsedated esophagoscopy via transnasal and transoral routes using a 4-mm video endoscope with conventional endoscopy with sedation. Endos-copy 2005;37:559–65.

28. Tanuma T, Morita Y, Doyama H. Current status of transnasal endoscopy worldwide using ultrathin videoscope for upper gastrointestinal tract. Dig Endosc 2016;28(Suppl 1):25–31.
29. Breiner SM. Preparation of the pediatric patient for invasive procedures. J Infus Nurs 2009;32:252–6.
30. Moriarty JP, Shah ND, Rubenstein JH, et al. Costs associated with Barrett's esophagus screening in the community: an economic analysis of a prospective randomized controlled trial of sedated versus hospital unsedated versus mobile community unsedated endoscopy. Gastrointest Endosc 2018;87:88–94.e2.
31. Watanabe H, Watanabe N, Ogura R, et al. A randomized prospective trial comparing unsedated endoscopy via transnasal and transoral routes using 5.5-mm video endoscopy. Dig Dis Sci 2009;54:2155–60.
32. Despott E, Baulf M, Bromley J, et al. OC-059 Scent: final report of the first UK prospective, randomised, head-to-head trial of transnasal vs oral upper gastrointestinal endoscopy. Gut 2010;59(Suppl 1):A24.
33. Uchiyama K, Ishikawa T, Sakamoto N, et al. Analysis of cardiopulmonary stress during endoscopy: is unsedated transnasal esophagogastroduodenoscopy appropriate for elderly patients? Can J Gastroenterol Hepatol 2014;28:31–4.
34. Koo S, Leinwand K, Panter S, et al. Transnasal gastrointestinal endoscopy. Pract Pediatr Gastrointest Endosc 2021;377–85.
35. Rees CJ, Fordham T, Belafsky PC. Transnasal balloon dilation of the esophagus. Arch Otolaryngol Head Neck Surg 2009;135:781–3.
36. Qin H, Lu XY, Zhao Q, et al. Evaluation of a new method for placing nasojejunal feeding tubes. World J Gastroenterol 2012;18:5295–9.
37. Zhihui T, Wenkui Y, Weiqin L, et al. A randomised clinical trial of transnasal endoscopy versus fluoroscopy for the placement of nasojejunal feeding tubes in patients with severe acute pancreatitis. Postgrad Med J 2009;85:59–63.
38. Mitchell RG, Kerr RM, Ott DJ, et al. Transnasal endoscopic technique for feeding tube placement. Gastrointest Endosc 1992;38:596–7.
39. Crews NR, Gorospe EC, Johnson ML, et al. Comparative quality assessment of esophageal examination with transnasal and sedated endoscopy. Endosc Int Open 2017;5:E340–4.
40. Rahmani K, Karimi S, Rezayatmand R, et al. Value-Based procurement for medical devices: A scoping review. Med J Islam Repub Iran 2021;35:134.
41. van der Wiel SE, Kuttner Magalhaes R, Rocha Goncalves CR, et al. Simulator training in gastrointestinal endoscopy - From basic training to advanced endoscopic procedures. Best Pract Res Clin Gastroenterol 2016;30:375–87.
42. Walsh CM, Cohen J, Woods KL, et al. ASGE EndoVators Summit: simulators and the future of endoscopic training. Gastrointest Endosc 2019;90:13–26.
43. Khan R, Plahouras J, Johnston BC, et al. Virtual reality simulation training in endoscopy: a Cochrane review and meta-analysis. Endoscopy 2019;51:653–64.
44. Benadom EM, Potter NL. The use of simulation in training graduate students to perform transnasal endoscopy. Dysphagia 2011;26:352–60.
45. Atar M, Kadayifci A. Transnasal endoscopy: Technical considerations, advantages and limitations. World J Gastrointest Endosc 2014;6:41–8.

Endoscopy in Pediatric Eosinophilic Esophagitis

Ramy Sabe, MBBCh[a], Girish Hiremath, MD, MPH[b], Kenneth Ng, DO[c],*

KEYWORDS

- Eosinophilic esophagitis • Food allergy • Dysphagia • Food impaction
- Esophageal dilation

KEY POINTS

- Eosinophilic esophagitis (EoE) is a chronic allergen-mediated clinicopathologic condition that currently requires esophagogastroduodenoscopy (EGD) with biopsies and histologic evaluation to diagnose and monitor treatment response.
- EGD plays a crucial therapeutic role for management of esophageal strictures and food impaction and related complications, including perforation and bleeding.
- There are multiple recent innovations that can facilitate the diagnosis of EoE through minimally invasive approaches and provide important complementary information to enhance an endoscopists' understanding of EoE disease activity for surveillance purposes.
- Newer therapeutic devices can aid in the endoscopic management of complications, enhancing the safety and efficiency of endoscopic therapy.

INTRODUCTION

Eosinophilic esophagitis (EoE) is a chronic immune-mediated disease affecting the esophagus. Once thought to be a rare disorder, the burden of EoE has increased over past three decades and is currently estimated to affect one in 2000 individuals in the United States.[1–4] It is known to affect Caucasian and males more commonly.[5,6]

Financial disclosure: G. Hiremath serves as a consultant to Allakos, Bristol Myer Squibb, Regeneron, and Sanofi. He has received speaker fees from Bristol Myer Squibb. Other authors report no conflict of interest.
Funding: G. Hiremath is supported by the 1K23DK131341 award by the National Institutes of Health.

[a] Division of Pediatric Gastroenterology, Hepatology, and Nutrition, Rainbow Babies and Children's Hospitals, Case Western Reserve University School of Medicine, 11100 Euclid Avenue, Cleveland, OH 44106, USA; [b] Division of Pediatric Gastroenterology, Hepatology, and Nutrition, Monroe Carell Jr. Children's Hospital at Vanderbilt, Vanderbilt University Medical Center, 11226, 2200 Children's Way, Nashville, TN 37232, USA; [c] Division of Pediatric Gastroenterology, Hepatology, and Nutrition, Johns Hopkins Children's Center, Johns Hopkins University School of Medicine, 600 North Wolfe Street, CMSC 2-116, Baltimore, MD 21287, USA
* Corresponding author.
E-mail address: kng13@jhmi.edu

As a major cause of upper gastrointestinal morbidity with a chronic and progressive course, EoE imposes a significant economic burden on the health care system. Recent estimates suggest that annual EoE-related health care costs in the United States are as much as $1.4 billion.[7,8] At an individual level, EoE can have a substantial impact on social and psychological functioning.[9–12]

Clinically, affected infants and young children usually present with vomiting, abdominal pain, and poor weight gain which can be indicative of the inflammatory phenotype of EoE (**Table 1**). A delay in diagnosis or prolonged suboptimally controlled eosinophilic inflammation can lead to progressive involvement of the deeper esophageal layers and result in fibrostenotic complications.[13,14] As such, teenagers and adults often present with chest pain, dysphagia, and esophageal food impaction. EoE is confirmed histologically by an intense eosinophilic infiltrate ($\geq$15 eosinophils per high power field [eos/hpf]) and related epithelial and subepithelial alterations in at least one of multiple esophageal biopsies.[15,16] Although empiric elimination of dietary allergen(s) and/or medications (including proton pump inhibitors and topical steroids) has remained the mainstay of EoE management, these are not approved by the US Food and Drug Administration (FDA). Only recently, Dupilumab, a humanized monoclonal antibody that inhibits the interleukin (IL)-4 receptor alpha chain augmenting IL-4 and IL-13 signaling, became the first US FDA-approved treatment for EoE in patients 12 years and older and weighing 40 kg or more.[17]

The diagnosis and surveillance of EoE currently relies heavily on repeated esophago-gastroduodenoscopy (EGD) to visualize the esophageal mucosa and obtain esophageal biopsies for histologic confirmation, assess treatment response, facilitate management of fibrostenotic complications, and monitor the course of disease.[18,19] In this state-of-the art review, the authors describe application of endoscopy as a diagnostic and a therapeutic tool for EoE. Furthermore, the authors outline minimally invasive tests which hold potential to advance the field. Finally, the authors discuss the potential endoscopy-related complications, strategies to manage them, and describe innovative advances that are poised to enhance endoscopic treatment safety and efficiency.

ROLE OF ENDOSCOPY IN THE DIAGNOSIS AND SURVEILLANCE OF EOSINOPHILIC ESOPHAGITIS
Endoscopic Features

Endoscopic signs, although relevant to EoE, are not pathognomonic of the disease. The EoE Endoscopic Reference Score (EREFS) has been developed to unify endoscopic reporting when evaluating EoE. This grading system assesses the presence and severity of edema, furrows, and white exudate which represent the inflammatory

Table 1 Characteristics of eosinophilic esophagitis phenotypes		
	Inflammatory	**Fibrostenotic**
Typical presentation	Childhood	Adulthood
Common symptoms	Nausea Vomiting Food aversions Abdominal pain	Dysphagia Swallowing difficulties Food impaction
Endoscopic findings	Edema Furrows Exudates	Rings Esophageal narrowing Strictures

phenotype as well as the presence of rings and strictures which are suggestive of the fibrostenotic phenotype.[20] EREFS has been shown to reliably differentiate EoE from other non-EoE conditions such as gastroesophageal reflux disease (GERD), predict treatment response, and assess disease activity.[21–23] Alternatively, a normal appearing esophagus on endoscopy does not eliminate a diagnosis of EoE, as this occurs in up to 32% of children, and a more recent study reported that nearly half of patients had a normal appearing esophagus.[24] This emphasizes the need for obtaining biopsies for histologic confirmation.[24–28]

Histologic Abnormalities

Given the patchy nature of the disease, current guidelines recommend collecting four to six biopsies from two or more locations in the esophagus to increase the yield of establishing a diagnosis.[16,25] Obtaining biopsies from three locations has been shown to be superior to two locations as it increases the probability of identifying patients with EoE, with distal esophageal biopsies having the highest diagnostic sensitivity.[29] Whenever possible, biopsies should be obtained from areas of abnormal mucosa such as longitudinal furrows and white exudates, where eosinophil counts tend to be the highest.

A threshold of 15 eos/hpf in esophageal epithelium is considered the key histologic feature of EoE. With the growing recognition of other epithelial and subepithelial features of the disease, the EoE Histologic Scoring system (EoEHSS) was developed to assess the global tissue involvement in EoE.[15,16] EoEHSS provides an objective framework to assess eosinophil infiltration, basal zone hyperplasia, the presence of eosinophilic abscesses, eosinophil surface layering, dilated intercellular spaces, surface epithelial alterations, dyskeratotic epithelial cells, and lamina propria fibrosis. A scale of 0 to 3 is used to classify the severity (grade) and the extent (stage) of the changes, with 24 being the maximum score for each biopsy for grade and stage. The ratio between the total of the scores for each item is divided by the maximum possible score to identify the final score, which ranges from 0 to 1. This validated approach can differentiate active from inactive disease.[30,31] However, it has been found to be less accurate in predicting active disease in children as compared with adults.[24] Unfortunately, its application in routine clinical practice has been limited due to the time required for interpretation, the complexity of the score, and the lack of a visual atlas to help pathologists who are not specialized in EoE to score specimens accurately.[32]

Surveillance

Currently, EGD with esophageal biopsies is recommended for monitoring disease activity and assessing treatment response given the lack of correlation between clinical symptoms and esophageal eosinophilic inflammation in patients with EoE. This is typically completed 6 to 12 weeks from the treatment change.[25,33] There are no guidelines on long-term endoscopic monitoring of EoE in asymptomatic disease, but close follow-up every 12 to 18 months has been associated with a lower probability of developing esophageal strictures and early detection of histologic relapse.[34]

Promising, less-invasive disease activity surveillance techniques have been pursued. An esophageal string test has been developed and studied in children and adults.[35] The test entails swallowing a weighted gelatin capsule which contains 90 cm of nylon string that remains in place for 1 hour to capture esophageal contents. It is then withdrawn and analyzed for eosinophil-associated proteins. This test was found to be safe and accurate in differentiating active and inactive EoE.[35] Another technique is the Cytosponge, which is also an ingestible gelatin capsule (20 mm long) that has been tested in the adult EoE population.[36] The capsule contains a compressed mesh sponge that is attached to a string. The sponge is designed to collect esophageal mucosal secretions from which one can measure the peak eosinophilic count. The cytosponge has been shown to be safe and accurate in assessing esophageal eosinophilia.[36] No studies have assessed the safety and accuracy of the cytosponge in children. Since both tests require the ability to swallow a larger pill-sized object, their utility will be limited to older children and adolescents with EoE.

Severity Assessment

A novel tool called the Index of Severity for Eosinophilic Esophagitis (I-SEE) was recently developed to help unify the assessment and monitoring of patients with EoE. It is composed of a combination of selected clinical symptoms, endoscopic findings, and histologic elements including fibrostenotic features that are thought to best evaluate the disease severity. This index score is awaiting validation and possible modification to help optimize and unify management of patients with EoE.[37]

THERAPEUTIC ROLE OF ENDOSCOPY IN EOSINOPHILIC ESOPHAGITIS

EGD plays a crucial therapeutic role in EoE.[38] Up to 31% of patients with EoE can present with an esophageal stricture, whereas up to 54% of affected patients can present with food impaction, especially in adolescence and adulthood.[25]

Management of Esophageal Strictures

In patients with EoE, strictures develop from progressive eosinophilic inflammation and involvement of deeper esophageal layers. They can be identified during an EGD and/or based on a barium esophagram, the latter being more sensitive in early stages of stricture development.[39,40] Strictures are graded as mild (>9 mm in diameter) and moderate to severe (<9 mm).[39] A goal esophageal caliber of at least 16 mm in adolescents and adults is reported to relieve dysphagia and decrease the likelihood of food impaction.[40]

Esophageal dilation, although commonly used, may not treat the underlying inflammation which led to the stricture development. Concomitant dietary or medical therapy for patients with EoE is paramount as it reduces inflammation, increases the esophageal caliber, and decreases the need for subsequent dilation.[40] As such, the North American Society of Pediatric Gastroenterology, Hepatology and Nutrition foreign body ingestion management guidelines published in 2015 recommended against dilating any identified strictures on the initial presentation with food impaction to allow for review of the biopsies to potentially confirm a diagnosis of EoE and provide medical treatment accordingly.[41]

The techniques and approaches for endoscopic dilation have evolved over the years, thereby making this procedure safer and better tolerated. In a recently published meta-analysis of 1820 esophageal dilations in adult and pediatric patients with a median of three sessions per patient, through the scope balloon dilators were the most commonly used dilators ($n = 768$) followed by Savary dilators ($n = 454$), and Maloney dilators ($n = 110$).[42,43] Older adult studies reported higher rates of deep mucosal tears (9.2%) and perforations (1%) in patients with EoE compared with those without.[44] However, more recent adult studies have showed reduced complication rates as deep mucosal tears or rents are considered an appropriate response to endoscopic dilation rather than a complication.[40] Likewise, pediatric studies have reported no perforations associated with stricture dilation in patients with EoE, including those who have not been treated for their EoE.[39,45,46] Currently, there are no guidelines or recommendations regarding what type of dilator is best to use. This largely depends on endoscopist's training, experience, preference, and comfort level.

Management of Esophageal Food Impaction

Esophageal food impaction is relatively common in adolescents and adults with EoE. It can be the presenting symptom of EoE in up to 55% of patients,[47,48] and a quarter of patients have recurrent food impactions.[47] An urgent or emergent flexible EGD to remove the lodged food is usually necessary depending on whether there is complete or near complete esophageal obstruction. Rigid esophagoscopy, which can be done by an otorhinolaryngologist if available, can be useful in the management of proximal esophageal impactions. Given the increased risk of aspiration, a patient who is unable to handle their oral secretions requires an emergent procedure (within 2 hours) regardless of their *nil per os* status.[41] Patients who can handle their oral secretions need to undergo an EGD with food disimpaction within 24 hours to decrease the chance of tissue necrosis and potential perforation.[41] This timeframe allows for potential spontaneous passage of the impacted food, thus negating the need for an endoscopic procedure. Otolaryngologists or surgeons may participate in managing such patients depending on the location and presence or absence of complications.[38]

En bloc, piece meal, cap-assisted, and push techniques are different methods used in managing esophageal food impaction.[49] Various tools have been described for removing the impacted food, including forceps (rat tooth, alligator, and biopsy forceps), snare, retrieval net, tripod grasper, basket, and suction. More than one tool and/or technique may be required in difficult cases. Using an overtube in older children should be considered to limit mucosal trauma if multiple passes are needed.[9,38,41] Endotracheal intubation should be done to protect the patient's airway.

The cap-assisted technique has been reported in esophageal foreign body extraction, including food impaction. It is performed using a transparent cap that is secured onto the tip of the endoscope, placed on top of the impacted food, and then with continuous suction applied to secure the bolus, the endoscope is withdrawn. This technique results in a shorter retrieval and total procedure time, a higher rate of en bloc removal, a higher procedure success rate, a lower risk of complications, and a lower cost.[50–52]

The push technique has been used in adults with a low risk of complications but has not been well described in children.[49] Herein, gentle pressure is applied to push the impacted food into the stomach. This should be performed with the highest level of caution as a distal stricture may be present and such action may result in esophageal injury including esophageal perforation.[38] Kriem and colleagues[53] described 39 cases of esophageal food impaction management in 23 children with different disorders, mainly EoE and repaired trachea-esophageal fistula. Twenty were treated using the push technique, whereas the pull (suction and/or removal) technique was used for the remainder. They reported that the push and pull techniques were equally safe and effective and can be complimentary to each other.[53]

Regardless of the tool(s) and/or technique(s) used to remove the impacted food, it is strongly recommended that multiple biopsies (away from the site of impaction) be obtained after removal, given the strong association between esophageal food impaction and EoE and the requirement for histologic confirmation of the diagnosis.[9]

POTENTIAL COMPLICATIONS AND MANAGEMENT
Perforation

Spontaneous esophageal perforation is a rare but serious complication of EoE, occurring in approximately 2% of cases.[54] Mucosal friability related to active inflammation, as well as esophageal remodeling, is thought to place individuals at an increased risk of perforation. Most perforations occur during removal of an impacted food bolus or secondary to dilation of esophageal strictures, suggesting that patients with fibrostenotic disease due to longer duration of symptoms are at increased risk.[54] Perforation can also happen secondary to recurrent retching or vomiting and may be the presenting sign of EoE. A systematic review found that EoE was diagnosed after a perforation in 73% of cases (51/76 perforations, patients aged 9–65 years).[55] Based on older studies, the rate of perforation secondary to esophageal stricture dilation in EoE was thought to be higher than in dilation for other stenotic esophageal disorders; however, more recent research has shown no difference.[54]

Esophageal perforation is usually managed conservatively by nil per os with parenteral nutrition, antibiotics, proton pump inhibitors, and analgesia. Partially and fully covered metal esophageal stents as well as endoscopic clips (through-the-scope or over-the-scope) can be used to manage esophageal perforation in patients with EoE. Some patients may require surgical interventions including thoracotomy with esophageal repair, laparotomy, and laparoscopy. No deaths have been reported related to either esophageal perforation or therapy.[55]

Bleeding

Spontaneous esophageal bleeding in patients with EoE is rare. A few case reports have described EoE patients with hematemesis as their initial presentation. Hematemesis resolved with conservative management without endoscopic intervention, and outcomes of those patients were favorable.[56–58] Hematemesis may also occur iatrogenically in a very small proportion of patients, for example, related to esophageal stricture dilation.[42,59]

EMERGING DIAGNOSTIC AND SURVEILLANCE TECHNIQUES

There are several emerging techniques that provide important complimentary information to enhance the gastroenterologist's understanding of EoE disease activity. These tools may be used in conjunction with follow-up endoscopies to monitor disease activity, providing additional data to gauge treatment response. Although helpful, they are not meant to directly replace an EGD. Access to these tools will vary from institution to institution and likely be impacted by the accessibility of a pediatric gastroenterologist trained in these techniques.[60]

Functional Lumen Imaging Probe

Endoluminal functional lumen imaging probe (EndoFLIP; Medtronic, Minneapolis, MN) measures the mechanical properties of the gastrointestinal lumen using high-resolution impedance planimetry (**Fig. 1**). During an EGD, a balloon catheter (referred to as the FLIP catheter), which contains 17 impedance sensors and a pressure transducer, is positioned at the area of interest. The endoscopist can choose from either an 8- or 16-cm long catheter. Through volume-controlled distension, the system generates key luminal parameters in real time, including diameter, cross-sectional area (CSA), compliance, pressure, and distensibility index (DI). The DI value is calculated by dividing the narrowest CSA by the pressure measured.[61] A topography module (commonly referred to as the "2.0" system) is also available. It converts the data from the base computer to generate contraction-like data analogous to high-resolution manometry (HRM). Esophageal distension by the FLIP catheter causes contractile feedback which is represented as either anterograde or retrograde contractions (secondary peristalsis). This dynamically generated topographic data can be used to screen for abnormal contraction.[62]

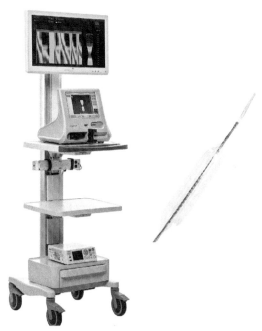

Fig. 1. Endoluminal functional lumen imaging probe (EndoFLIP; Medtronic, Minneapolis, MN) uses high-resolution impedance planimetry to evaluate the mechanical properties of the gastrointestinal lumen. (©2022 Medtronic. All rights reserved. Used with the permission of Medtronic.)

This tool has been safely used in both adult and pediatric patients with EoE.[63] In a prospective pediatric study, esophagogastric junction parameters and repetitive anterograde contractions (RACs) on FLIP correlated to improved bolus flow on high-resolution impedance manometry.[64] These investigators concluded that patients without RACs should undergo additional manometric evaluation with HRM to evaluate for esophageal dysmotility.[64] Whereas in manometry the patient is awake, EndoFLIP is performed while the patient is sedated during endoscopy which makes it a unique and valuable tool especially when caring for children that are unable to comply with the steps involved in a traditional manometry study such as young children or those with neurologic deficits.

The acquired data can also be useful in guiding treatment and assessing response during follow-up endoscopic evaluation.[65] Research has shown that active esophageal inflammation (>15 eos/hpf) has a low DI value and reduced compliance. Pediatric patients with EoE have been shown to have reduced distensibility, even after adjusting for age when compared with pediatric patients without EoE.[65]

EndoFLIP can also be used before and after esophageal dilation to assess luminal response. In this technique, the catheter is brought to the area of interest and serial measurements are taken. The catheter is then removed, and dilation is performed using a controlled radial expansion (CRE) balloon or mechanical dilators. Afterward, the dilation tool is removed, and comparative post-dilation measurements are taken to confirm treatment efficacy. This removes the need to use endoscopic tools (ie, width of biopsy forceps) or fluoroscopy to estimate the size of the stricture along with the treatment response.[61]

Endoscopic Ultrasound

Endoscopic ultrasound (EUS) uses an echoendoscope, which houses an ultrasound transducer at the tip of an endoscope. It has been shown to be safe in children over 15 kg and can evaluate the layers of the gastrointestinal lumen as well as neighboring structure, including the vasculature, pancreas, liver, biliary tree, kidney, mediastinum, and lymph nodes.[66,67] Although more commonly used in adults, it is being increasingly being used in the pediatric population. The radial echoendoscope provides a 360° view, perpendicular to the transducer, akin to axial images acquired on a computed tomography (CT) scan. A curvilinear array (CLA) echoendoscope provides a 120° to 180° view parallel to the transducer. There are also EUS probes that can be passed through the working channel of endoscopes, providing detailed imaging of the layers of the gastrointestinal lumen. The CLA echoendoscope has an elevator and working channel which allows for passage of therapeutic tools.[66,67]

EUS may play an important role in the evaluation of EoE. Among pediatric patients with EoE, EUS showed an increased total wall thickness (TWT), mucosa and submucosa, and muscularis propria thickness when compared with control subjects, highlighting the presence of esophageal remodeling.[68] It is believed that dysphagia symptoms may be secondary to mucosal and submucosal fibrosis as well as smooth muscle hypertrophy resulting in diminished esophageal compliance.[69] Rabinowitz and colleagues[70] measured the mid and distal esophagus in a cohort of children without EoE and demonstrated that TWT and the diameter of the individual esophageal layers correlated positively with age and height. This work may serve as an important guide when assessing a patient with possible EoE. Esophageal measurements can also potentially be used to assess treatment response and help plan for esophageal dilation.[71]

Transnasal Endoscopy

Unsedated transnasal endoscopy (TNE) uses an ultrathin endoscope (bronchoscope) with an outer diameter of 2.8 or 4 mm (1.2 or 2.0 mm working channel) to acquire esophageal biopsies. After the patient is given a topical nasal anesthetic, the endoscope is carefully passed through a patient's nostril where it is advanced to the stomach.[72] The procedure is performed in an outpatient setting without the need for sedation and takes up to 15 minutes allowing for fast turnover. In the pediatric population, this technique is commonly supported by members of Child Life, but it also takes advantage of modern technologies such as virtual reality goggles to keep patients in a relaxed state during the endoscopy.[73] In addition, parents often prefer TNE over EGD as they can be at the bedside during the procedure, enabling them to comfort their child.[74] The TNE process, including preprocedural wait time and minimal recovery period, translates to reduced time away from work and school. Rajitha and colleagues[75] expand on this topic in their article entitled *Pediatric Unsedated Transnasal Endoscopy* which can be found in this issue of the journal.

Narrow Band Imaging

Narrow band imaging (NBI) and the ability to magnify the endoscopic view are features found in various conventional gastroscopes. Combination of NBI magnifying endoscopy (NBI-ME) is a technique commonly performed to screen for gastrointestinal lesions, including malignancies.[76] In adult patients with EoE or lymphocytic esophagitis (LE), NBI-ME has been shown to demonstrate beige colored mucosa (normal mucosa has light green color), increased and congested intrapapillary capillary loop (IPCL), and absence of cyan-colored vessels when compared with patients with GERD.[76] In one study, 90% of participates aged 18 to 82 years (median: 39 years) with EoE or LE had all three features and 95.2% had at least one.[77] The other features were not seen in patients with GERD, asides from IPCLs which were observed in 30% of patients with GERD. EoE and LE were differentiated by histologic analysis.[77] NBI-ME was validated in a subsequent study and both abnormal IPCL and absent cyan vessels showed better sensitivity, specificity, and positive/negative predictive values compared with signs found on white-light endoscopy (rings, furrows, exudate, stenosis, edema).[76] Ayaki and colleagues[78] similarly showed that beige mucosa on NBI was indicative of active EoE and was associated with thinning of the superficial differentiated cell layer.

Raman Spectroscopy

Raman spectroscopy is used to profile the biochemical composition of tissue without requiring stains or dyes. In this technique, a monochromatic laser interacts with the chemical bonds of molecules within the specimen leading to detectable energy exchanges which are processed and reported as wavenumber shifts (Raman spectral plots). Each wavenumber shift is unique for individual molecules such as glycogen, proteins, and lipids, thus serving as a biochemical fingerprint.[79] Hiremath and colleagues[80] compared the *in vitro* Raman spectra from distal esophageal biopsies of children with active EoE, inactive EoE, and non-EoE controls. They showed that the glycogen content was lower, and the protein intensity was higher in children with active EoE compared with controls. Moreover, lipid intensity was higher in patients with inactive EoE compared with children with active EoE. Glycogen and lipid spectral peaks correlated inversely with eosinophilic inflammation and basal zone hyperplasia.[79] Efforts are underway to apply Raman spectroscopy through a flexible endoscope *in vivo*, in real time, to diagnose and monitor EoE in a non-biopsy-dependent manner.

Artificial Intelligence

There is a growing interest to apply computational analysis to improve medical care. Machine learning is a field of artificial intelligence that harnesses computer-based methods to elaborate data through complex algorithms.[81] Sallis and colleagues[82] designed a diagnostic probability score for EoE (pEoE) using esophageal messenger ribonucleic acid (mRNA) transcriptome from esophageal biopsies. The investigators showed a pEoE score of ≥ 25 detected EoE with a sensitivity of 91%, a specificity of 93%, and an area under the curve of 0.985. Moreover, this tool could also be used to monitor treatment response. This form of machine learning may have the potential to examine an individual's allergic sensitization status and identify EoE phenotypes.[82] Deep learning, which goes one step beyond machine learning, uses a network of systems (called neural networks) that work together to analyze raw data and detect a finding of interest automatically. Czyzewski and colleagues[83] created a system using deep convolutional neural networks and downscaling of esophageal biopsy images to differentiate active EoE from control images. This system, which was conducted using biopsy samples exclusively from pediatric patients, had a sensitivity of 82.5% and specificity of 87%.

EMERGING THERAPEUTIC TECHNIQUES

In this section, the authors explore three emerging therapeutic devices that are new alternatives for dilating strictures or removing food impaction. Although some techniques provide added data during the dilation process thereby improving precision, others may simplify the task at hand potentially saving time.

Functional Lumen Imaging Probe

EsoFLIP (Medtronic, Minneapolis, MN) is a variant of EndoFLIP that is used for luminal dilation and also provides luminal data (diameter and CSA) in real time (**Fig. 2**). Although the EndoFLIP balloon catheter is made of polyurethane, the EsoFLIP is a rigid hydraulic dilation balloon catheter used in a similar manner to a CRE balloon to dilate a stricture. The EsoFLIP catheter comes in either 20- or 30-mm diameter (both are 80 mm in length). The device is unique in that the endoscopist can see luminal change or the elimination of a luminal "waist" in real time on the FLIP computer without using fluoroscopy.[61] In a case report describing successful treatment of a pediatric patient with a benign stricture secondary to EoE using EsoFLIP, the stricture was dilated from approximately 10 to 15 mm, and the procedure was well tolerated.[84]

Over-the-Scope Dilation Cap

The BougieCap (Ovesco Endoscopy AG, Tübingen, Germany) is a single-use dome-shaped transparent hard plastic cap that can be used to dilate strictures caused by EoE (**Fig. 3**). The device comes in diameters ranging from 7 to 16 mm and can be mounted to the tip of the endoscope. The device contains a 1.1 mm orifice at its tip to allow passage of a guidewire when needed. The side of the device also has holes, allowing for insufflation and suction. In one series of 50 adult patients, 96% were successfully treated.[85] These investigators report the smallest endoscope used was an Olympus GIF-XP190N with an outer diameter of 5.4 mm. Another group examined the effectiveness of the BougieCap in adult patients with EoE and found that it was

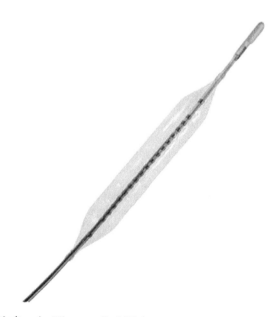

Fig. 2. EsoFLIP (Medtronic, Minneapolis, MN) is a variant of EndoFLIP used for luminal dilation while also providing luminal data (diameter and cross-sectional area) in real time. (©2022 Medtronic. All rights reserved. Used with the permission of Medtronic.)

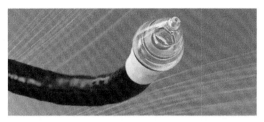

Fig. 3. The BougieCap (Ovesco Endoscopy AG, Tübingen, Germany) is a single-use dome-shaped transparent hard plastic cap used to dilate strictures. (*Courtesy of* Ovesco Endoscopy AG, Cary, NC; with permission.)

successful in all 50 patients in their series.[86] The investigators showed the median esophageal diameter increased from 12 to 16 mm, with improvements in clinical symptoms 2 weeks post-dilation. One benefit of the device is its proximity to the tip of the endoscope giving the endoscopist direct visualization of the stricture during treatment. Moreover, it may be easier to use when treating strictures in the upper esophagus as positioning a CRE balloon may be logistically challenging.[87]

Over-the-Scope Grasper

The over-the-scope grasper (OTSG), called the Xcavator (Ovesco Endoscopy AG, Tübingen, Germany), is a single-use, conical, transparent grasping device that can be attached to the tip of a standard endoscope (9.5–10.5 mm; **Fig. 4**). The maximum outer diameter in the closed position is 14.3 to 15.5 mm, and the device can open to a maximum width of 28 mm. The tool is connected to a sliding handgrip handle via a flexible shaft that runs along the endoscope and is controlled by the assistant who opens and closes the device like a biopsy forceps. It was shown to be effective in removal of large esophageal food boluses without complication in one case series.[88]

SUMMARY

EoE is an increasingly prevalent, allergen-mediated, clinicopathologic condition. In the absence of reliable noninvasive approaches, repeated EGD with biopsies is currently required to diagnose and monitor EoE. Furthermore, endoscopic maneuvers are increasingly being used to manage children with complicated EoE. The authors summarized the pathophysiology of EoE and reviewed the application of endoscopy as a diagnostic and therapeutic tool while outlining approaches to manage potential complications arising from therapeutic endoscopic interventions. Several recent

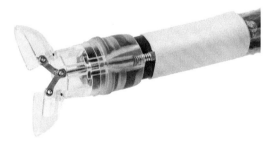

Fig. 4. The Xcavator (Ovesco Endoscopy AG, Tübingen, Germany) is a single-use, conical, transparent grasping device that can be attached to the tip of a standard endoscope. (*Courtesy of* Ovesco Endoscopy AG, Cary, NC; with permission.)

innovations have added to our ability to diagnose and monitor EoE with minimally invasive procedures and perform therapeutic maneuvers more safely and effectively, with anticipated continual growth in this area.

CLINICS CARE POINTS

- An esophagogastroduodenoscopy with multiple biopsies from at least two levels of the esophagus (>4–6 total) is required to diagnose eosinophilic esophagitis (EoE) in children and monitor treatment response.
- Although EoE can be managed with medical and dietary therapy, one must also be cognizant of the potential need for therapeutic endoscopic interventions (for management of esophageal strictures, food impaction, and related complications, including perforation and bleeding).
- Pediatric endoscopists need to be aware of innovative tools that can enhance the existing diagnostic and therapeutic modalities, including minimally invasive options that can be useful in all phases of EoE care.

REFERENCES

1. Furuta GT, Katzka DA. Eosinophilic esophagitis. N Engl J Med 2015;373(17): 1640–8.
2. Khalil MM, Ahmed F, Rahman MM, et al. Frequency of eosinophilic esophagitis among patients with gastroesophageal reflux symptoms in an academic hospital of bangladesh: a cross sectional study. Mymensingh Med J 2021;30(3):744–50.
3. Jimenez AC, López FF, Vilchez MJR, et al. Prospective observational study on the characteristics of eosinophilic esophagitis in south-east Spain. Allergol Immunopathol 2021;49(4):137–40.
4. Izquierdo ELO, Mahillo-Fernández I, Fernández SF, et al. Rising trend in p ediatric eosinophilic esophagitis incidence in Spain: Results of a prospective study 2014–16. Pediatr Allergy Immunol 2021;32(6):1307–15.
5. Dellon ES, Hirano I. Epidemiology and natural history of eosinophilic esophagitis. Gastroenterology 2018;154(2):319–32.e3.
6. Moawad FJ. Eosinophilic esophagitis incidence and prevalence. Gastrointest Endosc Clin N Am 2018;28(1):15–25.
7. Jensen ET, Kappelman MD, Martin CF, et al. Health-care utilization, costs, and the burden of disease related to eosinophilic esophagitis in the United States. Am J Gastroenterol 2015;110(5):626–32.
8. Lu M, Goodwin B, Vera-Llonch M, et al. Disease burden and treatment patterns associated with eosinophilic esophagitis in the United States. J Clin Gastroenterol 2022;56(2):133–40.
9. Hiremath G, Kodroff E, Strobel MJ, et al. Individuals affected by eosinophilic gastrointestinal disorders have complex unmet needs and frequently experience unique barriers to care. Clin Res Hepatol Gastroenterol 2018;42(5):483–93.
10. Taft TH, Guadagnoli L, Edlynn E. Anxiety and Depression in eosinophilic esophagitis: a scoping review and recommendations for future research. J Asthma Allergy 2019;12:389–99.
11. Reed CC, Ketchem CJ, Miller TL, et al. Psychiatric comorbidities are highly prevalent in nonesophageal eosinophilic gastrointestinal diseases. Clin Gastroenterol Hepatol 2022;20(4):e664–70.

12. Breslin G, Wills W, Bartington S, et al. Evaluation of a whole system approach to diet and healthy weight in the east of Scotland: Study protocol. PLoS One 2022; 17(3):e0265667.

13. Melgaard D, Westmark S, Laurberg PT, et al. A diagnostic delay of 10 years in the DanEoE cohort calls for focus on education - a population-based cross-sectional study of incidence, diagnostic process and complications of eosinophilic oeso-phagitis in the North Denmark Region. United European Gastroenterol J 2021; 9(6):688–98.

14. Lenti MV, Savarino E, Mauro A, et al. Diagnostic delay and misdiagnosis in eosin-ophilic oesophagitis. Dig Liver Dis 2021;53(12):1632–9.

15. Liacouras CA, Furuta GT, Hirano I, et al. Eosinophilic esophagitis: updated consensus recommendations for children and adults. J Allergy Clin Immunol 2011;128(1):3–20.e6.

16. Dellon ES, Liacouras CA, Molina-Infante J, et al. Updated international consensus diagnostic criteria for eosinophilic esophagitis: proceedings of the AGREE Con-ference. Gastroenterology 2018;155(4):1022–33.e10.

17. U.S. Food and Drug Administration. FDA Approves First Treatment for Eosino-philic Esophagitis, a Chronic Immune Disorder [Press release]. 2022. Available at: https://www.fda.gov/news-events/press-announcements/fda-approves-first-treatment-eosinophilic-esophagitis-chronic-immune-disorder (Accessed January 1, 2023).

18. Chehade M, Aceves SS. Treatment of eosinophilic esophagitis: diet or medica-tion? J Allergy Clin Immunol Pract 2021;9(9):3249–56.

19. Peterson K, Safroneeva E, Schoepfer A. Emerging therapies for eosinophilic gastrointestinal diseases. J Allergy Clin Immunol Pract 2021;9(9):3276–81.

20. Hirano I, Moy N, Heckman MG, et al. Endoscopic assessment of the oesophageal features of eosinophilic oesophagitis: validation of a novel classification and grading system. Gut 2013;62(4):489.

21. Dellon ES, Cotton CC, Gebhart JH, et al. Accuracy of the eosinophilic esophagitis endoscopic reference score in diagnosis and determining response to treatment. Clin Gastroenterol Hepatol 2016;14(1):31–9.

22. Ahuja N, Weedon J, Schwarz SM, et al. Applying the eosinophilic esophagitis endoscopic reference scores (EREFS) to different aged children. J Pediatr Gas-troenterol Nutr 2020;71(3):328–32.

23. Wechsler JB, Bolton SM, Amsden K, et al. Eosinophilic esophagitis reference score accurately identifies disease activity and treatment effects in children. Clin Gastroenterol Hepatol 2018;16(7):1056–63.

24. Hiremath G, Correa H, Acra S, et al. Correlation of endoscopic signs and mucosal alterations in children with eosinophilic esophagitis. Gastrointest Endosc 2020; 91(4):785–94.e1.

25. Lucendo AJ, Molina-Infante J, Arias Á, et al. Guidelines on eosinophilic esopha-gitis: evidence-based statements and recommendations for diagnosis and man-agement in children and adults. United European Gastroenterol J 2017;5(3): 335–58.

26. Kim HP, Vance RB, Shaheen NJ, et al. The prevalence and diagnostic utility of endoscopic features of eosinophilic esophagitis: a meta-analysis. Clin Gastroen-terol Hepatol 2012;10(9):988–96.e5.

27. Papadopoulou A, Koletzko S, Heuschkel R, et al. Management guidelines of eosinophilic esophagitis in childhood. J Pediatr Gastroenterol Nutr 2014;58(1): 107–18.

28. Bolton SM, Kagalwalla AF, Wechsler JB. Eosinophilic esophagitis in children: endoscopic findings at diagnosis and post-intervention. Curr Gastroenterol Rep 2018;20(1):4.

29. Wechsler JB, Bolton SM, Gray E, et al. Defining the patchy landscape of esophageal eosinophilia in children with eosinophilic esophagitis. Clin Gastroenterol Hepatol 2022;20(9):1971–6.e2.

30. Collins MH, Martin LJ, Alexander ES, et al. Newly developed and validated eosinophilic esophagitis histology scoring system and evidence that it outperforms peak eosinophil count for disease diagnosis and monitoring. Dis Esophagus 2016;30(3):1–8.

31. Cruz J, Irvine MA, Avinashi V, et al. Application of the eosinophilic esophagitis histology scoring system grade scores in patients at British Columbia Children's Hospital. Fetal Pediatr Pathol 2022;41(6):962–76.

32. COREOS Collaborators, Ma C, Schoepfer AM, Dellon ES, et al. Development of a core outcome set for therapeutic studies in eosinophilic esophagitis (COREOS). J Allergy Clin Immunol 2022;149(2):659–70.

33. Godwin B, Wilkins B, Muir AB. EoE disease monitoring where we are and where we are going. Ann Allergy Asthma Immunol 2020;124(3):240–7.

34. Bon L, Safroneeva E, Bussmann C, et al. Close follow-up is associated with fewer stricture formation and results in earlier detection of histological relapse in the long-term management of eosinophilic esophagitis. United European Gastroenterol J 2022;10(3):308–18.

35. Ackerman SJ, Kagalwalla AF, Hirano I, et al. One-hour esophageal string test: a nonendoscopic minimally invasive test that accurately detects disease activity in eosinophilic esophagitis. Am J Gastroenterol 2019;114(10):1614–25.

36. Katzka DA, Smyrk TC, Alexander JA, et al. Accuracy and safety of the cytosponge for assessing histologic activity in eosinophilic esophagitis: a two-center study. Am J Gastroenterol 2017;112(10):1538–44.

37. Dellon ES, Khoury P, Muir AB, et al. A clinical severity index for eosinophilic esophagitis: development, consensus, and future directions. Gastroenterology 2022;163(1):59–76.

38. Nguyen N, Kramer RE, Menard-Katcher C. Endoscopy in pediatric eosinophilic esophagitis. Front Pediatr 2021;9:713027.

39. Menard-Katcher C, Furuta GT, Kramer RE. Dilation of pediatric eosinophilic esophagitis: adverse events and short-term outcomes. J Pediatr Gastroenterol Nutr 2017;64(5):701–6.

40. Feo-Ortega S, Lucendo AJ. Evidence-based treatments for eosinophilic esophagitis: insights for the clinician. Therap Adv Gastroenterol 2022;15. 17562848211068664.

41. Kramer RE, Lerner DG, Lin T, et al. Management of ingested foreign bodies in children: a clinical report of the NASPGHAN Endoscopy Committee. J Pediatr Gastroenterol Nutr 2015;60(4):562–74.

42. Moawad FJ, Molina-Infante J, Lucendo AJ, et al. Systematic review with meta-analysis: endoscopic dilation is highly effective and safe in children and adults with eosinophilic oesophagitis. Aliment Pharmacol Ther 2017;46(2):96–105.

43. Lucendo AJ, Arias Á, Molina-Infante J, et al. The role of endoscopy in eosinophilic esophagitis: from diagnosis to therapy. Expert Rev Gastroenterol Hepatol 2017; 11(12):1135–49.

44. Jung KW, Gundersen N, Kopacova J, et al. Occurrence of and risk factors for complications after endoscopic dilation in eosinophilic esophagitis. Gastrointest Endosc 2011;73(1):15–21.

45. Al-Hussaini A. Savary dilation is safe and effective treatment for esophageal narrowing related to pediatric eosinophilic esophagitis. J Pediatr Gastroenterol Nutr 2016;63(5):474–80.
46. Robles-Medranda C, Villard F, Gall C le, et al. Severe dysphagia in children with eosinophilic esophagitis and esophageal stricture: an indication for balloon dilation&quest. J Pediatr Gastroenterol Nutr 2010;50(5):516–20.
47. Hiremath GS, Hameed F, Pacheco A, et al. Esophageal food impaction and eosinophilic esophagitis: a retrospective study, systematic review, and meta-analysis. Dig Dis Sci 2015;60(11):3181–93.
48. Pasha SF, DiBaise JK, Kim HJ, et al. Patient characteristics, clinical, endoscopic, and histologic findings in adult eosinophilic esophagitis: a case series and systematic review of the medical literature. Dis Esophagus 2007;20(4):311–9.
49. ASGE Standards of Practice Committee, Ikenberry SO, Jue TL, et al. Management of ingested foreign bodies and food impactions. Gastrointest Endosc 2011;73(6):1085–91.
50. Ooi M, Duong T, Holman R, et al. Comparison of cap-assisted vs conventional endoscopic technique for management of food bolus impaction in the esophagus: results of a multicenter randomized controlled trial. Am J Gastroenterol 2021;116(11):2235–40.
51. Smith CR, Miranda A, Rudolph CD, et al. Removal of impacted food in children with eosinophilic esophagitis using saeed banding device. J Pediatr Gastroenterol Nutr 2007;44(4):521–3.
52. Wahba M, Habib G, Mazny AE, et al. Cap-assisted technique versus conventional methods for esophageal food bolus extraction: a comparative study. Clin Endosc 2019;52(5):458–63.
53. Kriem J, Rahhal R. Safety and efficacy of the push endoscopic technique in the management of esophageal food bolus impactions in children. J Pediatr Gastroenterol Nutr 2018;66(1):e1–5.
54. Runge TM, Eluri S, Cotton CC, et al. Causes and outcomes of esophageal perforation in eosinophilic esophagitis. J Clin Gastroenterol 2017;51(9):805–13.
55. Arias-González L, Rey-Iborra E, Ruiz-Ponce M, et al. Esophageal perforation in eosinophilic esophagitis: a systematic review on clinical presentation, management and outcomes. Dig Liver Dis 2020;52(3):245–52.
56. Hommeida S, Grothe RM, Hafed Y, et al. Assessing the incidence trend and characteristics of eosinophilic esophagitis in children in Olmsted County, Minnesota. Dis Esophagus 2018;31(12):doy062.
57. Aydin E, Beşer ÖF. Profuse upper GI bleeding secondary to eosinophilic esophagitis. APSP J Case Rep 2017;8(4):24.
58. Ozdogan E, Caglayan LD, Mizikoglu O, et al. Upper gastrointestinal bleeding as the first presentation of eosinophilic gastrointestinal disease. JPGN Rep 2020;1(2):e017.
59. Moole H, Jacob K, Duvvuri A, et al. Role of endoscopic esophageal dilation in managing eosinophilic esophagitis. Medicine 2017;96(14):e5877.
60. McGowan EC, Keller JP, Muir AB, et al. Distance to pediatric gastroenterology providers is associated with decreased diagnosis of Eosinophilic Esophagitis (EoE) in rural populations. J Allergy Clin Immunol Pract 2021;9(12):4489–92.e2.
61. Ng K, Mogul D, Hollier J, et al. Utility of functional lumen imaging probe in esophageal measurements and dilations: a single pediatric center experience. Surg Endosc 2019;64(5):701–6.
62. Pannala R, Krishnan K, Watson RR, et al. Devices for esophageal function testing. VideoGIE 2021;7(1):1–20.

63. Hoskins B, Almazan E, Mogul D, et al. Endoluminal functional lumen imaging probe is safe in children under five years old. J Pediatr Gastroenterol Nutr 2022;74(6):e148–52.

64. Rosen R, Stayn Z, Garza JM, et al. The utility of functional luminal imaging probes measurements to diagnose dysmotility and their relationship to impaired bolus clearance. J Pediatr Gastroenterol Nutr 2022;74(4):523–8.

65. Menard-Katcher C, Benitez AJ, Pan Z, et al. Influence of age and eosinophilic esophagitis on esophageal distensibility in a pediatric cohort. Am J Gastroenterol 2017;2(suppl):61.

66. Piester TL, Liu QY. EUS in pediatrics: a multicenter experience and review. Front Pediatr 2021;9:709461.

67. Lakhole A, Liu QY. Role of endoscopic ultrasound in pediatric disease. Gastrointest Endosc Clin N Am 2016;26(1):137–53.

68. Fox VL, Nurko S, Teitelbaum JE, et al. High-resolution EUS in children with eosinophilic "allergic" esophagitis. Gastrointest Endosc 2003;57(1):30–6.

69. Gonsalves NP, Aceves SS. Diagnosis and treatment of eosinophilic esophagitis. J Allergy Clin Immunol 2020;145(1):1–7.

70. Rabinowitz SS, Grossman E, Feng L, et al. Predicting pediatric esophageal wall thickness: an EUS study. Endosc Ultrasound 2020;9(4):259–66.

71. Pytrus T, Akutko K, Kofla-Dłubacz A, et al. Endoscopic ultrasonography in children with eosinophilic esophagitis—a review. Pediatr Rep 2022;14(1):13–9.

72. Friedlander JA, DeBoer EM, Soden JS, et al. Unsedated transnasal esophagoscopy for monitoring therapy in pediatric eosinophilic esophagitis. Gastrointest Endosc 2016;83(2):299–306.e1.

73. Nguyen N, Lavery WJ, Capocelli KE, et al. Transnasal endoscopy in unsedated children with eosinophilic esophagitis using virtual reality video goggles. Clin Gastroenterol Hepatol 2019;17(12):2455–62.

74. Scherer C, Sosensky P, Schulman-Green D, et al. Pediatric patients' and parents' perspectives of unsedated transnasal endoscopy in eosinophilic esophagitis: a qualitative descriptive study. J Pediatr Gastroenterol Nutr 2020;72(4):558–62.

75. Venkatesh R, Leinwand K, Nguyen N. Pediatric Unsedated Transnasal Endoscopy. Gastrointest Endosc Clin N Am 2023.

76. Ichiya T, Tanaka K, Rubio C, et al. Evaluation of narrow-band imaging signs in eosinophilic and lymphocytic esophagitis. Endoscopy 2017;49(05):429–37.

77. Tanaka K, Rubio CA, Dlugosz A, et al. Narrow-band imaging magnifying endoscopy in adult patients with eosinophilic esophagitis/esophageal eosinophilia and lymphocytic esophagitis. Gastrointest Endosc 2013;78(4):659–64.

78. Ayaki M, Manabe N, Tomida A, et al. Beige mucosa observable under narrowband imaging indicates the active sites of eosinophilic esophagitis. J Gastroenterol Hepatol 2022;37(5):891–7.

79. Krafft C, Sergo V. Biomedical applications of Raman and infrared spectroscopy to diagnose tissues. J Spectrosc 2006;20(5–6):195–218.

80. Hiremath G, Locke A, Thomas G, et al. Novel insights into tissue-specific biochemical alterations in pediatric eosinophilic esophagitis using raman spectroscopy. Clin Transl Gastroenterol 2020;11(7):e00195.

81. Visaggi P, Bortoli N de, Barberio B, et al. Artificial intelligence in the diagnosis of upper gastrointestinal diseases. J Clin Gastroenterol 2022;56(1):23–35.

82. Sallis BF, Erkert L, Moñino-Romero S, et al. An algorithm for the classification of mRNA patterns in eosinophilic esophagitis: Integration of machine learning. J Allergy Clin Immunol 2018;141(4):1354–64.e9.

83. Czyzewski T, Daniel N, Rochman M, et al. Machine learning approach for biopsy-based identification of eosinophilic esophagitis reveals importance of global features. IEEE Open J Eng Med Biol 2021;2:218–23.

84. Lirio RA, Nazarey P, O'Dea J, et al. Sa1664 the first case report of esoflip for dilation of a pediatric esophageal stricture. Gastrointest Endosc 2015;81(5): AB299–300.

85. Walter B, Schmidbaur S, Rahman I, et al. The BougieCap – a new method for endoscopic treatment of complex benign esophageal stenosis: results from a multicenter study. Endoscopy 2019;51(09):866–70.

86. Schoepfer AM, Henchoz S, Biedermann L, et al. Technical feasibility, clinical effectiveness, and safety of esophageal stricture dilation using a novel endoscopic attachment cap in adults with eosinophilic esophagitis. Gastrointest Endosc 2021;94(5):912–9.e2.

87. Ramrakhiani H, Triadafilopoulos G. Negotiating Dire Straits with a BougieCap. Dig Dis Sci 2020;65(11):3107–10.

88. Brand M, Hofmann N, Ho C-N, et al. The over-the-scope grasper (OTSG). Endoscopy 2020;53(02):152–5.

Endoscopic Management of Congenital Esophageal Defects and Associated Comorbidities

Jessica L. Yasuda, MD[a], Michael A. Manfredi, MD[b],*

KEYWORDS

- Esophageal atresia • Congenital esophageal stricture • Dilation • Surveillance
- Esophagitis

KEY POINTS

- Esophageal atresia patients are at risk for multiple comorbid pathologies, which may be identified and treated endoscopically.
- Dilation is the cornerstone of endoscopic management of anastomotic and congenital esophageal strictures.
- The endoscopic toolbox for management of refractory strictures includes intralesional steroid injection, stenting, and endoscopic incisional therapy.
- Endoscopic approaches for recurrent tracheoesophageal fistula have been described with mixed results.
- Routine endoscopic surveillance for mucosal pathology is critical in patients with esophageal atresia.

INTRODUCTION

Congenital esophageal defects are rare, medically complex problems. The endoscopist plays a critical role in the surveillance and treatment of these complex disorders. This review focuses on esophageal atresia (EA) and congenital esophageal strictures (CESs) and, in particular, the endoscopic management of comorbidities related to these conditions, including anastomotic strictures, tracheoesophageal fistulas (TEFs), esophageal perforations, and esophagitis surveillance. Practical aspects of endoscopic techniques for stricture management are reviewed, including dilation,

[a] Division of Gastroenterology, Hepatology and Nutrition, Boston Children's Hospital, 300 Longwood Avenue, Boston, MA 02115, USA; [b] Division of Gastroenterology, Hepatology and Nutrition, Children's Hospital of Philadelphia, 3401 Civic Center Boulevard, Philadelphia, PA 19104, USA
* Corresponding author.
E-mail address: manfredim@chop.edu

Gastrointest Endoscopy Clin N Am 33 (2023) 341–361
https://doi.org/10.1016/j.giec.2022.11.005

intralesional steroid injection (ISI), stenting, and endoscopic incisional therapy. Endoscopic surveillance for mucosal pathology is essential in this population, as patients are at high risk of esophagitis and its late complications such as Barrett's esophagus.

ESOPHAGEAL ATRESIA

EA with or without TEF is the most common congenital anomaly of the esophagus. The overall incidence of EA/TEF ranges from one in every 2500 to 4500 live birth.[1] The first successful EA/TEF repair was performed by Dr Cameron Height in 1941.[2] Survival rates for patients with EA, with or without TEF, have improved greatly over the past two decades with technical advances in surgery and critical care medicine. The most recent survival rates have ranged from 91% to 97%.[3–6] The survival rates for infants born full-term with no associated congenital anomalies have been reported to approach 100%.[3,7] Although survival rates are quite high, patients with EA may deal with significant comorbidities postoperatively, both in the immediate postoperative period and later in life (**Box 1**). In this review, the authors focus on the endoscopic management and surveillance for some of these comorbidities.

Tracheoesophageal Fistula

Most children with EA are also born with an associated TEF. TEFs are typically surgically addressed in infancy. In some cases, congenital fistulas—especially proximal fistulas—may be missed during the initial surgical repair of EA and persist. In addition, recurrence after initial surgical division has been described in up to 10% of cases,[8] and acquired fistulas may occur after surgical leaks or perforations. TEFs can be difficult to diagnose and require a high index of suspicion, often requiring combinations of diagnostic modalities (eg, fluoroscopy, upper endoscopy, bronchoscopy) to detect them. For the gastroenterologist, a recently described method using capnography in an intubated patient while performing esophagoscopic insufflation with carbon dioxide can provide an additional method of identifying the presence of a TEF during upper endoscopy.[9]

There has been interest in endoscopic treatment of recurrent TEFs to potentially spare a patient the potential morbidity of an additional surgery. Various esophagoscopic and bronchoscopic methods for managing TEF have been described in case reports and case series, typically involving mechanical (eg, brushing), chemical (eg, polidocanol, aethoxysklerol), or thermal (eg, diathermy, laser) disruption of the fistula epithelium; application of an occlusive substance into the fistula tract (eg, fibrin adhesive, tissue adhesive); or both.[10–13] The bronchoscopic approach is more commonly reported. This approach may take advantage of additional stability offered by the use of rigid instruments and technically more straightforward access into the fistula tract, as typically TEFs have a downward angle of takeoff from the trachea toward the esophagus. Reported pooled success rates of endoscopic TEF closure attempts are 60%, requiring a mean of 2.1 endoscopic procedures, with low morbidity reported.[12,13] However, possible reporting bias in the literature may be inflating this statistic and in practice the durable success of endoscopic TEF closure is highly variable.

CONGENITAL ESOPHAGEAL STRICTURE

CESs are rare congenital anomalies of the esophagus, affecting approximately one in 25,000 to 50,000 live births.[14] CES may be present in isolation or in association with other anomalies of the esophagus, particularly EA.[15–17]

Three subtypes of CES include tracheobronchial remnants (TBR), fibromuscular thickening, or membranous webs and are differentiated by histopathological and anatomical configuration differences.[18] Response to endoscopic therapy (in particular, dilations) is felt by some practitioners to depend on the subtype, with TBR potentially more refractory to dilations.[15,18–22] Endoscopic ultrasound has been reported as an emerging tool for noninvasive subtype differentiation, though the ultrasonographic appearances in these reports are descriptively incongruous with each other (eg, cartilage reported as either hypo- and hyperechoic, depending on the report).[23–25] Additional study of endoscopic ultrasound with definitively histopathological correlation would be helpful in making ultrasound a more robust diagnostic tool in CES, though unlikely given its rarity as a condition.

Special Considerations for Management of Congenital Esophageal Stricture

Management of CES is often first attempted via endoscopic therapy for all subtypes, with surgical intervention reserved for refractory cases.[17–19,21,22,26,27] Dilation is considered first line, though potentially insufficient to produce durable response. Perforation rates for dilation of CES are high, reported anywhere from 9% to 44.4%.[15,19] Endoscopic electrocautery incisional therapy (EIT), in which electrocautery is used to incise the congenital stricture in a selective fashion to create controlled weak points in the thickened stricture tissue, in combination with stenting and conventional dilation, has been described to allow for successful endoscopic therapy and avoidance of surgery.[28] However, EIT is also high risk for perforation and should only be performed when the endoscopist is prepared to manage perforation with either endoscopic vacuum-assisted closure (EVAC) or with experienced surgical backup.[29–33] Surgical intervention with myotomy, stricture resection, or in some cases esophageal replacement may ultimately be necessary. Patients undergoing surgical intervention must be monitored and treated for symptoms of anastomotic stricture, which may occur in over half of surgically managed CES patients.[14,20]

ENDOSCOPIC MANAGEMENT OF COMORBIDITIES RELATED TO ESOPHAGEAL ATRESIA AND CONGENITAL ESOPHAGEAL STRICTURE
Esophageal Anastomotic Strictures

Surgical repair of congenital esophageal defects may be complicated by subsequent development of esophageal anastomotic stricture. The following sections describe the clinical presentation and endoscopic methods of treating anastomotic stricture.

Pathophysiology and incidence

Surgical creation of an esophageal anastomosis results in a wound, which heals by the natural process of granulation and scar tissue formation. During the tissue remodeling phase of wound healing, fibroblasts promote wound contraction.[34] Tissue contraction of open wounds is beneficial in order to close the injury; however, wound contraction in the setting of a circular end-to-end anastomosis creates narrowing. Therefore, it is quite common to see a degree of narrowing at the site of the esophageal anastomosis after EA repair (**Fig. 1**).

The reported incidence of anastomotic stricture after EA repair has varied in case series from as low as 9% to as high as 80%.[35–40] There are several factors implicated in the pathogenesis of anastomotic strictures, including creation of the esophageal anastomosis under excessive tension, ischemia at the ends of the esophageal pouches, creation of the anastomosis with two suture layers, use of silk suture material, anastomotic leak, esophageal gap length greater than 4 cm (long gap EA), and postoperative gastroesophageal reflux.[3,36,41,42]

> **Box 1**
> **Significant comorbidities associated with surgically repaired esophageal atresia**
>
> Esophageal stricture
>
> Esophageal leak or perforation
>
> Anastomosis dehiscence
>
> Recurrent tracheoesophageal fistula
>
> Gastroesophageal reflux disease
>
> Dysphagia
>
> Esophageal dysmotility
>
> Aspiration
>
> Peptic esophagitis
>
> Eosinophilic esophagitis
>
> Barrett's esophagus
>
> Esophageal cancer

Presentation

When a swallowed food bolus becomes too large to pass through the narrowed portion of the esophagus, symptoms of dysphagia will occur. Although a lumen size does not always correlate with symptoms,[43] esophageal lumen size at which dysphagia tends to occur in pediatric patients have been proposed based on expert opinion (**Table 1**).[44] Typical symptoms of an esophageal stricture include feeding difficulties, coughing and choking during feeds, food impaction, and regurgitation of undigested material. In younger children, apnea may be a presenting symptom as well as feeding refusal. If a patient with EA develops any of these symptoms, they should undergo a contrast fluoroscopy study and/or endoscopy to evaluate for a possible

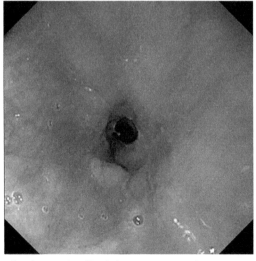

Fig. 1. An esophageal stricture visualized during upper endoscopy.

Table 1
Proposed age-based minimum esophageal lumen diameters

Age	Esophageal Lumen Diameter (mm)
Less than 9 mo	8
9 to 23 mo	10
24 mo to 5 y	12
Greater than 6 y	14

stricture. An esophageal stricture, therefore, is defined as an intrinsic luminal narrowing that leads to the patient becoming clinically symptomatic.[45] A complex esophageal stricture is defined in adult patients as having one or more of the following characteristics: length ≥ 2 cm, angulated, irregular surface, diameter ≤ 10 mm and the presence of diverticulum.[46]

Treatment

Dilation
The cornerstone of esophageal stricture treatment is dilation. The goal of esophageal dilation is to increase the luminal diameter of the esophagus while also improving dysphagia symptoms. This is achieved through circumferential stretching and splitting of the scar tissue within the stricture.[47,48] Even though there are many dilation techniques and a variety of available equipment, they fall into two main categories: mechanical (bougie or push-type) dilators or balloon-based dilators.

Mechanical (bougie) dilation
The basic technique of mechanical dilation involves the passage of a bougie dilator across the stricture (**Fig. 2**). This results in both longitudinal shearing force and radial force on the strictured area. The goal of mechanical dilation is to pass serial bougie dilators of incremental size across the stricture site. Although fluoroscopy is frequently recommended to confirm correct positioning as the bougie dilator is passed across the stricture, it is not mandatory in short strictures. It is generally recommended to use fluoroscopy in strictures longer than 1 cm and/or strictures that are angulated.

There are several different types of bougie-based dilators, the most common of which are guidewire-based. Presuming the wire position is checked frequently (using fluoroscopy or a fixed external landmark), this helps ensure the dilator will pass

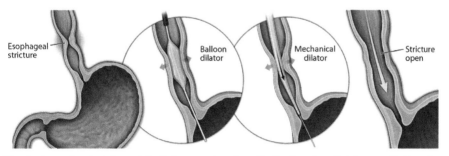

Fig. 2. A mechanical (bougie) dilator exerts a longitudinal and radial force, dilating the stricture proximal to distal, whereas a balloon dilator exerts a radial force delivered simultaneously across the entire stricture. (*Adapted from* Adler DG, Siddiqui AA. Endoscopic management of esophageal strictures. Gastrointest Endosc. 2017;86(1):35-43.)

correctly through the stricture. These dilators are tapered, cylindrical solid tubes made of polyvinyl chloride with a central channel to accommodate a guidewire.[49] These dilating tubes have varying lengths of tapering at the tip and also have radiopaque markers to permit fluoroscopic guidance (eg, Savary-Gilliard dilators, American Dilators, and SafeGuide). There are also non-guidewire mechanical dilators that are tungsten weighted to allow for gravity assistance when the patient is in a seated position. The two commonly used non-guidewire bougie dilators are Hurst and Maloney dilators.[49]

Another type of mechanical dilator is Tucker dilators, which are small, tapered silicone bougies with loops on each end. A string is attached to the loops to allow for the dilator to be pulled antegrade or retrograde across strictures. These dilators, therefore, require the patient to have a gastrostomy. Tucker dilators can remain inside the patient for periodic serial dilations.

Mechanical bougie dilation is a tactile technique.[37,45,50] As the bougie is advanced across the stricture site, a degree of resistance should be appreciated by the operator. The object is to feel, and then overcome, the resistance across the strictured area. Once moderate resistance is encountered with the bougie dilator, it is generally recommended passing no greater than three consecutive dilators in increments of 1 mm in a single session for a total of 3 mm. This approach, known as the "rule of 3," is a well-established approach for mechanical dilation.[51] Strict adherence to the rule is not always necessary and there may be occasions that one may dilate larger than 3 mm in a single session. Two studies, one adult and one pediatric, have shown that nonadherence to the "rule of 3" was not associated with increased adverse events.[52–54]

Balloon dilation

Balloons deliver equal radial force across the entire length of the stricture (see **Fig. 2**). They are designed to pass through the endoscope channel with or without a guidewire. Most commonly, they are 5 cm in length and 6 to 20 mm in diameter (some are multidiameter with increasing pressures). Through-the-scope (TTS) dilation allows the endoscopist to directly visualize the stricture during and immediately after the dilation. However, TTS balloon dilation requires the use of an adult gastroscope with a minimum working channel diameter of 2.8 mm, which is difficult to use in younger infants under 10 kg.

In smaller patients, the balloon can be passed over a guidewire under fluoroscopic guidance. This technique is performed by passing a 0.035-mm guidewire across the stricture through the endoscope working channel, followed by a wire exchange under fluoroscopy, leaving the wire in place as the scope is removed. The balloon is then passed over the wire and positioned across the stricture under fluoroscopic guidance.

When possible, TTS balloon dilation should be performed as it can provide direct visualization of the tissue during and immediately following the dilation and permit monitoring of the degree of developing mucosal disruption. It also allows the endoscopist to minimize fluoroscopy time as balloon placement can be done by endoscopic view. However, a balloon should not be passed blindly through a stricture if the scope cannot traverse the stricture beforehand and instead a wire should be used to prevent unintentional perforation from the tip of the dilator.

Dilating balloons expand by the injection of liquid (eg, water, radiopaque contrast) under pressure using a handheld inflation device. A manometer on the device will measure the fluid pressure in the balloon to allow for accurate radial expansion force.[49] Balloon dilators are either designed to inflate to a single target diameter or to allow for sequential inflation to multiple sizes (typically three incremental diameters per balloon, depending on the pressure delivered into the balloon).

The basic approach to balloon dilation is to first estimate the size of the stricture. This can be done by performing an intraoperative contrast esophagogram immediately before dilation to estimate stricture diameter, length, and possible underlying contraindicative pathology (eg, TEF or preexisting esophageal leak). To guide decision-making in regard to balloon size, further assessment of stricture size can be estimated by using a visual reference such as the biopsy forceps of known dimensions as a measurement tool and/or by estimating size based on the outer diameter of the endoscope and ability of the endoscope to pass the stricture.

Once the size is estimated, the "rule of 3" can similarly be applied to balloon dilators by choosing a balloon that will increase in size by increments of 1 mm in a single session for a total of 3 mm above the originally estimated stricture size. A recent pediatric study found that dilating up to 5 mm above the stricture diameter did not increase the risk of perforation compared with dilating only to 3 mm.[53] This study points out that these rules are meant as a guide rather than a replacement for clinical judgment based on inspection of the stricture post-dilation. It is important to carefully inspect the tissue in between dilations, and in situations, where the endoscopist notes an unsatisfactory response to standard dilation increments with no evidence of perforation, there is now precedent to support dilating further if indicated.

Before dilation, the balloon is advanced across the stricture either with endoscopic and/or fluoroscopic guidance. Ideally, the balloon should be positioned so that the middle of the balloon is centered across the stricture. Balloons are available with or without a wire. Our recommended approach is to have a wire passed across the stricture and typically into the stomach. The goal of the wire is to make certain that the tip of the balloon remains within the lumen of the esophagus, as the tip of the balloon is sharp, and it is possible for the tip to dissect through the esophageal wall if blindly passed without a guidewire.

Once the balloon is properly positioned, the balloon is inflated to the desired size. The optimal inflation time has not been established. Balloon inflation times of 30 to 60 seconds are generally accepted.[47] A randomized study of patients with strictures who underwent dilation using different balloon inflation times showed no significant difference in dilation effectiveness based on inflation time.[55] Therefore, it seems that the act of inflation, which tears the scar tissue, is more important than the duration of the balloon is inflated.

The use of fluoroscopy during balloon dilation is helpful. In the setting of a complex stricture, fluoroscopy is useful in advancing the wire and balloon safely across the stricture. In addition, inflating the balloon with contrast will allow the endoscopist to see if the stricture is being effectively dilated. It is useful to see the appearance of the stricture forming a waist around the balloon and the subsequent obliteration of a waist as the balloon is further inflated (**Fig. 3**). It is a practice of these authors to use fluoroscopy with our esophageal balloon-based stricture dilations. In addition, there is an added benefit of using fluoroscopy to conduct a post-dilation contrast study to evaluate for a post-dilation esophageal leak or perforation.

Comparative studies of mechanical and balloon dilation

There is little data comparing bougie (mechanical dilators) versus balloon dilators in both the pediatric and adult literature. In adult studies, there has been no significant difference in safety or efficacy between wire-guided bougie dilation and balloon dilation.[56–58] Pediatric studies show mixed results, although they are limited by small sample sizes. There have been two pediatric studies that favored balloon dilation over

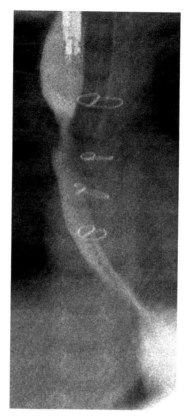

Fig. 3. An esophageal stricture visualized with fluoroscopy.

bougie in both safety and efficacy, whereas a third study only evaluated safety and found no difference between both groups.[59–61] Although further investigation is needed, the authors recommend based on the existing literature that the provider should use the technique with which they are most comfortable and experienced when performing a dilation. Wire-guided bougie dilation is generally recommend over non-wire-guided push bougie dilators in complex strictures due to higher rates of esophageal perforation without wire guidance.[46]

Refractory Strictures and Adjunct Treatments

Refractory strictures are defined in adults as a failure to remediate the stricture successfully up to diameter of 14 mm over five sessions at 2-week intervals as well as maintaining a satisfactory diameter for 4 weeks once the desired diameter has been achieved.[62] A modification for pediatrics has been suggested by the current authors, whereby a refractory stricture is defined as the inability to remediate the esophageal lumen with five dilatations performed within 5 months to the desired size for age.[45] Alternatively, a North American and European Societies of Pediatric Gastroenterology, Hepatology and Nutrition EA guideline report based on expert opinion defined three or more clinically relevant stricture relapses as a recurrent stricture.[50] There is a need for consensus around the definitions of refractory stricture to help standardize study outcomes and accurately evaluate the efficacy of different therapies.[63] Regardless of the definition, once a stricture becomes refractory to esophageal dilation, there are several treatment therapies available as adjuncts to dilation therapy that should be considered before surgical resection.

Intralesional steroid injection

ISIs are typically used in conjunction with dilation to facilitate larger post-dilation esophageal stricture diameter. The proposed mechanism of ISI in the treatment of esophageal strictures is to locally inhibit the inflammatory response that promotes collagen formation and scarring within a stricture.[64] Triamcinolone acetonide 40 and 10 mg/mL is commonly used. The authors prefer 10 mg/mL concentration as the 40 mg/mL is viscous and typically needs to be diluted before injection; dilution is not necessary with the 10 mg/mL concentration. ISI is administered via a sclerotherapy needle in 0.1 to 0.2 mL aliquots. Four quadrant injections are common; however, if the scar tissue is uneven a preponderance of steroid can be injected into targeted scar tissue areas. The dose of triamcinolone acetonide used is 1 to 2 mg/kg per dose, up to a maximum dose of 80 mg in adults. ISI may be injected before or after dilation therapy.

The efficacy of ISI in peptic strictures was demonstrated in a randomized double-blind placebo controlled trial in which patients received four quadrant injections of 0.5 mL of triamcinolone acetate (40 mg per mL) for total of 80 mg or a sham.[65] Two of 15 (13%, 95% CI 4%–38%) patients in the steroid group and 9 of 15 (60%, 95% CI 36%–80%) in the sham group required repeat dilation ($P = 0.021$).[65] There have been multiple studies that have shown the benefit of ISI in reducing recurrent stricture formation in other types of strictures. However, most reports are small uncontrolled studies evaluating strictures of diverse etiology.[66–69] In a multicenter double-blind placebo control trial involving 60 patients with benign esophagogastric anastomotic strictures, the authors reported no statistically significant decrease in frequency of repeat dilations with a median number of two dilations (range, 1–7) performed in the corticosteroid group compared with three dilations (range, 1–9) in the control group ($P = 0.36$).[70] A pediatric retrospective study evaluating 158 patients with anastomotic strictures showed that ISI combined with dilation was well tolerated with no increased incidence of perforation, and statistically significant improvement in stricture diameter was observed when compared with dilation alone. In addition, this study showed that the effectiveness of ISI injections appeared to peak at three injections, with no significant gains in diameter beyond three injection sessions.[71]

Potential complications of ISI include adrenal suppression. Therefore, some authors suggest surveillance for adrenal suppression.[37] However, this is currently not standard of care. In addition, there have been reports of increased Candida esophagitis.[70] Last, there has been one report of intralesional steroids contributing to the spontaneous rupture of a right aortic arch presumably secondary to the steroids weakening the arterial wall.[37]

Mitomycin C

Mitomycin C is an antineoplastic agent that disrupts base pairing of DNA molecules, inhibits fibroblast proliferation, and reduces fibroblastic collagen synthesis by inhibiting DNA-dependent RNA synthesis. It also induces apoptosis at higher doses by suppressing cellular proliferation during the late G1 and S phases.[72] It has been proposed as an adjunct treatment to manage esophageal strictures. Mitomycin C has been mainly placed topically in the literature; however, there are also reports of injection of mitomycin C.[73] There have been numerous described methods of topically placing mitomycin C, such as soaking pledgets or cotton swabs and placing them topically on the stricture area, dripping mitomycin C via an injection needle onto the affected area, or using a spray catheter.[73–76] The concentration of mitomycin C used in these studies is also variable, ranging from 0.004 to 1 mg/mL.[77]

The efficacy of mitomycin C has been a controversial topic in patients with EA. A recent study reported a 71% success rate in EA patients with the majority of them being type C, with success defined a priori as any reduction in the number of dilations over the same period from before to after the application.[78] This is in stark contrast to another study on EA patients that showed a 27% success rate with no significant difference in dilations compared with historical controls.[79] The lack of standardized definitions of refractory strictures and treatment success may contribute to different outcomes. In addition, the timing of treatment early or late in the course of dilations may also be a factor. Mitomycin C has been shown to be effective in some prospective studies looking at strictures secondary to caustic ingestion.[80–82] However, a recent meta-analysis looking at the efficacy of mitomycin C in caustic strictures did not show a statistical difference in the overall number of dilations in treatment and nontreatment groups.[83]

There is a hypothetical risk of secondary malignancy with mitomycin C, so this must be taken into account and should be discussed with the patient and caregivers before use.[84] There have been reports of de novo gastric metaplasia around the areas of the anastomosis in two of the six cases that received topical mitomycin C.[84] Therefore, long-term follow-up with esophageal biopsies at the site of mitomycin C application should be recommended.

Esophageal stents

The rationale for stenting strictures, in theory, seems sound. By applying dilation forces to the esophagus for prolonged periods of time, stenting may reduce the risk of recurrent stricture formation and thus may be an alternative treatment option to serial esophageal stricture dilations. The first externally removable stents were self-expandable plastic stents. These have largely been replaced by fully covered self-expandable metal stents (FCSEMSs). These stents are composed of a memory shape metal nitinol (an alloy of nickel and titanium) and are available in various diameters and lengths. Esophageal FCSEMSs are designed for adult patients and thus are too large for the majority of pediatric patients. For most children, either biliary or airway FCSEMSs can be used in the pediatric esophagus.

Stent deployment requires the use of radiography to ensure proper placement. Many experts suggest that vascular imaging should be done before stenting to look for an aberrant right subclavian artery as this may increase risk of complication.[37,85] Each stent has their own unique deployment mechanism that separates the stent from the housing sheath. As FCSEMS have a degree of foreshortening during deployment, the placement should be done under fluoroscopy in order to reposition the stent in real time, whereas it is deploying.

The utility of stent treatment for esophageal strictures is unclear. The success of esophageal stenting in the pediatric literature is also variable with rates ranging from 0 to 86% success.[86–89] A pooled analysis of seven pediatric studies with a total of 69 patients with esophageal strictures of multiple etiologies reported a pooled success rate of 52%.[90] A single-center pediatric study looking at 49 esophageal strictures secondary to EA reported clinical success in 41% of patients.[91] Patients whose procedures were successful underwent a median of 0.5 dilations (Interquartile range [IQR] 0, 1) during follow-up period, which was a median duration of 5 years (IQR 2–6). This study found the greatest predictor of stent success was the degree of re-stricturing seen at the time of follow-up endoscopy performed at a median of 2 weeks after stent removal, with shrinkage of the stricture $\geq$ 4 mm from the starting stent diameter predicting endoscopic treatment failure.[91] Although the utility of stenting to treat strictures is still debatable, it may serve as a bridge to surgery.[92]

Esophageal stenting has been associated with numerous adverse events, including life-threating events such as bleeding, perforation, and erosion into the vascular system or airway. There has also been reported mortality secondary to esophageal stenting.[85] Additional adverse events include stent migration, tracheal compression, gastroesophageal reflux, aspiration pneumonia, and new esophageal stricture development due to the edges of the stent or ischemia secondary to overly aggressive stent diameter selection.[91,93]

Endoscopic electrocautery incisional therapy

EIT is a technique based on understanding that not all strictures are symmetrical. Many strictures, particularly anastomotic strictures, are asymmetric with areas of varying degrees of scar tissue. Thickened scar tissue may have the appearance of bands or shelves of tissue. Dilation alone in an asymmetric stricture tends to tear the stricture at areas of thinner scar tissue, and thus may lead to a less effective dilation. EIT is a technique that involves applying electrocautery via a needle knife to make small incisions into the scar tissue at its thickest areas to create preferential weak points (**Fig. 4**). Once the incisions are made, a balloon dilation can then be performed to preferentially dilate the areas that were weakened by the incisions. This technique tends to be better for strictures less than 1 cm in length.[45]

In a pediatric study of 58 patients, EIT was successful in remediating the stricture in 76% of patients with 2 year follow-up.[94] In subgroup analysis of patients who met criteria for a refractory stricture, EIT was successful in 61% ($N = 36$) of patients. This same study reported a perforation rate of 2.3%. As EIT has a higher adverse event rate than balloon dilation, it should be performed by a highly skilled endoscopist who has access to fluoroscopy and surgical backup at the time of the procedure to recognize an adverse event.

Esophageal Perforation or Leak

Esophageal perforation or leak is a potentially life-threatening problem if not quickly diagnosed and treated appropriately (**Fig. 5**). The rate of developing an esophageal anastomotic leak after surgical EA repair has been reported to range from 11% to 16%.[95] In addition, esophageal perforation may occur after esophageal dilation or another endoscopic therapeutic intervention at a stricture. In a systematic review with pooled analysis of 5 pediatric studies comprising 139 patients and 401 dilations, the perforation rate was 1.8%.[53,71] A large single-center pediatric study of 284 patients with 1384 dilations reported an esophageal perforation rate of 1.6% for balloon dilation. Of note, steroid injection in combination with dilation had no statistically significant increase in perforation compared with dilation alone.[53,71] Traditional management of esophageal perforations or leaks in children includes making the patient nil per os, intravenous broad-spectrum antibiotics, and esophageal decompression with the placement of a nasoesophageal tube to low wall suction. External wound drainage with a chest tube is considered in the setting of a large fluid collection in the chest.

Esophageal stenting has been shown to be effective in adult patients with esophageal perforations and has become a first-line treatment, with a reported clinical success rate of 85% with a mean stent duration time of 6 to 8 weeks.[96] In pediatrics, the use of esophageal stents to treat esophageal leaks has a reported success rate from 64% to 100%.[97–100] The median number of days that stents were left in situ in the pediatric studies ranged from 8 to 36 days with the longer duration of stent time being associated with higher success.[97–100] In our experience, esophageal stents

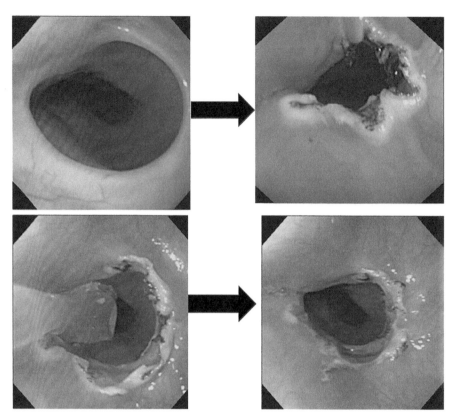

Fig. 4. Endoscopic incisional therapy involves incising the thickened scar bands of the stricture using electrocautery. After incisions are created, a balloon dilation is performed.

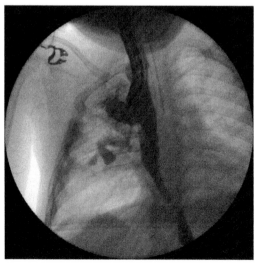

Fig. 5. A fluoroscopic image confirming extravasation of radiopaque contrast outside the lumen of the esophagus, consistent with esophageal leak.

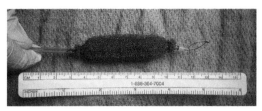

Fig. 6. A custom assembled endoscopic vacuum-assisted closure (EVAC) device to be placed in the esophageal lumen at a site of leak or perforation.

also have drawbacks, especially in children with a surgically repaired esophagus, as in the EA population. Esophageal stents may lead to local pressure necrosis of the esophagus, which may worsen the existing esophageal perforation and may lead to erosion into surrounding structures such as the airway and major blood vessels. Last, stenting does not facilitate drainage of the fluid collection around the esophagus and can in fact trap infection in the chest; thus, stents may facilitate abscess formation unless external drainage with a chest tube is initiated at the time of stent placement.[29]

EVAC is an adaptation of traditional vacuum-assisted closure devices (**Fig. 6**). It is based on the principles of negative pressure wound therapy, which stimulates wound healing by removal of fluid from the perforation site, source control for infection, reduction of tissue edema, and promotion of blood flow to the area stimulating granulation tissue formation.[101] In a pediatric study of 17 patients with EA who underwent EVAC therapy for esophageal perforation secondary to either postsurgical anastomotic leak or endoscopic therapy, the success rate of EVAC to seal all esophageal perforations was 88%.[29] The success rate was similar in both subgroups (surgical anastomotic leaks at 88% [7/8] and endoscopic therapy leaks at 89% [8/9]), with a median duration of EVAC treatment of 8 days. This same study compared EVAC with a cohort of esophageal perorations treated with esophageal stents ($n = 24$) and found a statistically significant difference in favor of EVAC in sealing surgical anastomotic perforations ($P = 0.032$); however, there was no statistical difference in sealing endoscopic therapy perforations ($P = 0.360$).

Endoscopic Surveillance for Mucosal Pathology

Long-term, patients with EA are at increased risk of esophagitis. Historically, most esophagitis in this population has been attributed to acid reflux; in recent years, increased attention has been paid to higher rates of allergic eosinophilic esophagitis in EA patients as well.[102,103] Dysmotility with poor esophageal clearance is also a likely contributor to long-term risk of esophageal mucosal pathology.[104,105] In the setting of higher rates of chronic esophageal inflammation and injury, individuals with EA have been noted to be at significantly higher risk of the precancerous condition Barrett's esophagus compared with the general population.[50,104,106] Chronic inflammation may also contribute to dysphagia and stricturing.

Chronic acid suppressive therapy is commonly prescribed and has been linked to lower odds of abnormal esophageal biopsy,[107] though optimal duration of treatment is uncertain and esophageal inflammation remains common even in those on acid suppression.[107] Thus, consensus guidelines advocate for endoscopic surveillance with multiple levels of esophageal biopsies, even in asymptomatic patients on acid suppression, to proactively monitor for esophagitis before its late complications such as Barrett's esophagus develop.[50] However, the optimal interval for surveillance has not been defined.[50] Current recommendations advocate for at least three endoscopies in childhood: one after stopping Proton Pump Inhibitior (PPI) therapy, one before age 10 years, and one on transition to adulthood.[50] In the authors' experience, this approach to surveillance may lead to delayed diagnosis of important pathology as the rate of endoscopic pathology in this patient population is high. Indeed, the authors have identified erosive esophagitis in 6% of patients and high rates of significant histologic esophagitis (>15 eosinophils/high-powered field) in over 25% of endoscopies as well as biopsy-confirmed Barrett's esophagus in patients as young as 5 years old, despite nearly 90% of endoscopies being performed on chronic acid suppressive therapy.[107]

Thus, the authors' current practice is to perform surveillance endoscopy every 1 to 3 years throughout childhood, with more frequent follow-up for patients with significant or refractory esophagitis, Barrett's esophagus, or other pathology; our initial surveillance endoscopy is performed around approximately 1 year after the surgical creation of the esophageal anastomosis.

SUMMARY

Dilation remains the first-line treatment for many types of esophageal strictures including anastomotic strictures that can develop after repair of EA. Adjunctive therapies such as ISI, mitomycin C application, stenting, and incisional therapy may be useful in treating strictures that do not adequately respond to dilation alone. CESs require special consideration and potentially referral to a center of expertise given the high risk of complications with all forms of endoscopic therapy. Dilation alone may be less effective in treating some congenital strictures and may be associated with relatively high rates of perforation. Esophageal perforations can often be managed via endoscopic means with stenting or EVAC devices. Rates of mucosal pathology in children with congenital esophageal defects are high, and routine endoscopic surveillance is warranted to prevent long-term complications of uncontrolled inflammation.

CLINICS CARE POINTS

- When performing dilation, the endoscopist should perform visual inspection to determine the degree of mucosal disruption. Some degree of mucosal disruption is expected and even desired in treating most strictures, though excessive or asymmetric mucosal disruption increases the risk of perforation.

- The use of real-time fluoroscopy during dilation allows the endoscopist to assess for obliteration of a radiographic "waist," which can aid in assessing anastomotic stricture response to dilation.

- In contrast, obliteration of the radiographic waist should not be the sole endpoint goal of a dilation session of a CES, which is high risk for perforation. CESs should be visually inspected frequently during the endoscopy session to assess for any evolving asymmetry in mucosal disruption that may indicate a region at risk for perforation should more aggressive dilation diameters be attempted.

- Asymmetric strictures often benefit from endoscopic incisional therapy to create select weakened points in the thicker scar bands to then more evenly spread the dilation force around the circumference of the stricture. Incisional therapy should only be attempted by a skilled endoscopist with appropriate backup plan in case of perforation (including availability of surgical backup, an intensive care unit bed, and an ability to place an endoscopic vacuum-assisted closure device or stent).

- Intralesional steroid injection may be performed in four quadrants around a stricture or can be focused in areas of apparent thickened scar tissue.

- Endoscopic treatment of esophageal perforation should be accompanied by medical management to address microbial contamination of the extraluminal space and should include broad spectrum intravenous antibiotics. In cases of persistent fevers or clinical deterioration, the addition of antifungal therapy should be considered.
- Surveillance endoscopy should be periodically performed in patients with history of EA, even if asymptomatic, as symptoms do not predict the presence of abnormal findings.

CONFLICTS OF INTEREST

The authors have no conflicts of interest or funding sources to disclose.

REFERENCES

1. Shaw-Smith C. Oesophageal atresia, tracheo-oesophageal fistula, and the VACTERL association: review of genetics and epidemiology. J Med Genet 2006; 43(7):545–54.
2. Pinheiro PFM, e Silva ACS, Pereira RM. Current knowledge on esophageal atresia. World J Gastroenterol 2012;18(28):3662–72.
3. Sistonen SJ, Pakarinen MP, Rintala RJ. Long-term results of esophageal atresia: Helsinki experience and review of literature. Pediatr Surg Int 2011;27(11): 1141–9.
4. Wang B, Tashiro J, Allan BJ, et al. A nationwide analysis of clinical outcomes among newborns with esophageal atresia and tracheoesophageal fistulas in the United States. J Surg Res 2014;190(2):604–12.
5. Sfeir R, Bonnard A, Khen-Dunlop N, et al. Esophageal atresia: data from a national cohort. J Pediatr Surg 2013;48(8). https://doi.org/10.1016/j.jpedsurg. 2013.03.075.
6. Evanovich DM, Wang JT, Zendejas B, et al. From the ground up: esophageal atresia types, disease severity stratification and survival rates at a single institution. Front Surg 2022;9:799052.
7. Pedersen RN, Calzolari E, Husby S, et al. Oesophageal atresia: prevalence, prenatal diagnosis and associated anomalies in 23 European regions. Arch Dis Child 2012;97(3). https://doi.org/10.1136/archdischild-2011-300597.
8. Ein SH, Stringer DA, Stephens CA, et al. Recurrent tracheoesophageal fistulas seventeen-year review. J Pediatr Surg 1983;18(4):436–41.
9. Yasuda JL, Staffa SJ, Ngo PD, et al. Comparison of detection methods for tracheoesophageal fistulae with a novel method: capnography with CO_2 insufflation. J Pediatr Gastroenterol Nutr 2020. https://doi.org/10.1097/MPG. 0000000000002647.
10. Lenz CJ, Bick BL, Katzka D, et al. Esophagorespiratory fistulas: survival and outcomes of treatment. J Clin Gastroenterol 2018;52(2):131–6.
11. Nazir Z, Khan MAM, Qamar J. Recurrent and acquired tracheoesophageal fistulae (TEF)-Minimally invasive management. J Pediatr Surg 2017;52(10): 1688–90.
12. Richter GT, Ryckman F, Brown RL, et al. Endoscopic management of recurrent tracheoesophageal fistula. J Pediatr Surg 2008;43(1):238–45.
13. Meier JD, Sulman CG, Almond PS, et al. Endoscopic management of recurrent congenital tracheoesophageal fistula: a review of techniques and results. Int J Pediatr Otorhinolaryngol 2007;71(5):691–7.

14. Michaud L, Coutenier F, Podevin G, et al. Characteristics and management of congenital esophageal stenosis: Findings from a multicenter study. Orphanet J Rare Dis 2013. https://doi.org/10.1186/1750-1172-8-186.

15. Kawahara H, Imura K, Yagi M, et al. Clinical characteristics of congenital esophageal stenosis distal to associated esophageal atresia. Surgery 2001. https://doi.org/10.1067/msy.2001.109064.

16. Mccann F, Michaud L, Aspirot A, et al. Congenital esophageal stenosis associated with esophageal atresia. Dis Esophagus 2015. https://doi.org/10.1111/dote.12176.

17. Romeo E, Foschia F, De Angelis P, et al. Endoscopic management of congenital esophageal stenosis. J Pediatr Surg 2011. https://doi.org/10.1016/j.jpedsurg.2011.02.010.

18. Nihoul-Fékété C, DeBacker A, Lortat-Jacob S, et al. Congenital esophageal stenosis: a review of 20 cases. Pediatr Surg Int 1987;2(2):86–92.

19. Amae S, Nio M, Kamiyama T, et al. Clinical characteristics and management of congenital esophageal stenosis: A report on 14 cases. J Pediatr Surg 2003. https://doi.org/10.1053/jpsu.2003.50123.

20. Suzuhigashi M, Kaji T, Noguchi H, et al. Current characteristics and management of congenital esophageal stenosis: 40 consecutive cases from a multicenter study in the Kyushu area of Japan. Pediatr Surg Int 2017;33(10):1035–40.

21. Yeung CK, Spitz L, Brereton RJ, et al. Congenital esophageal stenosis due to tracheobronchial remnants: A rare but important association with esophageal atresia. J Pediatr Surg 1992;27(7):852–5.

22. Neilson BIR, Croitoru DP, Guttman FM, et al. Distal congenital esophageal esophageal. J Pediatr Sur 1991;26(4):478–82.

23. Bocus P, Realdon S, Eloubeidi MA, et al. High-frequency miniprobes and 3-dimensional EUS for preoperative evaluation of the etiology of congenital esophageal stenosis in children (with video). Gastrointest Endosc 2011;74(1):204–7.

24. Kouchi BK, Yoshida H, Matsunaga T, et al. Endosonographic Evaluation in Two Children With. J Pediatr Surg 2002;37(6):934–6.

25. Quiros J, Hirose S, Patino M, et al. Esophageal tracheobronchial remnant , endoscopic ultrasound diagnosis, and surgical management. J Pediatr Gastroenterol Nutr 2013;56(3):31826.

26. Terui K, Saito T, Mitsunaga T, et al. Endoscopic management for congenital esophageal stenosis: a systematic review. World J Gastrointest Endosc 2015. https://doi.org/10.4253/wjge.v7.i3.183.

27. Takamizawa S, Tsugawa C, Mouri N, et al. Congenital esophageal stenosis: therapeutic strategy based on etiology. J Pediatr Surg 2002. https://doi.org/10.1053/jpsu.2002.30254.

28. Yasuda JL, Staffa SJ, Clark SJ, et al. Endoscopic incisional therapy and other novel strategies for effective treatment of congenital esophageal stenosis. J Pediatr Surg 2020. https://doi.org/10.1016/j.jpedsurg.2020.01.013.

29. Manfredi MA, Clark SJ, Staffa SJ, et al. Endoscopic esophageal vacuum therapy: a novel therapy for esophageal perforations in pediatric patients. J Pediatr Gastroenterol Nutr 2018. https://doi.org/10.1097/MPG.0000000000002073.

30. Laukoetter MG, Mennigen R, Neumann PA, et al. Successful closure of defects in the upper gastrointestinal tract by endoscopic vacuum therapy (EVT): a prospective cohort study. Surg Endosc Other Interv Tech 2017;31(6):2687–96.

31. Newton NJ, Sharrock A, Rickard R, et al. Systematic review of the use of endo-luminal topical negative pressure in oesophageal leaks and perforations. Dis Esophagus 2017;30(3):1–5.
32. Schniewind B, Schafmayer C, Voehrs G, et al. Endoscopic endoluminal vacuum therapy is superior to other regimens in managing anastomotic leakage after esophagectomy: A comparative retrospective study. Surg Endosc Other Interv Tech 2013;27(10):3883–90.
33. Manfredi MA, Clark SJ, Medford S, et al. Endoscopic electrocautery incisional therapy as a treatment for refractory benign pediatric esophageal strictures. J Pediatr Gastroenterol Nutr 2018;67(4):464–8.
34. Doillon CJ, Dunn MG, Bender E, et al. Collagen fiber formation in repair tissue: development of strength and toughness. Coll Relat Res 1985;5(6):481–92.
35. Baird R, Laberge JM, Lévesque D. Anastomotic stricture after esophageal atresia repair: a critical review of recent literature. Eur J Pediatr Surg 2013; 23(3). https://doi.org/10.1055/s-0033-1347917.
36. Rintala RJ, Pakarinen MP. Long-term outcome of esophageal anastomosis. Eur J Pediatr Surg 2013;23(3). https://doi.org/10.1055/s-0033-1347912.
37. Lévesque D, Baird R, Laberge JM. Refractory strictures post-esophageal atresia repair: What are the alternatives? Dis Esophagus 2013;26(4). https://doi.org/10.1111/dote.12047.
38. Engum SA, Grosfeld JL, West KW, et al. Analysis of morbidity and mortality in 227 cases of esophageal atresia and/or tracheoesophageal fistula over two de-cades. Arch Surg 1995;130(5):502–8 [discussion: 508-9. http://www.ncbi.nlm.nih.gov/pubmed/7748088.
39. Koivusalo AI, Pakarinen MP, Rintala RJ. Modern outcomes of oesophageal atresia: single centre experience over the last twenty years. J Pediatr Surg 2013;48(2):297–303.
40. Lal DR, Gadepalli SK, Downard CD, et al. Perioperative management and out-comes of esophageal atresia and tracheoesophageal fistula. J Pediatr Surg 2017;52(8). https://doi.org/10.1016/j.jpedsurg.2016.11.046.
41. Achildi O, Grewal H. Congenital anomalies of the esophagus. Otolaryngol Clin North Am 2007;40(1). https://doi.org/10.1016/j.otc.2006.10.010.
42. Kunisaki SM, Foker JE. Surgical advances in the fetus and neonate. esophageal atresia. Clin Perinatol 2012;39(2). https://doi.org/10.1016/j.clp.2012.04.007.
43. Krishnan U, Mousa H, Dall'Oglio L, et al. ESPGHAN-NASPGHAN guidelines for the evaluation and treatment of gastrointestinal and nutritional complications in children with esophageal atresia-tracheoesophageal fistula. J Pediatr Gastroen-terol Nutr 2016;63(5). https://doi.org/10.1097/MPG.0000000000001401.
44. Shahein AR, Krasaelap A, Ng K, et al. Esophageal dilation in children: a state of the art review. J Pediatr Gastroenterol Nutr 2022. https://doi.org/10.1097/MPG.0000000000003614.
45. Manfredi MA. Endoscopic management of anastomotic esophageal strictures secondary to esophageal atresia. Gastrointest Endosc Clin N Am 2016;26(1). https://doi.org/10.1016/j.giec.2015.09.002.
46. Hernandez LV, Jacobson JW, Harris MS, et al. Comparison among the perfora-tion rates of Maloney, balloon, and savary dilation of esophageal strictures. Gas-trointest Endosc 2000;51(4 Pt 1):460–2. https://doi.org/10.1016/s0016-5107(00)70448-2.
47. Lew RJ, Kochman ML. A review of endoscopic methods of esophageal dilation. J Clin Gastroenterol 2002;35(2). https://doi.org/10.1097/00004836-200208000-00001.

48. Abele JE. The physics of esophageal dilatation. Hepatogastroenterology 1992; 39(6):486–9.
49. Tokar JL, Barth B, Banarjee S, et al. Tools for endoscopic stricture dilation. Gastrointest Endosc 2013;78(3). https://doi.org/10.1016/j.gie.2013.04.170.
50. Krishnan U, Mousa H, Dall'Oglio L, et al. ESPGHAN-NASPGHAN guidelines for the evaluation and treatment of gastrointestinal and nutritional complications in children with esophageal atresia-tracheoesophageal fistula. J Pediatr Gastroenterol Nutr 2016;63(5):550–70. https://doi.org/10.1097/MPG.0000000000001401.
51. Siersema PD, de Wijkerslooth LR. Dilation of refractory benign esophageal strictures. Gastrointest Endosc 2009;70(5):1000–12.
52. Grooteman KV, Wong Kee, Song LM, Vleggaar FP, et al. Non-adherence to the rule of 3 does not increase the risk of adverse events in esophageal dilation. Gastrointest Endosc 2017;85(2):332–7.e1.
53. Clark SJ, Staffa SJ, Ngo PD, et al. Rules are meant to be broken: examining the "rule of 3" for esophageal dilations in pediatric stricture patients. J Pediatr Gastroenterol Nutr 2020;71(1):e1–5.
54. Yasuda JL, Ngo PD, Staffa SJ, et al. Commentary on "break the rule of three: critical thoughts from a tertiary care experience with bougie dilators. J Pediatr Gastroenterol Nutr 2021;72(1). https://doi.org/10.1097/MPG.0000000000002970.
55. Wallner O, Wallner B. Balloon dilation of benign esophageal rings or strictures: a randomized clinical trial comparing two different inflation times. Dis Esophagus 2014;27(2). https://doi.org/10.1111/dote.12080.
56. Saeed ZA, Winchester CB, Ferro PS, et al. Prospective randomized comparison of polyvinyl bougies and through-the-scope balloons for dilation of peptic strictures of the esophagus. Gastrointest Endosc 1995;41(3). https://doi.org/10.1016/S0016-5107(95)70336-5.
57. Scolapio JS, Pasha TM, Gostout CJ, et al. A randomized prospective study comparing rigid to balloon dilators for benign esophageal strictures and rings. Gastrointest Endosc 1999;50(1). https://doi.org/10.1016/S0016-5107(99)70337-8.
58. Cox JG, Winter RK, Maslin SC, et al. Balloon or bougie for dilatation of benign esophageal stricture? Dig Dis Sci 1994;39(4):776–81.
59. Chiu Y-C, Hsu C-C, Chiu K-W, et al. Factors influencing clinical applications of endoscopic balloon dilation for benign esophageal strictures. Endoscopy 2004;36(7):595–600.
60. Jayakrishnan VK, Wilkinson AG. Treatment of oesophageal strictures in children: a comparison of fluoroscopically guided balloon dilatation with surgical bouginage. Pediatr Radiol 2001;31(2). https://doi.org/10.1007/s002470000368.
61. Mark JA, Anderson BT, Pan Z, et al. Comparative analysis of adverse events after esophageal balloon and bougie dilations in children. J Pediatr Gastroenterol Nutr 2019;68(5):630–4.
62. Kochman ML, McClave SA, Boyce HW. The refractory and the recurrent esophageal stricture: A definition [5]. Gastrointest Endosc 2005;62(3). https://doi.org/10.1016/j.gie.2005.04.050.
63. O'Donnell JEM, Purcell M, Mousa H, et al. Clinician knowledge of societal guidelines on management of gastrointestinal complications in esophageal atresia. J Pediatr Gastroenterol Nutr 2021;72(2):232–8.
64. van Boeckel PGA, Siersema PD. Refractory esophageal strictures: what to do when dilation fails. Curr Treat Options Gastroenterol 2015;13(1). https://doi.org/10.1007/s11938-014-0043-6.

65. Ramage JI, Rumalla A, Baron TH, et al. A prospective, randomized, double-blind, placebo-controlled trial of endoscopic steroid injection therapy for recalcitrant esophageal peptic strictures. Am J Gastroenterol 2005;100(11). https://doi.org/10.1111/j.1572-0241.2005.00331.x.

66. Kochhar R, Makharia GK. Usefulness of intralesional triamcinolone in treatment of benign esophageal strictures. Gastrointest Endosc 2002;56(6). https://doi.org/10.1016/S0016-5107(02)70355-6.

67. Kochhar R, Ray JD, Sriram PV, et al. Intralesional steroids augment the effects of endoscopic dilation in corrosive esophageal strictures. Gastrointest Endosc 1999;49(4 Pt 1):509–13. Available at: http://www.ncbi.nlm.nih.gov/pubmed/10202068.

68. Miyashita M, Onda M, Okawa K, et al. Endoscopic dexamethasone injection following balloon dilatation of anastomotic stricture after esophagogastrostomy. Am J Surg 1997;174(4). https://doi.org/10.1016/S0002-9610(97)00116-5.

69. Gandhi RP, Cooper A, Barlow BA. Successful management of esophageal strictures without resection or replacement. J Pediatr Surg 1989;24(8):745–50. Available at: http://www.ncbi.nlm.nih.gov/pubmed/2769540.

70. Hirdes MMC, van Hooft JE, Koornstra JJ, et al. Endoscopic corticosteroid injections do not reduce dysphagia after endoscopic dilation therapy in patients with benign esophagogastric anastomotic strictures. Clin Gastroenterol Hepatol 2013;11(7). https://doi.org/10.1016/j.cgh.2013.01.016.

71. Ngo PD, Kamran A, Clark SJ, et al. Intralesional Steroid Injection therapy for esophageal anastomotic stricture following esophageal atresia repair. J Pediatr Gastroenterol Nutr 2019. https://doi.org/10.1097/MPG.0000000000002562.

72. Uhlen S, Fayoux P, Vachin F, et al. Mitomycin C: an alternative conservative treatment for refractory esophageal stricture in children? Endoscopy 2006;38(4):404–7. https://doi.org/10.1055/s-2006-925054.

73. Spier BJ, Sawma VA, Gopal DV, et al. Intralesional mitomycin C: successful treatment for benign recalcitrant esophageal stricture. Gastrointest Endosc 2009;69(1):152–3 [discussion: 153].

74. Bakken JC, Song LMWK, Groen PC De, et al. Use of a fully covered self-expandable metal stent for the treatment of benign esophageal diseases. Gastrointest Endosc 2010;72(4). https://doi.org/10.1016/j.gie.2010.06.028.

75. Chung J, Connolly B, Langer J, et al. Fluoroscopy-guided Topical Application of Mitomycin-C in a Case of Refractory Esophageal Stricture. J Vasc Interv Radiol 2010;21(1). https://doi.org/10.1016/j.jvir.2009.09.016.

76. Rosseneu S, Afzal N, Yerushalmi B, et al. Topical application of mitomycin-C in oesophageal strictures. J Pediatr Gastroenterol Nutr 2007;44(3). https://doi.org/10.1097/MPG.0b013e31802c6e45.

77. Berger M, Ure B, Lacher M. Mitomycin C in the therapy of recurrent esophageal strictures: hype or hope? Eur J Pediatr Surg 2012;22(2):109–16.

78. Ley D, Bridenne M, Gottrand F, et al. Efficacy and safety of the local application of mitomycin C to recurrent esophageal strictures in children. J Pediatr Gastroenterol Nutr 2019;69(5). https://doi.org/10.1097/MPG.0000000000002445.

79. Chapuy L, Pomerleau M, Faure C. Topical mitomycin-C application in recurrent esophageal strictures after surgical repair of esophageal atresia. J Pediatr Gastroenterol Nutr 2014;59(5). https://doi.org/10.1097/MPG.0000000000000352.

80. El-Asmar KM, Hassan MA, Abdelkader HM, et al. Topical mitomycin C can effectively alleviate dysphagia in children with long-segment caustic esophageal strictures. Dis Esophagus 2015;28(5). https://doi.org/10.1111/dote.12218.

81. Sweed AS, Fawaz SA, Ezzat WF, et al. A prospective controlled study to assess the use of mitomycin C in improving the results of esophageal dilatation in post corrosive esophageal stricture in children. Int J Pediatr Otorhinolaryngol 2015; 79(1). https://doi.org/10.1016/j.ijporl.2014.10.024.

82. Ghobrial CM, Eskander AE. Prospective study of the effect of topical application of Mitomycin C in refractory pediatric caustic esophageal strictures. Surg Endosc 2018;32(12). https://doi.org/10.1007/s00464-018-6253-6.

83. Flor MM, Ribeiro IB, Moura DTH De, et al. Efficacy of endoscopic topical mitomycin c application in caustic esophageal strictures in the pediatric population: A systematic review and meta-analysis of randomized controlled trials. Arq Gastroenterol 2021;58(2). https://doi.org/10.1590/S0004-2803.202100000-38.

84. Michaud L, Gottrand F. Anastomotic strictures: conservative treatment. J Pediatr Gastroenterol Nutr 2011;52(SUPPL. 1). https://doi.org/10.1097/MPG. 0b013e3182105ad1.

85. Lo A, Baird R, Angelis P De, et al. Arterioesophageal fistula after stenting for esophageal atresia. J Pediatr Gastroenterol Nutr 2013;56(5). https://doi.org/ 10.1097/MPG.0b013e31824ffd7f.

86. Best C, Sudel B, Foker JE, et al. Esophageal stenting in children: indications, application, effectiveness, and complications. Gastrointest Endosc 2009; 70(6). https://doi.org/10.1016/j.gie.2009.07.022.

87. Broto J, Asensio M, Vernet JM. Results of a new technique in the treatment of severe esophageal stenosis in children: poliflex stents. J Pediatr Gastroenterol Nutr 2003;37(2):203–6. Available at: http://www.ncbi.nlm.nih.gov/pubmed/ 12883312.

88. Zhang C, Yu JM, Fan GP, et al. The use of a retrievable self-expanding stent in treating childhood benign esophageal strictures. J Pediatr Surg 2005;40(3): 501–4.

89. Fallon BP, Overman RE, Geiger JD, et al. Efficacy and risk profile of self-expandable stents in the management of pediatric esophageal pathology. J Pediatr Surg 2019;54(6). https://doi.org/10.1016/j.jpedsurg.2019.02.025.

90. Tandon S, Burnand KM, Coppi P De, et al. Self-expanding esophageal stents for the management of benign refractory esophageal strictures in children: a systematic review and review of outcomes at a single center. J Pediatr Surg 2019;54(12). https://doi.org/10.1016/j.jpedsurg.2019.08.041.

91. Baghdadi O, Yasuda J, Staffa S, et al. Predictors and outcomes of fully covered stent treatment for anastomotic esophageal strictures in esophageal atresia. J Pediatr Gastroenterol Nutr 2022;74(2). https://doi.org/10.1097/MPG. 0000000000003330.

92. Slater BJ, Pimpalwar A, Wesson D, et al. Esophageal stents in children: bridge to surgical repair. Indian J Radiol Imaging 2018;28(2). https://doi.org/10.4103/ ijri.IJRI_313_17.

93. van Halsema EE. Clinical outcomes of self-expandable stent placement for benign esophageal diseases: a pooled analysis of the literature. World J Gastrointest Endosc 2015;7(2). https://doi.org/10.4253/wjge.v7.i2.135.

94. Manfredi MA, Clark SJ, Medford S, et al. Endoscopic electrocautery incisional therapy as a treatment for refractory benign pediatric esophageal strictures. J Pediatr Gastroenterol Nutr 2018. https://doi.org/10.1097/MPG. 0000000000002008.

95. Zimmer J, Eaton S, Murchison LE, et al. State of play: eight decades of surgery for esophageal atresia. Eur J Pediatr Surg 2019;29(1):39–48.

96. van Boeckel PGA, Sijbring A, Vleggaar FP, et al. Systematic review: temporary stent placement for benign rupture or anastomotic leak of the oesophagus. Aliment Pharmacol Ther 2011;33(12):1292–301.
97. Rollins MD, Barnhart DC. Treatment of persistent esophageal leaks in children with removable, covered stents. J Pediatr Surg 2012;47(10):1843–7.
98. Manfredi MA, Jennings RW, Anjum MW, et al. Externally removable stents in the treatment of benign recalcitrant strictures and esophageal perforations in pediatric patients with esophageal atresia. Gastrointest Endosc 2014;80(2):246–52.
99. Lange B, Demirakca S, Kähler G, et al. Experience with fully covered self-expandable metal stents for esophageal leakage in children. Klin Padiatr 2020;232(1):13–9.
100. Chauvet C, Bonnard A, Mosca A, et al. Postsurgical perforation of the esophagus can be treated using a fully covered stent in children. J Pediatr Gastroenterol Nutr 2017;64(2):e38–43.
101. Huang C, Leavitt T, Bayer LR, et al. Effect of negative pressure wound therapy on wound healing. Curr Probl Surg 2014;51(7):301–31.
102. Dhaliwal J, Tobias V, Sugo E, et al. Eosinophilic esophagitis in children with esophageal atresia. Dis Esophagus 2014;27(4):340–7.
103. Krishnan U. Eosinophilic esophagitis in esophageal atresia. Front Pediatr 2019; 7:497.
104. Sistonen SJ, Koivusalo A, Nieminen U, et al. Esophageal morbidity and function in adults with repaired esophageal atresia with tracheoesophageal fistula: A population-based long-term follow-up. Ann Surg 2010;251(6):1167–73.
105. Yasuda JL, Staffa SJ, Nurko S, et al. Pharmacogenomics fail to explain proton pump inhibitor refractory esophagitis in pediatric esophageal atresia. Neurogastroenterol Motil 2022;34(1):e14217.
106. Taylor ACF, Breen KJ, Auldist A, et al. Gastroesophageal reflux and related pathology in adults who were born with esophageal atresia: a long-term follow-up study. Clin Gastroenterol Hepatol 2007;5(6):702–6.
107. Yasuda JL, Clark SJ, Staffa SJ, et al. Esophagitis in pediatric esophageal atresia: acid may not always be the issue. J Pediatr Gastroenterol Nutr 2019; 69(2):163–70.

Endoscopy and Pediatric Pancreatitis

Amit S. Grover, MD[a], Roberto Gugig, MD[b], Monique T. Barakat, MD, PhD[b,c],*

KEYWORDS

- Pancreatitis • Endoscopy • Endoscopic retrograde cholangiopancreatography
- Endoscopic ultrasound • Training • Safety

KEY POINTS

- Pancreatic disease is increasingly common in children and adolescents.
- The endoscopic approaches to the diagnosis and management of pancreatic diseases have emerged as effective and safe for pediatric patients.
- The further evolution of endoscopic approaches to manage pancreatic disease in children and adolescents is on the horizon, with the potential to substantially improve patient care.

INTRODUCTION

Historically, interventional endoscopic procedures which can benefit patients with pancreatitis, such as endoscopic retrograde cholangiopancreatography (ERCP) and endoscopic ultrasonography (EUS), were performed by adult gastroenterologists with advanced endoscopic training. Adult physicians certainly have adequate training to perform the procedures, but they often lack formal training in caring for pediatric patients or pediatric pancreatitis. Adult advanced endoscopists are typically employed by facilities that care exclusively for adults and will either travel to pediatric institutions to perform procedures in an unfamiliar setting or perform pediatric procedures in an adult-focused facility. This approach, when executed well, can be very successful and provide excellent patient care. However, issues can arise in using this model due to limited physician availability, timeliness of care and procedures, and challenges in communication among all involved parties, including pediatric providers, adult proceduralists, and families. In an ideal setting, children should be treated at a center that offers patient- and family-centered endoscopic services, including availability of pediatric-specific monitoring and resuscitation equipment, age, size, and

[a] Division of Gastroenterology, Hepatology and Nutrition, Boston Children's Hospital, Boston, MA 02115, USA; [b] Division of Pediatric Gastroenterology, Lucille Packard Children's Hospital at Stanford University Medical Center, Stanford, CA 94305, USA; [c] Division of Gastroenterology, Stanford University Medical Center, Stanford, CA 94305, USA
* Corresponding author. 300 Pasteur Drive, Mail Code #5244, Stanford, CA 94305.
E-mail address: mbarakat@stanford.edu

Gastrointest Endoscopy Clin N Am 33 (2023) 363–378
https://doi.org/10.1016/j.giec.2022.11.002
1052-5157/23/© 2022 Elsevier Inc. All rights reserved.

weight appropriate endoscopic equipment, trained specialized nursing staff, pediatric anesthesia service providers, behavioral and child life specialists, and pediatric surgical and intensive care expertise if needed.[1,2]

Over the last 15 years, pediatric gastroenterologists have increasingly pursued training in interventional endoscopy. Pediatric ERCP, EUS, and other advanced endoscopic procedures are now performed safely and effectively in specialized centers by pediatric providers worldwide.[3,4] In conjunction with advancements in interventional endoscopy, pediatric pancreatology continues to evolve through increased recognition of acute and chronic pancreatitis (CP) and collaborative approaches to research.[5] It is increasingly important that providers managing children with pancreatitis are aware of the indications for endoscopic evaluations and interventions for pancreatitis, the benefits and risks involved, and when endoscopic therapy is no longer warranted.[6] In this state-of-the art review, the authors discuss the role of ERCP and EUS for pancreatic indications in pediatrics, with a focus on the range of indications for these procedures and the role of equipment, training, and volume on performance of ERCP and EUS for pancreatic indications in pediatric patients.

ENDOSCOPIC RETROGRADE CHOLANGIOPANCREATOGRAPHY IN PEDIATRIC PANCREATITIS

ERCP was first introduced in the 1960s in adults, and the range of applications and the capacity for endoscopic intervention during ERCP has expanded over the intervening decades.[7-9] ERCP is now the mainstay of pancreaticobiliary evaluation and therapy in adult patients, with biliary surgical interventions such as bile duct exploration and some interventional radiology interventions being phased out of the management of some biliary disorders.[10]

ERCP in the pediatric population has lagged somewhat relative to the adult experience, with the first pediatric ERCP performed in the 1970s. Still, early studies have been conducted and attest to the feasibility, safety, and diagnostic utility of ERCP in children and adolescents.[11-13] When ERCP was first introduced in pediatrics, it was almost exclusively performed by high-volume fellowship trained advanced endoscopists who primarily focus on performing the procedure in adult patients. As the utility of pediatric ERCP has expanded, it has become clear that ERCP is ideally performed by high-volume advanced endoscopists in a tertiary care setting with highly trained and specialized staff supporting the technical aspects of the procedure.

Some factors which have limited utilization of ERCP in children include patient size, limitations in pediatric endoscopist training, and the fact that the pediatric population is smaller relative to the adult population, with an understandably lower prevalence of pancreaticobiliary disorders in children.

Equipment Size Considerations

Challenges associated with the mismatch between adult-designed duodenoscopes and ERCP devices and pediatric-sized patients are notable. With respect to patient size, standard-sized duodenoscopes have been used in children heavier than 15 kg.[14,15] For infants, the infant duodenoscope manufactured by Olympus (Olympus Corp, Center Valley, PA, USA) with a 7.5-mm outer diameter and a 2-mm working channel that was typically used for the smallest children is being withdrawn from use, without a clear replacement scope on the horizon. This severely limits the performance of ERCP in the infants with biliary indications for ERCP. Other duodenoscopes used for smaller children, including the "diagnostic" duodenoscope (JF-140R, Olympus) with an outer diameter of 11 mm and a working channel size of 3.2 mm, have limited availability and technical utility for ERCP and are being phased out due to concerns associated with their closed elevator and potential for harboring and propagation of duodenoscope-transmitted infection.

Training in Pediatric Endoscopic Retrograde Cholangiopancreatography

In terms of training, pathways for gaining expertise in performing pediatric ERCP are not well-defined. This has limited utilization of pediatric ERCP—particularly performance of ERCP by pediatric gastroenterologists. Unlike adult advanced endoscopy fellowships, which are characterized by a formal applicant/institution match program sponsored by the American Society for Gastrointestinal Endoscopy (ASGE), training opportunities for pediatric advanced endoscopists are less formally organized.[16–19] Most pediatric advanced endoscopists practicing today received their training from adult advanced endoscopists, often outside of the United States. These training pathways are often in the form of a preceptorship, and sometimes involve a partnership between an advanced adult endoscopist and an aspiring pediatric advanced endoscopist at the same institution. Although some institutions have initiated pediatric-specific advanced endoscopy training programs, this remains a limited and very recently introduced pathway for training and most pediatric advanced endoscopists are trained through the more ad hoc approaches described above. In addition, although ERCP curricula and competency assessment tools have been developed for adult ERCP and competence thresholds (ie, recommended minimum volume of procedures before competence can be reliably assessed and for maintenance of competence) have been defined, this has not been the case in Pediatrics.[20–22] Competency thresholds related to pediatric ERCP is lacking, and whether volume standards for initial assessment of competency and maintenance of competence should differ for adult and pediatric patients, remains an area of debate.

Of note, challenges associated with pediatric ERCP training do not end when a fully ERCP-trained pediatric gastroenterologist enters practice. In those institutions where pediatric ERCP is performed, it is often not performed in volumes high enough to support optimal technical competency of those trained in pediatric ERCP or to support the training of other providers. The future of pediatric advanced endoscopy training and practice remains uncertain and may include partnership with adult endoscopists, coupled with a few high-volume tertiary care pediatric centers of excellence where the most complex pediatric endoscopy procedures are performed.

Associated Adverse Events and Safety

Outcome studies of pediatric ERCP, until recently, largely comprise single-center experiences and voluntary reporting of procedure outcomes in multicenter databases.[23–26] As pediatric ERCP differs in both most common indications and patient/endoscopist characteristics relative to adult ERCP, practice patterns of pediatric ERCP in North America were, until recently, largely uncharacterized. Some work has been conducted to evaluate pediatric ERCP safety in the United States, including a recent all-capture population-level study of pediatric ERCP procedures performed in the United States, free from endoscopist, single-center or region-level bias, which affirmed the overall safety of ERCP.[27] This study also identified some patient characteristics that were associated with increased odds of readmission following the ERCP hospitalization, including patients with a history of liver transplant, patients between 0 and 4 year old, of male gender and with a medical history notable for obesity.[27] Furthermore, patients in both urban teaching and urban hospitals had much lower odds than those in rural hospitals for prolonged length of stay associated with ERCP. The urban setting is often used as a surrogate for tertiary/academic medical centers, and these urban centers tend to be the highest volume centers. A volume-outcomes relationship has been well established for adult ERCP, with higher volume centers and providers performing ERCP more successfully and safely, with higher technical success rates and lower adverse event rates.[28] These pediatric population level data represent an initial suggestion that the same volume–outcomes relationship is likely true for pediatric ERCP.

Pancreatitis-Associated Endoscopic Retrograde Cholangiopancreatography Indications

Acute recurrent pancreatitis

Acute pancreatitis (AP) is a common gastrointestinal indication for hospitalization in both adults and children, with over 285,000 annual hospitalizations.[29–33] AP causes severe pain and carries the risk of permanent morbidity and mortality.[32,33] About one-quarter of patients with AP develop acute recurrent pancreatitis (ARP), and a subset of these patients progress to CP, which is also associated with substantial longer term morbidity.[34,35] Following workup for genetic etiologies of pancreatitis, and evaluation for other physiologic triggers of pancreatitis, ERCP performance is part of the standard of care in children with ARP to evaluate and treat factors that may be contributing to recurrent pancreatitis. Some of these contributing factors may include microlithiasis leading to intermittent biliary obstruction and anatomic variation in the pancreatic ductal anatomy that results in the relative obstruction of outflow of pancreatic fluid. For most people, pancreatic fluid is drained from the pancreas by the main pancreatic duct through the major papilla.

For those with pancreas divisum, by contrast, the minor pancreatic duct drains most of the pancreatic parenchyma through its tiny orifice—the minor papilla and this has been hypothesized to lead to a backup of pancreatic fluid with a concomitant increase in intraductal pressures.[36,37] There is some controversy surrounding the role of pancreas divisum in ARP, in part stemming from the fact that pancreas divisum is a common congenital variant that is present in roughly 7% of the general population.[38,39] However, recent reports in children and adults show an estimated twofold increased prevalence of pancreas divisum among patients with pancreatitis.[38,40,41] ERCP with minor papilla endoscopic sphincterotomy (miES) is often performed to relieve obstruction of pancreatic fluid outflow—a practice that is supported by adult and pediatric case series',[42–46] and a small published clinical trial in the adult literature.[47] However, it must be stressed that miES remains a high risk intervention given that it is associated with one of the highest rates of post-ERCP pancreatitis.

Because the practice of ERCP with miES remains controversial, investigation of the role of ERCP with miES in patients with pancreas divisum is underway. In 2018, a sham-controlled, single-blinded, multicenter, randomized clinical trial of ERCP with miES for the treatment of ARP in the setting of PD was initiated and is enrolling adult patients (Sphincterotomy for Acute Recurrent Pancreatitis , NCT03609944, co-led by Greg Cote, MD and Dhiraj Yadav, MD).[48,49] Although data from this trial may inform pediatric practice to some extent, the phenotype of children with pancreatitis distinctly differs from that of adults with pancreatitis. Genetic risk factors for pancreatitis are more common in children than adults, sometimes concomitant with another pancreatitis risk factor.[50–53] The role of ERCP in pediatric patients with ARP and ARP patients with pancreas divisum remains an area in need of further intensive study.

Gallstone pancreatitis

Biliary disease, including gallstones and microlithiasis, is the most common cause of AP in children, accounting for up to 30% of cases.[54] The mainstay of initial therapy for all types of AP remains supportive with aggressive fluid resuscitation, adequate analgesia, nutritional support, and close observation.[55] The early diagnosis of gallstone pancreatitis, however, remains crucial in regard to management as a proportion of cases in pediatrics, albeit small, can go on to develop a more severe phenotype and associated complications, namely necrotizing pancreatitis and/or cholangitis.

The basis for early ERCP with endoscopic sphincterotomy (ES) in gallstone pancreatitis stems from classic reports in the literature, which have suggested that the duration of ampullary obstruction is a major factor in determining the severity of pancreatitis in adults, with severe disease being more likely when obstruction lasts greater than 48 hours.[56,57] Substantial literature exists examining role of early or urgent ERCP and ES in acute biliary pancreatitis (ABP) in adults. While the indication for ERCP in the setting of cholangitis is well established, the use of this interventional strategy in its absence remains controversial. This is underscored in pediatrics, as there has been a dearth of research in this population. The importance of early identification of ABP has been addressed in pediatrics,[58] along with the predictors of choledocholithiasis.[59] Despite this, however, studies have also suggested that choledocholithiasis in children, albeit frequent, may resolve spontaneously, obviating ERCP with ES in the ABP pre-cholecystectomy scenario.[60]

Currently, no pediatric consensus guidelines exist as to the role of ERCP in ABP or the optimal timing.[55] The most current American Gastroenterological Association guideline recommend against the use of urgent ERCP in the setting of ABP without cholangitis.[61] In addition, the ASGE guideline on the management of choledocholithiasis also strongly recommend against early ERCP in those with gallstone pancreatitis without cholangitis or biliary obstruction, given the lack of benefit and potential for increased procedure-related harm.[62] Despite these consensus guidelines, it remains unclear whether urgent ERCP with ES improves the outcome of patients with severe ABP without concomitant cholangitis.[63] To address this, a recent multicenter randomized controlled superiority trial[64] concluded that in adult patients with severe gallstone pancreatitis, but without cholangitis, when compared with conservative management ERCP with ES did not reduce mortality. Although data are limited in pediatrics, extrapolating from adult literature it seems that if the episode of ABP is mild, early ERCP with sphincterotomy can be avoided unless the patient progresses to develop worsening signs of necrotizing pancreatitis or cholangitis. Whether or not to intervene in severe biliary pancreatitis in pediatrics, however, warrants further study and investigation.

Chronic pancreatitis and pancreatic duct stones

ERCP and EUS are the principal endoscopic methods to assess patients with CP and complement radiologic methods (computed tomography [CT] scans, MRI, and magnetic resonance cholangiopancreatography [MRCP]). Although ERCP can establish the diagnosis of CP,[7] ERCP should be reserved for patients in whom the diagnosis is still unclear after noninvasive pancreatic function testing or other noninvasive (CT, MRI) or less invasive (EUS) imaging studies have been performed.[65] ERCP has a sensitivity of 71% to 93% and a specificity of 89% to 100% for establishing the diagnosis of CP.[66] ERCP is highly effective in visualizing ductal findings and enables detection of pancreatic duct changes, including ductal dilation, strictures, abnormal side branches, communicating pseudocysts, pancreatic duct stones, and pancreatic duct leaks. The Cambridge Classification, which assesses the main pancreatic duct and side branches, is a widely accepted system for scoring ductal findings seen on ERCP.[66]

Unfortunately, pancreatography is imperfect and care should be taken not to over interpret minor findings seen on ERCP. Conversely, ERCP may not detect changes of less advanced CP. Although ERCP can be used to obtain information about ductal anatomy to define the level and degree of obstruction and the presence of strictures and stones, it does not provide information regarding the surrounding pancreatic parenchyma. EUS, alternatively, can provide high-resolution images of both the ductal structures and parenchyma.[67] There is good interobserver agreement in the diagnosis of CP by EUS in adult patients, and EUS may detect early CP in a reliable manner compared with ERCP.[68]

Pancreatic duct stones

Obstructing pancreatic duct stones may contribute to abdominal pain or attacks of AP in patients with underlying CP. ERCP provides direct access to the pancreatic duct for evaluation and treatment of symptomatic pancreatic duct stones. In one randomized trial comparing endoscopic and surgical therapy, surgery was superior for long-term pain reduction in patients with painful obstructive CP.[69] However, because of its lower degree of invasiveness, endotherapy may be preferred, reserving surgery as second-line therapy for patients in whom endoscopic therapy fails or is ineffective.

Pancreatic stone removal can be challenging. Frequently the stone configuration and size, coupled with pancreatic duct strictures, occlude the lumen. Adjuvant endoscopic approaches such as stricture dilation, intraductal lithotripsy and pancreatic sphincterotomy may be needed. Even when accessible, pancreatic duct stones (which are often dense and hardened) may be impacted, requiring extracorporeal shock wave lithotripsy to fragment the stones before endoscopic removal can be achieved.[70] Intraductal lithotripsy guided by pancreatoscopy has also been used to fragment pancreatic stones.

Most series have shown improvement in pain with pancreatic endotherapy. Some encouraging short-term results and long-term 5 years follow-up results showing improvements in pain (77%–100% and 54%–86%, respectively) have been reported in adults.[71] Although modest, these success rates are acceptable in the context of traditionally difficult to manage groups of patients.

Pancreatic duct leaks

Pancreatic duct disruptions or leaks can occur secondary to severe AP or CP. The causes of the disruption are usually severe inflammation or obstruction of the duct or severe pancreatic necrosis. Pancreatic leaks can result in pancreatic ascites, pleural effusions, pseudocyst formation, and internal and external pancreatic fistulas. Pancreatic duct leaks can often be treated with endoscopic placement of transpapillary stents in a similar manner to the use of biliary stents for closing bile duct leaks.[72] Endoscopic therapy is successful in closing the leaks in approximately 60% of patients in adult studies. Factors associated with a better outcome in duct disruption include a partial disruption, successfully bridging the disruption with a stent and longer duration of stent placement (approximately 6 weeks). There are no comparative studies of surgical, medical, and endoscopic therapy for treatment of pancreatic duct leaks.

A novel treatment approach using endoscopic injection of N-butyl-2-cyanoacrylate to achieve closure of the fistula has also been reported in adult patients.[73] Inadvertent injection of the cyanoacrylate into the pancreatic duct at the time of glue injection into a pancreatic fistula can be associated with chemical or obstructive pancreatitis. In contrast, the injection of glue to completely fill a disconnected ductal system usually results in glandular atrophy and has been used to avoid surgical resection in high-risk patients by some institutions.[74]

Pancreatic trauma and duct disruption

The pancreas is the least commonly injured solid organ following blunt abdominal trauma in children, with reported injury rates ranging from 0.12% to 0.7%; therefore, many centers have limited experience managing these complicated injuries.[75] Management of blunt pancreatic trauma hinges on the ability of the trauma team to accurately diagnose and manage pancreatic ductal disruption. In general, nonoperative management is favored for low-grade pancreatic injury (American Association for the Surgery of Trauma grades I and II injuries which do not involve injury to the pancreatic duct). However, there is a lack of consensus regarding the optimal management of high-grade injuries involving the pancreatic duct, especially grade III injuries which involve the pancreatic body.[75]

In these cases, either operative or nonoperative strategies can be used. Unfortunately, differentiating a grade II injury from a grade III injury requires demonstration of pancreatic duct disruption on cross-sectional imaging. The sensitivity of 16 and 64 multidetector CT imaging to detect duct injury is reported at 54% and 52%, respectively, making their use limited for the diagnosis of pancreatic duct injuries, especially in small children with small glands.[76] In addition, serum chemistries (amylase and lipase) have not been shown to correlate directly with duct injury, and therefore are not generally helpful when grading injuries.[77]

ERCP provides a method of diagnosing pancreatic duct integrity. Its use has also been described for therapeutic purposes using stent placement to attempt to decrease pancreatic duct leak.[78] ERCP utilization for diagnosis and treatment of pancreatic injuries in the pediatric population is based mainly on retrospective, small, single-center studies.

The use of ERCP for pancreatic trauma was first suggested in 1986 based on a series by Hall and colleagues, in which he identified four pancreatic duct injuries using ERCP. ERCP has been shown to be safe and effective in diagnosing ductal injuries in pediatric patients, and several studies have shown that ERCP has a role in the diagnosis and management of pancreatic injuries.[79,80] In pediatric patients, the diagnosis of pancreatic injuries can be challenging, especially when determining whether duct injury has occurred. Timely and accurate diagnosis and treatment can improve morbidity and mortality and are therefore essential.[81] Compared with cross-sectional imaging modalities, ERCP is the most accurate method in the diagnosis of ductal injuries.[82]

In one of the largest series evaluating the use of ERCP in pediatric pancreatic injuries, Houben and colleagues described 15 children with traumatic pancreatic injuries from 1999 to 2004 who all had delayed presentations (48 hour from injury). Nine received stents owing to ductal injury or development of a symptomatic fluid collection.[79] Two patients were unable to have a stent placed owing to technical difficulties. Four patients required a second endoscopy to exchange stents to a larger caliber. Four required external drainage of a pseudocyst owing to continued pain, and two required cystogastrostomy despite pancreatic stent placement. Minor complications noted after ERCP included transient increases in serum amylase ($n = 5$) and an exacerbation in epigastric pain for up to 48 hours ($n = 2$).[79]

Rosen and colleagues reported an overall complication rate of 10% following ERCP in a series of 215 pediatric patients, with higher rates in children less than 4 year old, those undergoing a sphincterotomy, or after pancreatic duct cannulation.[83] Additional described complications of stent placement include stricture, occlusion, migration, duodenal erosion, and infection. Furthermore, unsuccessful duct cannulation (up to 14% in published pediatric series) can be considered to be a complication, as it required an unnecessary anesthetic and potential risk of ERCP.[83] This is likely owing to severe inflammation causing duodenal distortion and is certainly a consideration when ERCP is only performed for diagnostic indications, as MRCP may be an alternative in these cases.

ENDOSCOPIC ULTRASONOGRAPHY IN PEDIATRIC PANCREATITIS

As noted earlier, similar factors to those described for pediatric ERCP have limited broad utilization of EUS in children and adolescents. These factors include patient size, limitations in pediatric endoscopist training, and the smaller pediatric population with lower prevalence of pancreaticobiliary disorders in children. These factors will be briefly discussed here in the context of EUS.

Equipment Size Considerations

With respect to patient size, available standard-sized echoendoscopes (12.1–14.6 mm outer diameter) have been used in children as young as 2 year old and may be reasonably used for patients over 15 kg, so EUS is highly likely to be feasible in fairly young patients even with existing equipment.[4,14,15] Introduction and development of newly available ultra-slim echoendoscopes as well as compatible accessories carry the potential to facilitate EUS-based diagnosis and intervention in even younger and smaller children in coming years.

Training in Pediatric Endoscopic Ultrasonography

Pediatric endoscopy training limitations represent a very significant challenge to integration of EUS into mainstream pediatric gastroenterology practice. Most pediatric gastroenterologists—even those who are pediatric advanced endoscopists—did not learn endosonography in their training and do not have access to appropriate equipment to perform the procedure or a well-trained endoscopy technician support to successfully execute the procedure. EUS is currently performed even less frequently than ERCP in pediatrics and is only performed at a subset of pediatric institutions.[84] These challenges surrounding pediatric EUS volume and training necessitate creative approaches for successful performance of EUS by pediatric endoscopists. These creative approaches may include training abroad, establishment of dedicated pediatric endoscopy training programs in partnership with adult endoscopy programs, partnership with adult endoscopists and/or simulation and digital training approaches for EUS training and maintenance of competency.

Associated Adverse Events and Safety

It is worthwhile underscoring the fact that diagnostic EUS procedures are quite safe. A recent population level study evaluating safety and quality metrics of EUS procedures in adult patients found that EUS was safely performed in all community and academic contexts evaluated, including in low-volume settings.[85] This study found, however, that the quality metrics for EUS improved with higher institutional EUS volume (operationalized as need for re-biopsy after initial attempted biopsy of a lesion with EUS).[85] Therapeutic EUS performed, for example, for management of pancreatic fluid collections and necrosis, is associated with higher risk that varies based on factors that may include clinical context/indication, patient comorbidities, and endoscopist experience. Therapeutic EUS risk is less likely to be generalizable from adult to pediatric patients.

In the largest pediatric EUS series to date, a total of 306 diagnostic and therapeutic EUS procedures were analyzed.[4] Among these procedures, there were no major EUS-associated adverse events. Technical success of diagnostic and therapeutic EUS procedures was over 95%. These high rates of success and low rates of adverse events are reassuring, though they underscore that pediatric EUS is largely being performed when the success of these procedures is nearly certain.[4] Ideally, as familiarity and comfort with EUS in pediatrics expands, novel and more ambitious EUS applications could be considered and attempted in pediatric patients, leading to overall expansion of EUS utilization, but with understandable reduction in technical success rates and potential modest increase in adverse event rates.

Pancreatitis-Associated Diagnostic Endoscopic Ultrasonography

The utility of both diagnostic and therapeutic EUS in pancreaticobiliary disorders is well established. As there has been a rising incidence in pediatric pancreatic disorders in the past decade,[5] it is no surprise that the role of diagnostic EUS has also grown in the pediatric population. EUS provides a detailed anatomic evaluation of not only the pancreas and liver but also surrounding organs and tissues as well as the layered walls of the gastrointestinal tract.[86,87] Sampling of tissue to aid in diagnosis of pancreaticobiliary disease or malignancy can also be performed with fine needle aspiration or core biopsy. EUS has also been demonstrated to be safe and effective in the care of children.[88]

Two types of EUS imaging exist, radial and curvilinear. A radial echoendoscope provides a 360° view perpendicular to the tissue, analogous to an axial CT scan but does not allow for submucosal tissue sampling, whereas a curvilinear array echoendoscope provides a 180° view, parallel to the transducer and offers the ability to sample submucosal tissue.[89] Although the indications for EUS are varied and extensive, the largest indication in pediatrics has remained for the evaluation and management of pancreaticobiliary diseases.[88,89] Although cystic and malignant pancreatic lesions are rare, there is a role for EUS in pediatric patients with both AP and more often CP.

Common findings in CP on noninvasive imaging studies, such as CT and MRI, include parenchymal calcifications, ductal changes, or pancreatic atrophy.[90] The benefit of EUS, however, stems in its capacity to identify subtle parenchymal or ductal alterations not picked up on conventional radiographic imaging.[6] Characteristic findings of CP identifiable on EUS include focal or diffuse changes in the pancreatic parenchyma (echogenic foci or stranding, small cystic cavities, lobularity, heterogeneous parenchyma, calcifications) and/or pancreatic duct (dilation, irregularity, hyperechoic walls, side-branch ectasia, echogenic foci, or stones).[86] The combination of these findings are what make up the Rosemount Criteria, the most recognized classification system for the diagnosis of CP via EUS in adults.[91] Although debate exists as to the criterion standard for the diagnosis of CP, a recent meta-analysis concluded that the combination of EUS (and ERCP) outperform MRI, CT, and transabdominal US in imaging modalities. Diagnostic EUS also compares favorably to histologic data and pancreatic function testing.[86] Despite the various adult criterion used in the diagnosis of CP, currently no pediatric EUS criteria exist.

Autoimmune pancreatitis (AIP), a distinct type of pancreatitis, occurs in children and has characteristic findings on radiographic imaging, often presenting with pancreatic head enlargement, or nonencapsulated mass-like lesions.[92] As treatment of AIP consists of corticosteroid therapy, it is imperative that AIP is differentiated from similar appearing pancreatic malignant tumors seen in children, namely pancreatoblastoma or solid pseudopapillary epithelial neoplasm or lymphoma, before initiating steroids. The efficacy of EUS with fine-needle biopsy in the diagnosis of AIP has been demonstrated[93] and herein lies a prime example demonstrating the utility of EUS in pediatric pancreatic disorders. A child who presents with radiographic imaging equivocal for AIP can now undergo EUS with fine-needle biopsy, which may confirm or rule out a diagnosis thereby avoiding what would have been, in the past, a more invasive surgical biopsy and/or resection in favor of medical therapy.

Pancreatitis-Associated Therapeutic Endoscopic Ultrasonography

As pediatric EUS continues to grow, so do the indications. Concomitant advances in technology, improvements echoendoscope scope size and smaller devices/accessories that allow for more therapeutic interventions are now becoming available to the practicing pediatric advanced endoscopist.

Therapeutic EUS interventions in pediatric patients have predominantly focused on transluminal drainage of pancreatic fluid collections. Although heterogeneity exists in the types of fluid collection based on contents and timing relative to the inciting event,[94] symptomatic pediatric patients will often require drainage of these collections. Percutaneous interventions are still widely accepted; however, endoscopic-based drainage is now the first line for symptomatic or infected pseudocysts or walled off necrotic collections in adults. Pediatric reports have also demonstrated the safety and feasibility of endoscopic drainage procedures.[95] The general consensus is that intervention should be delayed until a mature wall has developed around the fluid collection.[96,97] Using the curvilinear echoendoscope within either the stomach or duodenum, the location, size, and wall maturity of the pancreatic fluid collection can be identified. Overlying Doppler flow can identify any intervening vasculature structures during the creation of a cyst gastrostomy or cyst duodenostomy. Both plastic and metal stents have been used to facilitate drainage as reported in the pediatric literature;[98,99] and more recently there has been a shift toward the usage of lumen apposing metal stents for fluid drainage of larger collections.[100] Although many case reports and small sample studies exist, there remains a dearth of comparative prospective studies in pediatrics examining the various methods of transluminal cyst drainage.

EUS has also been used in pain management for CP through EUS-guided celiac plexus block/neurolysis. The aim is to deliver local anesthetic along with corticosteroid to the celiac plexus, which normally transmits visceral pain signals from upper abdominal organs including the pancreas. Unfortunately, adult data supporting the benefit of celiac plexus block are lacking.[101] Recent reports in pediatrics, however, have reported positive results with celiac plexus block/neurolysis for management of chronic pain.[4] Knowing that pediatric and adult pathophysiology differs, the role of EUS-guided celiac plexus block warrants further study in the pediatric population with CP.

SUMMARY

The incidence of pancreatic disease in children has grown over the past decade, and the scope of diagnostic and treatment options has paralleled. Once an unheard of disease in children, pancreatitis is more recognized now that it has ever been. Most pediatric centers across North America have programs devoted to pancreatic care; and although management remains predominantly medical, complex disease is associated with complex outcomes and complications. This has concurrently fueled the growth of advancement and innovation in pediatric endoscopy. Looking to our adult counterparts, the fields of endoscopy and pancreatic disease not only overlap but also exist in an intertwined state. One does not exist without the other, and growth, advancement, and innovation cannot occur without the other. There has been a shift in pediatric endoscopic training, with more trainees interested in pancreatic disorders as well as therapeutic endoscopy. We are just at the tip of the iceberg in regard to the growing field of pediatric advanced endoscopy and pancreatic disorders and it is clear the future looks bright.

CLINICS CARE POINTS

- Pediatric interventional endoscopic procedures have become more widely available for children and adolescents with pancreatitis and other pancreatic disorders.
- The safety and efficacy of these endoscopic procedures—particularly endoscopic retrograde cholangiopancreatography (ERCP) and endoscopic ultrasound (EUS) —are increasingly studied.
- Studies to date support the safety of both ERCP and EUS for pediatric patients in the context of pancreatic disorders.

DISCLOSURE

None of the authors have any conflicts of interest pertaining to the study to disclose.

REFERENCES

1. Troendle DM, Barth BA. ERCP can be safely and effectively performed by a pediatric gastroenterologist for choledocholithiasis in a pediatric facility. J Pediatr Gastroenterol Nutr 2013;57(5):655–8.
2. Lightdale JR, et al. Pediatric endoscopy quality improvement network quality standards and indicators for pediatric endoscopy facilities: a joint NASP-GHAN/ESPGHAN guideline. J Pediatr Gastroenterol Nutr 2022;74(S1 Suppl 1):S16–29.
3. Troendle DM, Barth BA. Pediatric considerations in endoscopic retrograde cholangiopancreatography. Gastrointest Endosc Clin N Am 2016;26(1):119–36.
4. Barakat MT, Cagil Y, Gugig R. Landscape of pediatric endoscopic ultrasound in a united states tertiary care medical center. J Pediatr Gastroenterol Nutr 2022;74(5):657–61.
5. Uc A, Husain SZ. Pancreatitis in Children. Gastroenterology 2019;156(7):1969–78.
6. Liu QY, et al. The Roles of endoscopic ultrasound and endoscopic retrograde cholangiopancreatography in the evaluation and treatment of chronic pancreatitis in children: a position paper from the north american society for pediatric gastroenterology, hepatology, and nutrition pancreas committee. J Pediatr Gastroenterol Nutr 2020;70(5):681–93.
7. Adler DG, et al. ASGE guideline: the role of ERCP in diseases of the biliary tract and the pancreas. Gastrointest Endosc 2005;62(1):1–8.
8. Cotton PB. Cannulation of the papilla of Vater by endoscopy and retrograde cholangiopancreatography (ERCP). Gut 1972;13(12):1014–25.
9. Cotton PB, Beales JS. The role of endoscopic retrograde cholangiopancreatography (ERCP) in patients with jaundice. Acta Gastroenterol Belg 1973;36(12):689–92.
10. Huang RJ, et al. Evolution in the utilization of biliary interventions in the United States: results of a nationwide longitudinal study from 1998 to 2013. Gastrointest Endosc 2017;86(2):319–26.e5.

11. Buckley A, Connon JJ. The role of ERCP in children and adolescents. Gastrointest Endosc 1990;36(4):369–72.
12. Varadarajulu S, et al. Technical outcomes and complications of ERCP in children. Gastrointest Endosc 2004;60(3):367–71.
13. Bang JY, Varadarajulu S. Pediatrics: ERCP in children. Nat Rev Gastroenterol Hepatol 2011;8(5):254–5.
14. Asge Technology C, et al. Echoendoscopes. Gastrointest Endosc 2007;66(3): 435–42.
15. Committee AT, et al. Equipment for pediatric endoscopy. Gastrointest Endosc 2012;76(1):8–17.
16. Bisschops R, et al. Correction: European Society of Gastrointestinal Endoscopy (ESGE) curricula development for postgraduate training in advanced endoscopic procedures: rationale and methodology. Endoscopy 2019;51(10):C6.
17. Bisschops R, et al. European Society of Gastrointestinal Endoscopy (ESGE) curricula development for postgraduate training in advanced endoscopic procedures: rationale and methodology. Endoscopy 2019;51(10):976–9.
18. Committee AT, et al. Endoscopic retrograde cholangiopancreatography (ERCP): core curriculum. Gastrointest Endosc 2016;83(2):279–89.
19. Qayed E, et al. Advanced endoscopy fellowship training in the United States: recent trends in American Society for Gastrointestinal Endoscopy advanced endoscopy fellowship match, trainee experience, and postfellowship employment. Gastrointest Endosc 2021;93(6):1207–1214 e2.
20. Wani S, et al. Competence in Endoscopic Ultrasound and Endoscopic Retrograde Cholangiopancreatography, From Training Through Independent Practice. Gastroenterology 2018;155(5):1483–1494 e7.
21. Siau K, et al. ERCP assessment tool: evidence of validity and competency development during training. Endoscopy 2019;51(11):1017–26.
22. Wani S, et al. Setting minimum standards for training in EUS and ERCP: results from a prospective multicenter study evaluating learning curves and competence among advanced endoscopy trainees. Gastrointest Endosc 2019;89(6): 1160–1168 e9.
23. Yildirim AE, et al. The safety and efficacy of ERCP in the pediatric population with standard scopes: Does size really matter? Springerplus 2016;5:128.
24. Giefer MJ, Kozarek RA. Technical outcomes and complications of pediatric ERCP. Surg Endosc 2015;29(12):3543–50.
25. Halvorson L, et al. The safety and efficacy of therapeutic ERCP in the pediatric population performed by adult gastroenterologists. Dig Dis Sci 2013;58(12): 3611–9.
26. Issa H, Al-Haddad A, Al-Salem AH. Diagnostic and therapeutic ERCP in the pediatric age group. Pediatr Surg Int 2007;23(2):111–6.
27. Barakat MT, et al. Nationwide evolution of pediatric endoscopic retrograde cholangiopancreatography indications, utilization, and readmissions over time. J Pediatr 2021;232:159–165 e1.
28. Huang RJ, et al. Unplanned hospital encounters after endoscopic retrograde cholangiopancreatography in 3 large north American States. Gastroenterology 2019;156(1):119–129 e3.
29. Brindise E, et al. Temporal trends in incidence and outcomes of acute pancreatitis in hospitalized patients in the United States From 2002 to 2013. Pancreas 2019;48(2):169–75.
30. Garg SK, et al. Incidence, admission rates, and predictors, and economic burden of adult emergency visits for acute pancreatitis: data from the national

emergency department sample, 2006 to 2012. J Clin Gastroenterol 2019;53(3): 220–5.

31. Sellers ZM, et al. Nationwide trends in acute and chronic pancreatitis among privately insured children and non-elderly adults in the United States, 2007-2014. Gastroenterology 2018;155(2):469–478 e1.

32. Peery AF, et al. Burden of gastrointestinal, liver, and pancreatic diseases in the United States. Gastroenterology 2015;149(7):1731–1741 e3.

33. Yadav D, Lowenfels AB. The epidemiology of pancreatitis and pancreatic cancer. Gastroenterology 2013;144(6):1252–61.

34. Bang UC, et al. Mortality, cancer, and comorbidities associated with chronic pancreatitis: a Danish nationwide matched-cohort study. Gastroenterology 2014;146(4):989–94.

35. Sankaran SJ, et al. Frequency of progression from acute to chronic pancreatitis and risk factors: a meta-analysis. Gastroenterology 2015;149(6):1490–1500 e1.

36. Cotton PB. Congenital anomaly of pancreas divisum as cause of obstructive pain and pancreatitis. Gut 1980;21(2):105–14.

37. Pezzilli R. Pancreas divisum and acute or chronic pancreatitis. JOP 2012;13(1): 118–9.

38. Lin TK, et al. Pancreas Divisum in Pediatric Acute Recurrent and Chronic Pancreatitis: Report From INSPPIRE. J Clin Gastroenterol 2019;53(6):e232–8.

39. Gursoy Coruh A, et al. Frequency of bile duct confluence variations in subjects with pancreas divisum: an analysis of MRCP findings. Diagn Interv Radiol 2018; 24(2):72–6.

40. Gonoi W, et al. Pancreas divisum as a predisposing factor for chronic and recurrent idiopathic pancreatitis: initial in vivo survey. Gut 2011;60(8):1103–8.

41. Coyle WJ, et al. Evaluation of unexplained acute and acute recurrent pancreatitis using endoscopic retrograde cholangiopancreatography, sphincter of Oddi manometry and endoscopic ultrasound. Endoscopy 2002;34(8):617–23.

42. Gerke H, et al. Outcome of endoscopic minor papillotomy in patients with symptomatic pancreas divisum. Jop 2004;5(3):122–31.

43. Attwell A, et al. Endoscopic pancreatic sphincterotomy for pancreas divisum by using a needle-knife or standard pull-type technique: safety and reintervention rates. Gastrointest Endosc 2006;64(5):705–11.

44. Chacko LN, Chen YK, Shah RJ. Clinical outcomes and nonendoscopic interventions after minor papilla endotherapy in patients with symptomatic pancreas divisum. Gastrointest Endosc 2008;68(4):667–73.

45. Borak GD, et al. Long-term clinical outcomes after endoscopic minor papilla therapy in symptomatic patients with pancreas divisum. Pancreas 2009;38(8): 903–6.

46. Crino SF, et al. Efficacy of endoscopic minor papilla sphincterotomy for symptomatic santorinicele. Clin Gastroenterol Hepatol 2017;15(2):303–6.

47. Lans JI, et al. Endoscopic therapy in patients with pancreas divisum and acute pancreatitis: a prospective, randomized, controlled clinical trial. Gastrointest Endosc 1992;38(4):430–4.

48. Available at: https://clinicaltrials.gov/ct2/show/NCT03609944. Accessed October 19, 2022.

49. Cote GA, et al. SpHincterotomy for acute recurrent pancreatitis randomized trial: rationale, methodology, and potential implications. Pancreas 2019;48(8): 1061–7.

50. Bertin C, et al. Pancreas divisum is not a cause of pancreatitis by itself but acts as a partner of genetic mutations. Am J Gastroenterol 2012;107(2):311–7.

51. Ballard DD, et al. Evaluating adults with idiopathic pancreatitis for genetic predisposition: higher prevalence of abnormal results with use of complete gene sequencing. Pancreas 2015;44(1):116–21.

52. Garg PK, et al. Association of SPINK1 gene mutation and CFTR gene polymorphisms in patients with pancreas divisum presenting with idiopathic pancreatitis. J Clin Gastroenterol 2009;43(9):848–52.

53. DiMagno MJ, Dimagno EP. Pancreas divisum does not cause pancreatitis, but associates with CFTR mutations. Am J Gastroenterol 2012;107(2):318–20.

54. Bai HX, Lowe ME, Husain SZ. What have we learned about acute pancreatitis in children? J Pediatr Gastroenterol Nutr 2011;52(3):262–70.

55. Abu-El-Haija M, et al. Management of acute pancreatitis in the pediatric population: a clinical report from the north american society for pediatric gastroenterology, hepatology and nutrition pancreas committee. J Pediatr Gastroenterol Nutr 2018;66(1):159–76.

56. Acosta JM, et al. Effect of duration of ampullary gallstone obstruction on severity of lesions of acute pancreatitis. J Am Coll Surg 1997;184(5):499–505.

57. Acosta JM, Pellegrini CA, Skinner DB. Etiology and pathogenesis of acute biliary pancreatitis. Surgery 1980;88(1):118–25.

58. Abu-El-Haija M, et al. Predictive biomarkers for acute gallstone pancreatitis in the pediatric population. Pancreatology 2018;18(5):482–5.

59. Fishman DS, et al. A prospective multicenter analysis from the Pediatric ERCP Database Initiative: predictors of choledocholithiasis at ERCP in pediatric patients. Gastrointest Endosc 2021;94(2):311–317 e1.

60. Vrochides DV, et al. Is there a role for routine preoperative endoscopic retrograde cholangiopancreatography for suspected choledocholithiasis in children? Arch Surg 2005;140(4):359–61.

61. Crockett SD, et al. American Gastroenterological Association Institute Guideline on Initial Management of Acute Pancreatitis. Gastroenterology 2018;154(4):1096–101.

62. Committee ASoP, et al. ASGE guideline on the role of endoscopy in the evaluation and management of choledocholithiasis. Gastrointest Endosc 2019;89(6):1075–1105 e15.

63. van Geenen EJ, et al. Lack of consensus on the role of endoscopic retrograde cholangiography in acute biliary pancreatitis in published meta-analyses and guidelines: a systematic review. Pancreas 2013;42(5):774–80.

64. Schepers NJ, et al. Urgent endoscopic retrograde cholangiopancreatography with sphincterotomy versus conservative treatment in predicted severe acute gallstone pancreatitis (APEC): a multicentre randomised controlled trial. The Lancet 2020;396(10245):167–76.

65. Albert JG, Riemann JF. ERCP and MRCP–when and why. Best Pract Res Clin Gastroenterol 2002;16(3):399–419.

66. Sai JK, et al. Diagnosis of mild chronic pancreatitis (Cambridge classification): comparative study using secretin injection-magnetic resonance cholangiopancreatography and endoscopic retrograde pancreatography. World J Gastroenterol 2008;14(8):1218–21.

67. Buscail L, et al. Endoscopic ultrasonography in chronic pancreatitis: a comparative prospective study with conventional ultrasonography, computed tomography, and ERCP. Pancreas 1995;10(3):251–7.

68. Wallace MB, Hawes RH. Endoscopic ultrasound in the evaluation and treatment of chronic pancreatitis. Pancreas 2001;23(1):26–35.

69. Dite P, et al. A prospective, randomized trial comparing endoscopic and surgical therapy for chronic pancreatitis. Endoscopy 2003;35(7):553–8.
70. Mergener K, Kozarek RA. Therapeutic pancreatic endoscopy. Endoscopy 2005; 37(3):201–7.
71. Rosch T, et al. Endoscopic treatment of chronic pancreatitis: a multicenter study of 1000 patients with long-term follow-up. Endoscopy 2002;34(10):765–71.
72. Bracher GA, et al. Endoscopic pancreatic duct stenting to treat pancreatic ascites. Gastrointest Endosc 1999;49(6):710–5.
73. Seewald S, et al. Endoscopic sealing of pancreatic fistula by using N-butyl-2-cyanoacrylate. Gastrointest Endosc 2004;59(4):463–70.
74. Haber GB. Tissue glue for pancreatic fistula. Gastrointest Endosc 2004;59(4): 535–7.
75. Canty TG, Sr , Weinman D. Management of major pancreatic duct injuries in children. J Trauma 2001;50(6):1001–7.
76. Phelan HA, et al. An evaluation of multidetector computed tomography in detecting pancreatic injury: results of a multicenter AAST study. J Trauma 2009; 66(3):641–6 ; discussion 646-7.
77. Matsuno WC, et al. Amylase and lipase measurements in paediatric patients with traumatic pancreatic injuries. Injury 2009;40(1):66–71.
78. Mattix KD, et al. Pediatric pancreatic trauma: predictors of nonoperative management failure and associated outcomes. J Pediatr Surg 2007;42(2):340–4.
79. Houben CH, et al. Traumatic pancreatic duct injury in children: minimally invasive approach to management. J Pediatr Surg 2007;42(4):629–35.
80. Hall RI, Lavelle MI, Venables CW. Use of ERCP to identify the site of traumatic injuries of the main pancreatic duct in children. Br J Surg 1986;73(5):411–2.
81. Snajdauf J, et al. Surgical management of major pancreatic injury in children. Eur J Pediatr Surg 2007;17(5):317–21.
82. Telford JJ, et al. Pancreatic stent placement for duct disruption. Gastrointest Endosc 2002;56(1):18–24.
83. Rosen JD, et al. Success and safety of endoscopic retrograde cholangiopancreatography in children. J Pediatr Surg 2017;52(7):1148–51.
84. Barakat MT, Triadafilopoulos G, Berquist WE. Pediatric endoscopy practice patterns in the united states, canada, and mexico. J Pediatr Gastroenterol Nutr 2019;69(1):24–31.
85. Huang RJ, et al. Quality metrics in the performance of EUS: a population-based observational cohort of the United States. Gastrointest Endosc 2021;94(1): 68–74 e3.
86. Committee ASoP, et al. Role of EUS. Gastrointest Endosc 2007;66(3):425–34.
87. Lin TK, et al. Specialized imaging and procedures in pediatric pancreatology: a north american society for pediatric gastroenterology, hepatology, and nutrition clinical report. J Pediatr Gastroenterol Nutr 2017;64(3):472–84.
88. Scheers I, et al. Diagnostic and therapeutic roles of endoscopic ultrasound in pediatric pancreaticobiliary disorders. J Pediatr Gastroenterol Nutr 2015; 61(2):238–47.
89. Lakhole A, Liu QY. Role of endoscopic ultrasound in pediatric disease. Gastrointest Endosc Clin N Am 2016;26(1):137–53.
90. Freeman AJ, et al. Medical management of chronic pancreatitis in children: a position paper by the north american society for pediatric gastroenterology, hepatology, and nutrition pancreas committee. J Pediatr Gastroenterol Nutr 2021;72(2):324–40.

91. Catalano MF, et al. EUS-based criteria for the diagnosis of chronic pancreatitis: the Rosemont classification. Gastrointest Endosc 2009;69(7):1251–61.
92. Scheers I, et al. Autoimmune pancreatitis in children: characteristic features, diagnosis, and management. Am J Gastroenterol 2017;112(10):1604–11.
93. Fujii LL, et al. Pediatric pancreatic EUS-guided trucut biopsy for evaluation of autoimmune pancreatitis. Gastrointest Endosc 2013;77(5):824–8.
94. Banks PA, et al. Classification of acute pancreatitis–2012: revision of the Atlanta classification and definitions by international consensus. Gut 2013;62(1):102–11.
95. Jazrawi SF, Barth BA, Sreenarasimhaiah J. Efficacy of endoscopic ultrasound-guided drainage of pancreatic pseudocysts in a pediatric population. Dig Dis Sci 2011;56(3):902–8.
96. Working Group, IAP/APA.APG. IAP/APA evidence-based guidelines for the management of acute pancreatitis. Pancreatology 2013;13(4 Suppl 2):e1–15.
97. Tenner S, et al. American College of Gastroenterology guideline: management of acute pancreatitis. Am J Gastroenterol 2013;108(9):1400–15.
98. Nabi Z, et al. Endoscopic ultrasound-guided drainage of walled-off necrosis in children with fully covered self-expanding metal stents. J Pediatr Gastroenterol Nutr 2017;64(4):592–7.
99. Nabi Z, et al. Endoscopic drainage of pancreatic fluid collections: Long-term outcomes in children. Dig Endosc 2017;29(7):790–7.
100. Costa PA, et al. Use of lumen-apposing metal stents for endoscopic drainage of intra-abdominal fluid collections in pediatric patients. J Pediatr Gastroenterol Nutr 2020;70(2):258–60.
101. Strand DS, et al. AGA clinical practice update on the endoscopic approach to recurrent acute and chronic pancreatitis: expert review. Gastroenterology 2022;163(4):1107–14.

Pediatric Neurogastroenterology and Motility Disorders
What Role Does Endoscopy Play?

Julie Khlevner, MD[a],*, Dhiren Patel, MBBS, MD[b],
Leonel Rodriguez, MD, MS[c]

KEYWORDS

- Pediatrics • Neurogastroenterology and motility • GI motility
- Gastrointestinal endoscopy • Functional lumen imaging probe (FLIP)
- Peroral endoscopic myotomy (POEM) • Volvulus • Colonic manometry

KEY POINTS

- Pediatric neurogastroenterology and motility (PNGM) disorders are prevalent and often challenging to diagnose and treat.
- The field of PNGM has made remarkable progress in the last decade, including novel diagnostic and therapeutic techniques.
- Gastrointestinal endoscopy has emerged as a valuable tool in the management of PNGM disorders.
- Novel modalities such as functional lumen imaging probe, peroral endoscopic myotomy (POEM), gastric-POEM, and electrocautery incisional therapy have added to the armamentarium of endoscopic diagnostic and treatment options.
- We summarize the emerging role of therapeutic and diagnostic endoscopy in esophageal, gastric, small bowel, colonic, and anorectal disorders and disorders of gut brain axis interaction.

[a] Division of Pediatric Gastroenterology, Hepatology and Nutrition, Columbia University Vagelos College of Physicians and Surgeons, Gastrointestinal Motility Center, NewYork Presbyterian Morgan Stanley Children's Hospital, 622 West 168th Street, PH 17, New York, NY 11032, USA; [b] Division of Pediatric Gastroenterology, Hepatology and Nutrition, Department of Pediatrics, Saint Louis University School of Medicine, SSM Cardinal Glennon Children's Medical Center, 1465 South Grand Boulevard, St Louis, MO 63104, USA; [c] Division of Pediatric Gastroenterology, Hepatology and Nutrition, Department of Pediatrics, Yale New Haven Children's Hospital, Yale School of Medicine, 333 Cedar Street, New Haven, CT 06510, USA
* Corresponding author.
E-mail address: jk3065@cumc.columbia.edu

Gastrointest Endoscopy Clin N Am 33 (2023) 379–399
https://doi.org/10.1016/j.giec.2022.10.004
1052-5157/23/© 2022 Elsevier Inc. All rights reserved.

Video content accompanies this article at http://www.giendo.theclinics.com.

INTRODUCTION

Although pediatric neurogastroenterology and motility (PNGM) disorders are prevalent, often debilitating, and remain challenging to diagnose and treat, this field has made remarkable progress in the last decade. Diagnostic and therapeutic gastrointestinal endoscopy emerged as a valuable tool in the management of PNGM disorders. Novel modalities such as functional lumen imaging probe (FLIP), per-oral endoscopic myotomy (POEM), gastric-POEM, and electrocautery incisional therapy have changed the diagnostic and therapeutic landscape of PNGM. In this review, the authors highlight the emerging role of diagnostic and therapeutic endoscopy in esophageal, gastric, small bowel, colonic, and anorectal disorders and disorders of gut–brain interaction (DGBI). A summary of the utility of endoscopy on motor disorders and DGBIs is depicted in **Table 1**A, B.

Gastroesophageal Reflux Disease and Esophageal Motor Disorders (Achalasia and Cricopharyngeal Dysfunction)

The role of endoscopy in gastroesophageal reflux disease (GERD) and esophageal motor disorders can be divided into 2 main indications—diagnostic and therapeutic—and then further subdivided into the following categories:

1. Diagnostic utility
   a. General role in evaluation of gastroesophageal reflux symptoms and dysphagia
   b. Wireless pH monitoring device
   c. Functional lumen imaging probe (FLIP)
   d. Posttherapeutic evaluation
2. Therapeutic
   a. Facilitate passage of nutrients through the esophagus
      i. Endoscopic electrocautery incisional therapy (EIT)
      ii. Botulinum toxin injection
      iii. Endoscopic cricopharyngeal myotomy (CPM)
      iv. Balloon dilation including EsoFlip
      v. Peroral endoscopic myotomy (POEM)

Diagnostic role of endoscopy

Gastroesophageal reflux disease. GERD is when gastroesophageal reflux (GER) causes troublesome symptoms that affect daily functioning and/or leads to complications. Symptoms of GERD are often similar to those of esophageal dysmotility, including regurgitation, emesis, cough, throat clearing, difficulty eating, and wet voice. The primary role of upper endoscopy in children with esophageal symptoms is to diagnose erosive esophagitis, microscopic esophagitis, and rule out other conditions that mimic GERD including Crohn disease and infectious and eosinophilic esophagitis. There is insufficient evidence to support the use of esophagogastroduodenoscopy (EGD) for the diagnosis of GERD in infants and children, as GERD may be present based on clinical symptoms despite normal endoscopic appearance of the esophageal mucosa as well as in the absence of histological abnormalities.[1,2] Recently published NASPGHAN-ESPGHAN GERD clinical practice guidelines concluded that there is lack of evidence to support routine use of pH-metry for diagnosis of GERD in infants and children.[2] However, endoscopic placement of a wireless pH device can be helpful to correlate troublesome symptoms with GER events and clarify the role of reflux in the

Table 1
Role of diagnostic and therapeutic endoscopy in pediatric neurogastroenterology and motility disorders

A. Disorders of foregut							
	Diagnostic			Therapeutic			
	EGD	Wireless pH Monitoring	FLIP	Botox	PD	EIT	POEM
GERD	+	++	X	X	X	X	X
Cricopharyngeal dysfunction	+	X	X	***	***	X	X
Achalasia	+	X	++	**	***	X	***
Esophageal peptic stricture	++	+	++	X	***	**	X

	Diagnostic			Therapeutic				
	EGD	ADM	Enteral Tube Placement	IPBI	PBD	G-POEM	Temporary GES	TSP
Gastroparesis	X	+	***	**	*	**	**	*
PIPO	X	+++	***	*	*	*	*	*
DGBI of foregut not classified otherwise	+	+	*	*	*	X	*	X

B. Disorders of Hindgut				
	Diagnostic		Therapeutic	
	Colonoscopy	CM	Endoscopic Cecostomy	Endoscopic Detorsion
Functional constipation	+	+	**	*
Colonic inertia/dysmotility	+	+++	***	*
Sigmoid volvulus	+	+	*	**

Diagnostic (+): +++ gold standard, ++ useful adjunct, + rule out alternative diagnoses and/or provide supporting evidence, X not useful or lack of evidence.

Therapeutic (*): *** clear evidence for its use, ** viable treatment option, * lack of pediatric evidence, X no role in therapy.

Abbreviations: ADM, antroduodenal manometry; CM, colonic manometry; DGBI, disorder of brain gut interaction; EGD, esophagogastroduodenoscopy; EIT, electrocautery incisional therapy; FLIP, functional lumen imaging probe; GERD, gastroesophageal reflux disease; GES, gastric electric stimulation; G-POEM, gastric peroral endoscopic myotomy; IPBI, intrapyloric botulinum toxin injection; PD, pneumatic dilation; PD, pneumation dilation; PIPO, pediatric intestinal pseudo obstruction; POEM, peroral endoscopic myotomy; TPS, transpyloric stent.

Adapted from Miller J, Khlevner J, Rodriguez L. Upper Gastrointestinal Functional and Motility Disorders in Children. Pediatr Clin North Am. 2021;68(6):1237-1253.

cause of esophagitis and other signs or symptoms suggestive of GERD. It can also be helpful in assessing efficacy of acid suppression therapy.[2]

EGD can also be useful to evaluate for complication of GERD including hemorrhage, esophageal peptic strictures, and Barrett esophagus. Adult guidelines recommend that patients undergo endoscopy off of acid suppression therapy so not to miss proton pump inhibitor–responsive eosinophilic esophagitis or subclass of GERD including nonerosive reflux disease, esophageal hypersensitivity, and functional heartburn.[3]

Cricopharyngeal dysfunction/achalasia. Cricopharyngeal dysfunction/achalasia (CPA) is a rare condition characterized by an incomplete relaxation of the upper esophageal sphincter (UES) or by lack of coordination of the UES opening with pharyngeal contractions. Infants and children with CPA can present with feeding difficulties, dysphagia, choking, coughing, pooling of secretions, aspiration, nasopharyngeal regurgitation, or even sudden death. Diagnosis of cricopharyngeal dysfunction is typically made with video fluoroscopic swallow study, with the support of esophageal manometry. The exact role of upper endoscopy in diagnosing CPA remains unclear. Endoscopy may be helpful to rule out mucosal disease, congenital esophageal web/stenosis, and tracheoesophageal fistula. One pediatric study used endoscopy to rule out vascular anomalies affecting upper esophagus and UES. The same study used air insufflation technique to confirm failure of UES relaxation before therapeutic approach.[4] Another study used rigid endoscope to assess for hypertrophic cricopharyngeal muscle as a sign of CPA,[5] although prominent CP muscle is rarely visualized in practice. Botulin toxin (BoT) injection to the CP muscle during endoscopy can be a useful diagnostic tool to confirm CPA[6] in the setting of symptom improvement after the injection.

Achalasia. Achalasia, a rare esophageal motor disorder, is characterized by degeneration of the inhibitory myenteric neurons in the esophageal body and lower esophageal sphincter (LES), resulting in disordered peristalsis and incomplete or absent LES relaxation on deglutition. The exact cause and molecular pathology of achalasia is not fully elucidated but autoimmune, genetic, and infectious causes have been implicated.[7] Children with achalasia usually present with obstructive symptoms including progressive dysphagia, regurgitation, and vomiting, leading to weight loss. Chest pain and recurrent food impaction have also been reported. Younger children often have atypical presentation including pneumonia, nocturnal cough, aspiration, hoarseness, feeding difficulties, food refusal, and undernutrition.[8]

High-resolution esophageal manometry is the gold standard for diagnosing and subtyping achalasia into type 1 or classic, type II, and type III or spastic. EGD is often performed in the assessment of the esophageal dysphagia, although limited evidence exists on its utility. Although the main purpose is to evaluate for mechanical obstruction, and mucosal abnormalities such as reflux and eosinophilic esophagitis, an assessment of esophageal function can be attempted at the time of endoscopy to guide further testing. A careful endoscopic assessment of the esophageal body and esophagogastric junction can be helpful in managing children with suspected esophageal motor disorders. Normally there is no visible narrowing or increased resistance at the LES during scope passage. In achalasia, the LES tone is increased and based on experience, a narrowing can sometimes be appreciated en face, with passage requiring a light forward pressure with the endoscope. Presence of a hiatal hernia can also be assessed on retroflexion maneuver. Esophageal body contractility is difficult to accurately assess endoscopically. Dilated esophageal lumen with retention of liquid and/or solids can suggest an esophageal dysmotility but is not diagnostic of a motility disorder.

The functional lumen imaging probe (FLIP) is a newer modality that can be performed during endoscopy and has emerged as an important tool in the evaluation of esophageal motor disorders. It is a catheter-based system that uses impedance planimetry to measure esophageal distensibility as a function of pressure and cross-sectional area and allows the assessment of distension-induced esophageal contractility.[9] Studies in adult population have shown utilization of FLIP as an adjunct modality to diagnose achalasia subtypes,[10] provide intraoperative feedback during Heller myotomy,[11] and evaluate EGJ distensibility after treatment. Although its use in pediatric patients with achalasia has not been validated, studies in children showed that FLIP offers an adjunct assessment of motor function during endoscopy and can be used during POEM[12] and intraoperative esophagomyotomy to assess geometry of LES and guide myotomy length.[13]

Endoscopic evaluation of patients with achalasia after therapeutic intervention can be useful in identifying complications of treatment. Patients may develop reflux esophagitis, peptic stricture, or stricture from postmyotomy fibrosis. If a patient has undergone a fundoplication the wrap could be tight, slipped, or herniated causing obstruction or wrap breakdown. Anatomical deformities present before intervention may persist and even worsen if there is ongoing outflow obstruction. Deformities such as a pseudodiverticulum at the myotomy site may also develop and can be visualized during endoscopy.

Therapeutic role of endoscopy

Gastroesophageal reflux disease. Peptic esophageal strictures are a rare complication of GERD in children and is usually found in the lower third of the esophagus. The exact treatment is controversial ranging from endoscopic dilation (balloon passed over a wire or advanced thought the endoscope channel vs bougies) to surgical resection (**Fig. 1**). There is no pediatric consensus regarding the duration and frequency of dilations or the diameter that should be achieved. Before planning an intervention, the esophageal stricture morphology should be endoscopically assessed for length, type, and location. More novel approaches such as endoscopic steroid injection therapy,[14] topical application of mitomycin C,[15] and stenting[16] for refractory strictures have been reported. Given the rarity of peptic strictures in children, the abovementioned techniques are mostly described in the setting of anastomotic or corrosive esophageal strictures. Each has its own limitations and are not universally successful.

Endoscopic electrocautery incisional therapy (EIT) has emerged as a promising alternative tool for recalcitrant esophageal strictures when used by an experienced endoscopist. The procedure is technically challenging, requires direct endoscopic visualization, and involves the use of a needle knife (standard or insulated tip, approximately 5 mm cutting length, and requires a 2 mm working channel) to radially incise the stricture at its most dense points and cut off of the stenotic rim (**Fig. 2**). The length of the stricture should typically be less than 1 cm.[17] Balloon dilation usually follows incisional therapy to cause preferential tearing at incision sites. In the largest pediatric retrospective chart review using EIT with balloon dilation in patients with refractory strictures (youngest patient was 3 months old), the median number of dilations

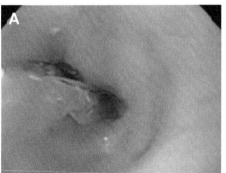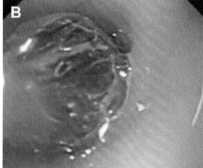

Fig. 1. (*A*) Balloon dilator passed via endoscopic channel through the esophageal stricture. (*B*) Inflated balloon dilator. (*Courtesy of* Michael Manfredi, MD, Boston, MA and Diana Lerner, MD, Milwaukee, MI.)

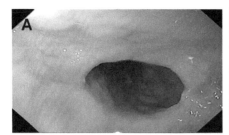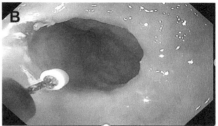

Fig. 2. (*A*) Refractory esophageal stricture. (*B*) Application of endoscopic electrocautery therapy to the stricture. (*Courtesy of* Michael Manfredi, MD, Boston, MA and Diana Lerner, MD, Milwaukee, MI.)

decreased from 8 to 2 within the subsequent 2 years. The investigators also reported a 61% rate of treatment success at 2 years after EIT, defined by no need for surgical resection, and less than 7 dilation sessions required after EIT to maintain appropriate esophageal diameter. Esophageal leak was reported in 5.3% resulting from free perforation or contained fluid leaks[18]; this highlights that EIT carries a similar or slightly higher risk of perforation than balloon dilation. Although most of the pediatric experience with EIT is in the setting of anastomotic strictures, similar principles can be applied to refractory peptic strictures.

Cricopharyngeal dysfunction/achalasia. The treatment experience of CPA in pediatric population is mostly limited to small case series or case reports. Recent studies advocate less invasive endoscopic approaches, including pneumatic dilation (PD), CPM, and BoT injections to the CP muscle.[19] These techniques have shown success although no clear recommendations exist regarding exact therapeutic approach, frequency and number of PDs, balloon inflation times, and frequency, and dose of BoT injections.

The appeal of a definitive cure with minimal recurrence risk has led some providers to recommend CPM as an early therapeutic consideration. In the literature, most of the endoscopic CPM are performed by otorhinolaryngologist using an endoscopic laser-assisted approach with reported success in infants as young as 6 months.[5] The risks of open CPM (hemorrhage, infection, pharyngocutaneous fistula, and esophageal or recurrent laryngeal nerve damage) have long been recognized, although an endoscopic approach may alleviate some of these.[5] A systematic review in adults found higher success rate with CPM as compared with BoT injections, and significantly higher endoscopic (84%) versus open (71%) CPM success rates, with fewer complications (2% vs 11%, respectively).[20]

Achalasia. The treatment goal for achalasia is to relieve outflow obstruction at the LES and improve symptoms and quality of life. Multiple therapeutic options exist, including Botox injection, PD, POEM, and surgery. Although treatment of patients with achalasia has evolved in recent years with new therapeutic techniques added to the armamentarium, there are no available evidence-based therapeutic recommendations for children with achalasia.

BoT injections to LES has limited use in pediatrics. Despite a reported high response rate among children, studies have shown its effect is short lived and those who responded require further procedures shortly after.[21] As a result, BoT injections should be reserved as a diagnostic tool in equivocal cases and for temporary relief in children who are poor candidates for more definite therapeutic options.

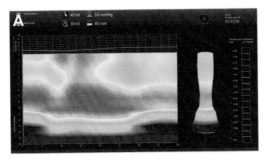

Pre-dilation

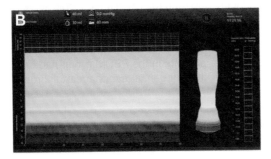

Post second dilation

Fig. 3. Functional lumen imaging probe (FLIP) image of patient with esophageal achalasia; (*A*) before dilation and (*B*) after dilation; note the increase in lumen caliber after dilation.

A number of pediatric and adult studies evaluated the use of PD in achalasia. In one pediatric prospective study, patients who underwent PD with 6-year follow-up had 67% success rate, and overall success rate after a maximum of 3 PDs was 87%. The investigators concluded that multiple dilatations may be required for optimal results, PD may be technically difficult in younger patients (<7 years), and some patients may ultimately require surgery.[22]

EsoFlip, a novel tool that integrates its diagnostic counterpart the FLIP's high-resolution impedance planimetry system technology into a balloon dilation catheter, has emerged as a valuable technique in adults. The balloon dilator is capable of dilating between 10 and 30 mm via controlled volumetric distention under direct endoscopic visualization with ability to assess esophageal dimensions before and after treatment[23] (**Fig. 3**). Although EsoFlip represents an appealing addition to the treatment toolbox of achalasia, studies in pediatric population are needed to evaluate its utilization.

POEM, where an endoscopic submucosal tunnel is created using triangle tip needle knife or hybrid knife, recently emerged as a minimal invasive option for children with achalasia irrespective of the achalasia subtype or prior treatments[24] (**Fig. 4**). A recent systemic review and meta-analysis of 146 pediatric patients who underwent POEM for the treatment of achalasia showed a significant postprocedure reduction in Eckardt score and LES pressure.[25] In addition, at least 93% had improvement or resolution of symptoms both short and long term, with a small number of patients experiencing adverse events including mucosal injury, esophageal tear or leak, pneumoperitoneum, pneumothorax, pneumonitis, or subcutaneous emphysema.[25] GER remains the most

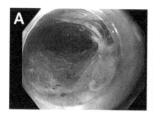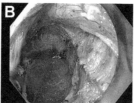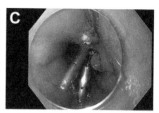

Fig. 4. Highlighting key steps in peroral endoscopic myotomy (POEM) procedure. (*A*) Creation of submucosal tunnel. (*B*) Myotomy, circumferential, and full thickness. (*C*) Mucosotomy closure with clips. (*Courtesy of* Amrita Sethi, MD, New York, NY.)

common long-term concern and requires close endoscopic surveillance for esophagitis,[24] although no clear recommendations on frequency of surveillance endoscopy exists. A retrospective pediatric study comparing the efficacy of POEM and PD showed significant improvement in long-term outcomes in the POEM group. In addition, unlike in the PD group, none of the patients in the PEOM group had recurrence.[26]

The role of endoscopy in the congenital esophageal disorders is discussed in a separate article in this volume.[27]

Stomach and Small Bowel Disorders of Gut–Brain Interaction Disorders: Gastroparesis, Pediatric Intestinal Pseudo-Obstruction, Functional Abdominal Pain Disorders

The role of endoscopy in DGBI including gastrointestinal motor abnormalities can be divided into 2 main indications—diagnostic and therapeutic—and then further subdivided into the following categories:

1. Diagnostic utility
   a. General role in evaluation of UGI symptoms
   b. Placement of diagnostic catheters (antroduodenal manometry)
2. Therapeutic
   a. Enteral tube placement
      i. Nasoduodenal/jejunal, gastrostomy, gastroduodenal/jejunal, and jejunostomy tubes
   b. Facilitate passage of nutrients through pylorus
      i. Intrapyloric botulinum toxin injection (IPBI)
      ii. Pyloric balloon dilation
      iii. Transpyloric stent placement
      iv. Gastric POEM (G-POEM)
   c. Stimulate/increase fundic accommodation, antral motility, and antro-pylorus-duodenal coordination and/or improve visceral sensitivity
      i. Temporary gastric pacing

Diagnostic role of endoscopy

Gastroparesis and pediatric intestinal pseudo-obstruction. Gastroparesis and pediatric intestinal pseudo-obstruction (PIPO) are DGBI that present with chronic symptoms such as nausea, vomiting, and abdominal pain associated with difficulty in tolerating enteral feeds. EGD can be used primarily to rule out organic conditions that may present in a similar fashion as DGBI, such as eosinophilic and collagenous gastropathy, Crohn disease, as well as anatomical problems missed on imaging studies such as pyloric webs. However, in terms of assisting in the diagnosis of DGBIs, its utility is not

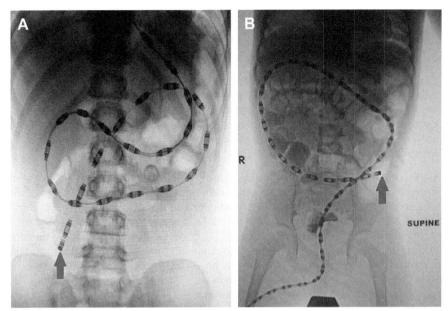

Fig. 5. (*A*) Abdominal film depicting the final position of an antroduodenal motility catheter; note the most distal port is in the proximal jejunum (*arrow*). (*B*) Abdominal film showing a colon motility catheter after endoscopic and fluoroscopic placement. The most proximal port is located within the terminal ileum (*arrow*).

well defined. Some have reported the yield of abnormal endoscopic gross and histologic findings in pediatric patients with gastroparesis (abnormal gastric emptying study by scintigraphy) is no different than controls, is poorly correlated with symptoms and other diagnostic studies, and concordance between gross and histologic findings is low at 50%,[28] whereas others have reported that those with gastroparesis are less likely to have histologic gastritis.[29] There are reports outlining the use of endoscopic mucosal resection, followed by creation of a pseudo-polyp by deploying a clip on the exposed muscle layer, which is then resected to obtain tissue from deeper layers of stomach that would not be obtained with a simple biopsy forceps.[30] However, the utility of this technique in pediatrics is not well established.

The presence of food residue in the stomach can be found in 3% of EGDs in adults,[31] and some have suggested it can be a predictor of delayed gastric emptying. One study showed that 26% of patients with delayed gastric emptying by scintigraphy demonstrated gastric food retention, with greater scintigraphic gastric retention at 4 hour in individuals with food retention compared with those without retention.[32] Another recent study also reported significantly high odds ratio (4.8) of finding food retention during endoscopy in those with gastroparesis, with a positive predictive value of retained gastric food ranging from 32%, for those without any risk factors, to 79% in those with type I diabetes, and 55% for delayed gastric emptying.[31]

Diagnostic catheter placement. Endoscopy can be very useful in the placement of catheters to evaluate antroduodenal motility; such tubes can be also placed blindly with fluoroscopy alone. Endoscopy can be advantageous in technically difficult cases and also to minimize radiation exposure (**Fig. 5A**).

Therapeutic role of endoscopy

Enteral tube placement. Enteral tubes may be required for nutrition support and/or venting (stomach) when patients do not tolerate oral intake. Enteral tubes may be required temporarily but in certain cases those may be required for long term.

Nasojejunal tube Transpyloric tubes/catheters can be placed blindly or with fluoroscopic assistance, and endoscopy can be invaluable in the placement of such tubes when they are unable to be placed conventionally.[33] The advent of transnasal endoscopy has also facilitated the placement of such tubes, with the capability of passing a guidewire transnasally directly into the small bowel and then placing the tube using the guidewire and with fluoroscopy assistance, with minimal complications.[34,35]

Gastrostomy/gastrojejunostomy tube To provide nutritional support and to assist with venting the stomach, many patients benefit from enteral routes such as a gastrostomy and/or a gastrojejunostomy. Such tubes can be placed surgically, with fluoroscopy by interventional radiology, and percutaneously with endoscopic assistance (percutaneous endoscopic gastrostomy [PEG]).[36] Although there is ample literature of their utility and complications for feeding disorders, there are no studies reporting the utility of PEG in gastroparesis. Others have also reported the placement of a PEG with jejunal extension to assist with feeds resulting on feeding tolerance improvement in around 50% in adults with gastroparesis.[37]

Jejunostomy tube Jejunostomy tubes are primarily used to provide nutritional support when gastric feeds are not tolerated. These tubes can be placed surgically, with fluoroscopy by interventional radiology, and percutaneously with endoscopic assistance (percutaneous endoscopic jejunostomy),[36,38] although complication rates for jejunostomy may be higher than gastrostomy.[39]

Facilitating passage of nutrients through the pylorus

Intrapyloric botulinum toxin injection Since the first reports of the use of IPBI in adults,[40–42] many other open-label studies in adults[43–46] and children[47] have reported important symptomatic improvement; however, 2 randomized controlled trials did not show a benefit from the IPBI,[48,49] although a concern has been raised about the possibility that both studies were not sufficiently powered (**Table 2**). Some centers have reported the utility of endoscopic ultrasound in guiding the location of the IPBI.[50] The pyloric distensibility (measured with EndoFLIP) has been reported as useful in predicting clinical response to IPBI,[51] and the IPBI response may be useful to predict response to pyloroplasty for gastroparesis in adults.[52] The largest pediatric study of the isolated use of IPBI in 45 children with gastroparesis reported success in 30 patients, with a mean response to first injection of 3.0 months (1.2–4.8 months 95% confidence interval). Only one patient reported side effects, which included a short-lived increase in vomiting that resolved completely after a week.[47] A recent study evaluating the potential effect of IPBI on feeding difficulties in children younger than 5 years (most receiving feeds via enteral tubes) reported an improvement in oral feeding, and patients were less likely to require postpyloric feeds.[53] A recent retrospective study found no difference between IPBI and pyloric balloon dilation (PBD) in children.[54]

The recommended dose for the botulinum toxin is 6 units/kg up to a total of 100 units. The technique for IPBI includes the dilution of the botulinum toxin in 1 to 2 cc of normal saline, an application of a quarter of the dose in each quadrant with the use of a sclerotherapy needle (Video 1). IPBI is indicated for patients failing medical therapy and not tolerating enteral feedings; it can be used alone or in combination with pyloric balloon dilation and can be used as a predictor for those requiring further surgical interventions.

Table 2
Studies reporting the clinical utility of isolated use of intrapyloric botulinum toxin injection in both adults and children with gastroparesis

Study	N	Study Type	Symptom Improvement		Follow-up (Weeks)	Effect Duration (Months)	4h Solid GET[a] Improvement
			Symptom Score	Patient Reported			
Ezzedine 2002[40]	6 (Diabetic)	Open	55%	—	6	—	52%
Lacy 2002[41]	3 (Idiopathic)	Open	—	100%	—	—	—
Miller 2002[42]	10 (Idiopathic)	Open	38%	—	4	—	70%
Lacy 2004[95]	8 (Diabetic)	Open	56%	—	12	—	33%
Bromer 2005[43]	63	Open	—	43%	12	5	—
Arts 2006[44]	20	Open	29%	—	4	—	36%
Arts 2007[48]	23 (12 IPBI and 11 Placebo)	DBPC[b]	35% IPBI vs 11% Placebo (p = 0.07)	—	4	—	No difference with placebo
Friedenberg 2008[49]	32 (16 IPBI and 16 placebo)	DBPC	37.5% IPBI and 56.3% Placebo, not significant	—	4	—	No difference from placebo
Coleski 2009[96]	179	Open	—	51%	16	—	—
Reddymasu 2009[48]	11 (PS[c])	Open	44%	70%	48	6	—
Rodriguez 2012[47]	45	Open	—	67%	—	3	—
Reichenbach 2020[45]	34	Open	—	64%	24	6	—

a GET, gastric emptying time.
b DBPC, double-blind placebo controlled.
c PS, post-surgical.

Pyloric balloon dilation PBD has been reported as useful in adults with gastroparesis, but little information is available in regard to its use in children. A study including patients undergoing IPBI or PBD showed a response to PBD increasing with consecutive dilations: 50% with first and second dilations and increasing to 70% success rate at the third dilation.[55] The most recent and largest retrospective study evaluating PBD in 47 adults with gastroparesis reported a significant clinical improvement in 53% at 2 months, 40% at 6 months, and 32% at 2 years.[56] There are also reports of the utility of PBD after failed pyloromyotomy in adults with gastroparesis, demonstrating not only symptomatic improvement but also pyloric distensibility.[57] The first study reporting utility PBD in 19 children with delayed gastric emptying showed a complete resolution of symptoms in 13 patients and transient improvement in 5 others lasting 4 to 8 weeks; no complications were reported.[58] A recent retrospective study in 24 children with gastroparesis comparing PBD with IPBI showed no difference in symptomatic improvement between both techniques, with an overall response rate of 76%.[54] Another retrospective study comparing IPBI with PBD with conventional therapy alone (medications and dietary and behavioral interventions) also showed a partial or complete response in 76% of patients compared with 49% in those receiving conventional therapy.[59] PBD can be used alone or in combination with IPBI in children failing medical therapy and before surgical interventions.

Transpyloric stenting The clinical utility of transpyloric stents in adult patients with gastroparesis has been reported primarily for postsurgical causes[60,61] but also for diabetic and idiopathic gastroparesis.[62] The largest study in adults reported the use of stents (48 procedures) in 30 patients with gastroparesis for different indications, resulting in symptom improvement in 75% of patients and improving gastric emptying in 69%.[63] A recent study highlighted the potential complications associated to the use of stents for gastroparesis, including migration, bleeding, perforation, and obstruction.[13] The use of stenting for functional gastric disorders should be viewed as a temporary measure (reported in selected adult cases) to facilitate the passage of nutrients through pylorus or to assess the need for other permanent interventions, including surgery. To date, no pediatric cases have been reported, and no information is available to recommend its use, although it could be considered in selected postsurgical cases with narrowed lumen.

Gastric peroral endoscopic myotomy Advances in combining endoscopic and surgical procedures allow for therapy for conditions such as esophageal achalasia and more recently for gastroparesis refractory to medical and other endoscopic interventions mentioned earlier. A variation of the original POEM for esophageal achalasia, the G-POEM, includes the following steps: creation of a submucosal bleb in the gastric antrum with saline injection, followed by a cut through bleb to access submucosal space and dissection through the submucosal space and locate pyloric ring, proceeded with pyloromyotomy, and finalized with closure of the submucosal tunnel with endoclips. Since the first report of a G-POEM on 2013,[64] multiple studies have reported a high successful completion rate with important symptomatic improvement and minimal complications. The most recent systematic review and meta-analysis, which included 10 studies (482 patients), reported a modest symptomatic improvement on the gastroparesis cardinal symptom index score at 1 year (61%) that correlates with pyloric distensibility (evaluated with EndoFLIP) and an 8% complication rate.[65] A recent study reported no increase in morbidity when patients were discharged on the same day of the procedure.[66] Studies including long-term outcomes are needed, and there are currently no reports of G-POEM being performed in children.

Stimulating/increasing fundic accommodation, antral motility, antro-pylorus-duodenal coordination, and/or improving visceral sensitivity
Temporary gastric electric stimulation. Gastric pacing has been reported to improve symptoms in adults with gastroparesis without a significant improvement on the gastric emptying. It is indicated for gastroparesis and selected cases of functional dyspepsia/nausea that failed medical treatment and before placement of permanent GES. The concept of temporary GES has been evaluated in adults and deemed to be a good predictor of response to permanent GES.[67] Temporary leads can be placed nasally or through a gastrostomy tube and fixed endoscopically to the antral mucosa with endoclips. Recently, a miniature GES placed endoscopically has been trialed in animals.[68] Since the initial report of temporary GES in children,[69] additional reports have been published that describe good symptom control.[70]

Colonic/Anorectal Disorders: Refractory Constipation/Colonic Dysmotility, Sigmoid Volvulus

The role of endoscopy in colonic and anorectal disorders can be divided into 2 main indications—diagnostic and therapeutic—and then further subdivided into the following categories:

a. Diagnostic utility
   i. General role in evaluation of constipation
   ii. Placement of diagnostic catheter (colonic manometry)
b. Therapeutic
   i. Placement of tube for antegrade colonic enemas
   ii. Colonic decompression and detorsion

Diagnostic role
Constipation is among the most common DGBI disorders, affecting around 15% of adults and 9% of children.[71,72] Diagnosis is clinical, based on history and physical examination. Usually, there is no further need for additional testing for the diagnosis, but at times, other tests may be recommended to further understand the pathophysiology and to potentially guide therapy. In general, routine colonoscopy is not warranted for functional constipation in the absence of alarming symptoms. However, American Society for Gastrointestinal Endoscopy (ASGE) recommends for adult patients that colonoscopy should be performed in patients with constipation who presents with rectal bleeding, iron deficiency anemia of unknown cause, heme-positive occult stool, or significant weight loss to exclude organic disease.[73] Also in adults, colonoscopy may be indicated to rule out malignant causes also allowing dilation of benign colonic stricture when appropriate.[74,75] Although these indications are extremely rare in children, they must be considered in presence of alarm signs. Colonoscopy has no role in routine bowel fecal disimpaction and is highly discouraged.[73] Some patients with medically refractory constipation in whom surgery is being considered may benefit from performing more advanced studies to evaluate colon motility and potentially guide therapy. Intraluminal manometry is the gold-standard test for motility disorders affecting the anorectum and colon. Colon manometry is performed to evaluate the neuromuscular integrity of the colon and primarily assess high amplitude propagating contractions and gastrocolonic response to the meal. Placement of the catheter requires colonoscopy to advance the catheter directly (by pulling a suture attached to the tip of the catheter) to the proximal colon (cecum as much as possible), and when unable to proceed that way, a guidewire is advanced and then the catheter is advanced via the guidewire and with fluoroscopy assistance[76–78] or fluoroscopy alone by an

interventional radiologist[79] but the latter may require larger radiation doses and the success rate to place it directly into the cecum is lower than colonoscopy-assisted placement. The use of colonoscopy for the catheter placement offers the advantages of being able to obtain tissue for diagnosis and visualize tortuosity and redundancy of the colon, particularly the rectosigmoid area. Hemostatic clips have been described to secure the catheter to prevent migration and displacement[80] (**Fig. 5B**).

Therapeutic role
Placement of cecostomy tube for antegrade colonic enemas. Patients with medically refractory constipation may benefit from surgical interventions aiming to improve stool evacuation, including antegrade colonic enemas. Similar to the PEG to assist with feeds and gastric venting, cecostomy tubes to provide antegrade colonic irrigations were initially placed using endoscopy in isolation. However, complications emerged related to sigmoid damage (piercing and perforation) during the blind placement of the needle guide due to proximity of redundant sigmoid colon in patients with refractory constipation, requiring urgent conversion to laparoscopic or open surgery. Laparoscopy was added to allow placement of the needle directly into the cecum under direct laparoscopic visualization to avoid sigmoid damage. Since the first description of the laparoscopic assisted endoscopy percutaneous cecostomy for antegrade enemas,[81] some modifications have been added to enable placement of a low-profile skin-level cecostomy tube at the initial procedure.[82] The procedure is successfully completed in up to 95% of patients with minimal complications.[83]

Colonic decompression and detorsion. Sigmoid volvulus is extremely uncommon in children, usually associated to chronic constipation, Hirschsprung disease, colonic pseudo-obstruction, or neuromuscular abnormalities.[84,85] Given high morbidity (12%) and mortality rates (8%–23%),[86] early diagnosis and a high index of suspicion are key to prevent further complications such as bowel perforation, sepsis, necrosis, hemodynamic instability, and fatality.[84,85,87–89] All information available in pediatrics consists of case series and single-center experiences. However, most agree that emergent surgery is indicated with signs of perforation, peritonitis, or bowel ischemia[86] or when endoscopic management fails to detorsion the sigmoid loop. A twisted spiral sphincter appearance 15 to 25 cm from the anus and difficulty in passing the scope in a twisted proximal loop could serve as guiding findings to establish the diagnosis before attempting endoscopic reduction.[85–87] For uncomplicated volvulus, the gentle insertion of the endoscope with clockwise torque beyond the rectosigmoid and very limited air insufflation is recommended while performing the procedure.[86] Once the descending colon is reached, the endoscopic reduction is achieved by clockwise rotation; shortening of the endoscope; and simultaneous suction of air, gas, and fluid (**Fig. 6**).

Some studies have suggested the insertion of a rectal tube after detorsion of the sigmoid loop to avoid immediate recurrence.[90,91] This procedure also reduces the risk of early relapse of the volvulus.[84] This is a very difficult procedure plagued by complications such as shaft-induced large perforation due to excessive looping, tip perforation, and excessive air pressure–induced perforation, although the latter is highly uncommon in pediatric patients.[92,93] In addition to detorsion of the loop, the bowel mucosa should be evaluated for any signs of ischemic damage that may prompt surgical evaluation for potential immediate bowel resection.

The recurrence rate for volvulus is high in adult series and reported in around 4.5% of cases.[87] However, due to minimal experience in children[84,94] it is suggested to perform a definitive surgery (sigmoid resection/primary anastomosis/sigmoidopexy)

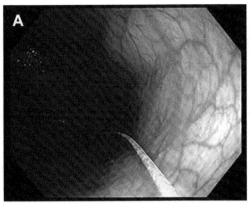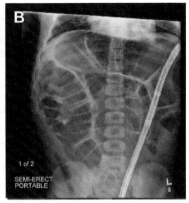

Fig. 6. (*A*) Radiographic image and (*B*) colonoscopy view during colonoscopic detorsion of sigmoid volvulus.

during the same hospital admission within a 48 to 72 hours interval. The role of percutaneous endoscopic sigmoidopexy has been discussed and was described in 1998.[92] However, this technique has minimal utility in adults, and no experience with pediatric sigmoid volvulus has been reported except for a very small number of patients in whom the risk of anesthesia for an elective open surgery for volvulus was exceedingly high for.[85]

SUMMARY

The last decade has observed numerous advances in diagnostic and therapeutic endoscopic modalities used for the improved assessment of gastrointestinal function and motility. Use of diagnostic endoscopy can identify relevant pathologies that may guide management, and novel therapeutic technologies allow for better outcomes in children with NGM.

CLINICS CARE POINTS

- Role of diagnostic endoscopy is limited in pediatric upper and lower gastrointestinal motility and functional disorders but may help with antroduodenal and colonic catheter placement and rule out organic diagnoses.

- Functional lumen imaging probe (FLIP) and EsoFLIP emerged as important diagnostic and therapeutic tools in the evaluation and management of esophageal motor disorders.

- Intrasphincteric botulinum toxin injections may provide temporary symptomatic relief and/ or help confirm diagnoses such as cricopharyngeal dysfunction, achalasia, and gastroparesis.

- Pneumatic dilation is a useful therapeutic modality in variety of upper gastrointestinal disorders including peptic strictures, cricopharyngeal dysfunction, achalasia, and gastroparesis but there is lack of pediatric consensus regarding duration and frequency of dilations or diameter that should be achieved.

- Although there are multiple novel therapeutic modalities including peroral endoscopic myotomy (POEM), gastric-POEM, transpyloric stenting, and electrocautery incisional therapy, there is a lack of evidence-based guidelines for pediatric use.

- Diagnostic and therapeutic gastrointestinal endoscopy has emerged as a valuable tool in the management of pediatric neurogastroenterology and motility (PNGM) disorders.

- Although novel modalities such as functional lumen imaging probe (FLIP), peroral endoscopic myotomy (POEM), gastric-POEM, and electrocautery incisional therapy have changed the landscape of PNGM, caution must be exercised, as these have important limitations such as the requirement of an experienced endoscopist and the paucity of pediatric data.
- *POEM* is an effective alternative to pneumatic dilatation and Heller's myotomy in *pediatric* achalasia although gastroesophageal reflux remains the most common long-term concern and requires close endoscopic surveillance for esophagitis.
- As compared with blind fluoroscopic approach, endoscopic placement of manometric catheters to evaluate antroduodenal and colonic motility can be advantageous to minimize the radiation dose in technically difficult cases, also allowing for simultaneous evaluation of mucosal disease and anatomical problems.
- Endoscopic placement of enteral tubes is an option for nutrition support (and/or venting the stomach) when patients do not tolerate oral intake (ie, in the setting of gastroparesis, pediatric pseudo-obstruction).
- Intrapyloric botulinum toxin injection (IPBI) is an option for pediatric patients with gastroparesis or feeding difficulties who are failing medical therapy and not tolerating enteral feedings. IPBI can be used alone or in combination with pyloric balloon dilation and as a predictor for those requiring further surgical interventions.

DISCLOSURE

All authors report no conflict of interest for this article and have nothing to disclose. No funding has been obtained for this scholarly work.

SUPPLEMENTARY DATA

Supplementary data related to this article can be found online at https://doi.org/10.1016/j.giec.2022.10.004.

REFERENCES

1. Arasu TS, Wyllie R, Fitzgerald JF, et al. Gastroesophageal reflux in infants and children comparative accuracy of diagnostic methods. J Pediatr 1980;96(5):798–803.
2. Rosen R, Vandenplas Y, Singendonk M, et al. Pediatric Gastroesophageal reflux clinical practice guidelines: joint recommendations of the north american society for pediatric gastroenterology, hepatology, and nutrition and the european society for pediatric gastroenterology, hepatology, and nutrition. J Pediatr Gastroenterol Nutr 2018;66(3):516–54.
3. Katz PO, Gerson LB, Vela MF. Guidelines for the diagnosis and management of gastroesophageal reflux disease. Am J Gastroenterol 2013;108(3):308–28 [quiz: 329].
4. Gollu G, Demir N, Ates U, et al. Effective management of cricopharyngeal achalasia in infants and children with dilatation alone. J Pediatr Surg 2016;51(11):1751–4.
5. Basler KJ, Swanson C, Andreoli SM. Endoscopic cricopharyngeal myotomy in infants. Int J Pediatr Otorhinolaryngol 2019;116:15–7.
6. Scholes MA, McEvoy T, Mousa H, et al. Cricopharyngeal achalasia in children: botulinum toxin injection as a tool for diagnosis and treatment. Laryngoscope 2014;124(6):1475–80.

7. Ruiz-de-León A, Mendoza J, Sevilla-Mantilla C, et al. Myenteric antiplexus antibodies and class II HLA in achalasia. Dig Dis Sci 2002;47(1):15–9.

8. Franklin AL, Petrosyan M, Kane TD. Childhood achalasia: a comprehensive review of disease, diagnosis and therapeutic management. World J Gastrointest Endosc 2014;6(4):105–11.

9. Carlson DA, Kou W, Lin Z, et al. Normal values of esophageal distensibility and distension-induced contractility measured by functional luminal imaging probe panometry. Clin Gastroenterol Hepatol 2019;17(4):674–81.e1.

10. Carlson DA, Kou W, Rooney KP, et al. Achalasia subtypes can be identified with functional luminal imaging probe (FLIP) panometry using a supervised machine learning process. Neurogastroenterol Motil 2021;33(3):e13932.

11. Su B, Callahan ZM, Novak S, et al. Using impedance planimetry (EndoFLIP) to evaluate myotomy and predict outcomes after surgery for achalasia. J Gastrointest Surg 2020;24(4):964–71.

12. Wood LS, Chandler JM, Portelli KE, et al. Treating children with achalasia using per-oral endoscopic myotomy (POEM): Twenty-one cases in review. J Pediatr Surg 2020;55(6):1006–12.

13. Gapp J, Crigler C, Ansari Z, et al. Transpyloric Lumen-Apposing Metal Stent for Gastroparesis Is Associated with Significant Complications. J Gastrointest Surg 2022;26(10):2212–4.

14. van Hal ARL, Pulvirenti R, den Hartog FPJ, et al. The safety of intralesional steroid injections in young children and their effectiveness in anastomotic esophageal strictures-a meta-analysis and systematic review. Front Pediatr 2021;9:825030.

15. Berger M, Ure B, Lacher M. Mitomycin C in the therapy of recurrent esophageal strictures: hype or hope? Eur J Pediatr Surg 2012;22(2):109–16.

16. Manfredi MA, Jennings RW, Anjum MW, et al. Externally removable stents in the treatment of benign recalcitrant strictures and esophageal perforations in pediatric patients with esophageal atresia. Gastrointest Endosc 2014;80(2):246–52.

17. Samanta J, Dhaka N, Sinha SK, et al. Endoscopic incisional therapy for benign esophageal strictures: Technique and results. World J Gastrointest Endosc 2015;7(19):1318–26.

18. Manfredi MA, Clark SJ, Medford S, et al. Endoscopic electrocautery incisional therapy as a treatment for refractory benign pediatric esophageal strictures. J Pediatr Gastroenterol Nutr 2018;67(4):464–8.

19. Huoh KC, Messner AH. Cricopharyngeal achalasia in children: indications for treatment and management options. Curr Opin Otolaryngol Head Neck Surg 2013;21(6):576–80.

20. Kocdor P, Siegel ER, Tulunay-Ugur OE. Cricopharyngeal dysfunction: a systematic review comparing outcomes of dilatation, botulinum toxin injection, and myotomy. Laryngoscope 2016;126(1):135–41.

21. Hurwitz M, Bahar RJ, Ament ME, et al. Evaluation of the use of botulinum toxin in children with achalasia. J Pediatr Gastroenterol Nutr 2000;30(5):509–14.

22. Di Nardo G, Rossi P, Oliva S, et al. Pneumatic balloon dilation in pediatric achalasia: efficacy and factors predicting outcome at a single tertiary pediatric gastroenterology center. Gastrointest Endosc 2012;76(5):927–32.

23. Baumann AJ, Carlson DA. EsoFLIP for esophageal dilation: proposed advantages. Curr Opin Gastroenterol 2020;36(4):329–35.

24. Nabi Z, Ramchandani M, Basha J, et al. POEM is a durable treatment in children and adolescents with achalasia cardia. Front Pediatr 2022;10:812201.

25. Lee Y, Brar K, Doumouras AG, et al. Peroral endoscopic myotomy (POEM) for the treatment of pediatric achalasia: a systematic review and meta-analysis. Surg Endosc 2019;33(6):1710–20.

26. Tan Y, Zhu H, Li C, et al. Comparison of peroral endoscopic myotomy and endoscopic balloon dilation for primary treatment of pediatric achalasia. J Pediatr Surg 2016;51(10):1613–8.

27. Yasuda J, Manfredi M. Endoscopic Management of Congenital Esophageal Defects. Gastrointest Endosc Clin N Am 2023;33(2):465–85.

28. Altepeter TA, Shaffer S. Yield of endoscopy in pediatric gastroparesis. J Pediatr Gastroenterol Nutr 2017;65(1):22–5.

29. Wong GK, Shulman RJ, Chiou EH, et al. Decreased relative diagnostic yield of esophagogastroduodenoscopy in children with gastroparesis. J Clin Gastroenterol 2014;48(3):231–5.

30. Rajan E, Gostout CJ, Wong Kee Song LM, et al. Innovative gastric endoscopic muscle biopsy to identify all cell types, including myenteric neurons and interstitial cells of Cajal in patients with idiopathic gastroparesis: a feasibility study (with video). Gastrointest Endosc 2016;84(3):512–7.

31. Bi D, Choi C, League J, et al. Food residue during esophagogastroduodenoscopy is commonly encountered and is not pathognomonic of delayed gastric emptying. Dig Dis Sci 2021;66(11):3951–9.

32. Coleski R, Baker JR, Hasler WL. Endoscopic gastric food retention in relation to scintigraphic gastric emptying delays and clinical factors. Dig Dis Sci 2016;61(9):2593–601.

33. Stark SP, Sharpe JN, Larson GM. Endoscopically placed nasoenteral feeding tubes. Indications and techniques. Am Surg 1991;57(4):203–5.

34. Zhang L, Huang YH, Yao W, et al. Transnasal esophagogastroduodenoscopy for placement of nasoenteric feeding tubes in patients with severe upper gastrointestinal diseases. J Dig Dis 2012;13(6):310–5.

35. Mahadeva S, Malik A, Hilmi I, et al. Transnasal endoscopic placement of nasoenteric feeding tubes: outcomes and limitations in non-critically ill patients. Nutr Clin Pract 2008;23(2):176–81.

36. Jazayeri A, McConnie RM, Ross AM, et al. Postpyloric feeding access in infants and children: a state of the art review. J Pediatr Gastroenterol Nutr 2022;75(3):237–43.

37. Strijbos D, Keszthelyi D, Smeets FGM, et al. Therapeutic strategies in gastroparesis: results of stepwise approach with diet and prokinetics, Gastric Rest, and PEG-J: a retrospective analysis. Neurogastroenterol Motil 2019;31(6):e13588.

38. Toussaint E, Van Gossum A, Ballarin A, et al. Percutaneous endoscopic jejunostomy in patients with gastroparesis following lung transplantation: feasibility and clinical outcome. Endoscopy 2012;44(8):772–5.

39. McCann C, Cullis PS, McCabe AJ, et al. Major complications of jejunal feeding in children. J Pediatr Surg 2019;54(2):258–62.

40. Ezzeddine D, Jit R, Katz N, et al. Pyloric injection of botulinum toxin for treatment of diabetic gastroparesis. Gastrointest Endosc 2002;55(7):920–3.

41. Lacy BE, Zayat EN, Crowell MD, et al. Botulinum toxin for the treatment of gastroparesis: a preliminary report. Am J Gastroenterol 2002;97(6):1548–52.

42. Miller LS, Szych GA, Kantor SB, et al. Treatment of idiopathic gastroparesis with injection of botulinum toxin into the pyloric sphincter muscle. Am J Gastroenterol 2002;97(7):1653–60.

43. Bromer MQ, Friedenberg F, Miller LS, et al. Endoscopic pyloric injection of botulinum toxin A for the treatment of refractory gastroparesis. Gastrointest Endosc 2005;61(7):833–9.

44. Arts J, van Gool S, Caenepeel P, et al. Influence of intrapyloric botulinum toxin injection on gastric emptying and meal-related symptoms in gastroparesis patients. Aliment Pharmacol Ther 2006;24(4):661–7.

45. Reichenbach ZW, Stanek S, Patel S, et al. Botulinum toxin A improves symptoms of gastroparesis. Dig Dis Sci 2020;65(5):1396–404.

46. Reddymasu SC, Singh S, Sankula R, et al. Endoscopic pyloric injection of botulinum toxin-A for the treatment of postvagotomy gastroparesis. Am J Med Sci 2009;337(3):161–4.

47. Rodriguez L, Rosen R, Manfredi M, et al. Endoscopic intrapyloric injection of botulinum toxin A in the treatment of children with gastroparesis: a retrospective, open-label study. Gastrointest Endosc 2012;75(2):302–9.

48. Arts J, Holvoet L, Caenepeel P, et al. Clinical trial: a randomized-controlled crossover study of intrapyloric injection of botulinum toxin in gastroparesis. Aliment Pharmacol Ther 2007;26(9):1251–8.

49. Friedenberg FK, Palit A, Parkman HP, et al. Botulinum toxin A for the treatment of delayed gastric emptying. Am J Gastroenterol 2008;103(2):416–23.

50. Bhutani MS. EUS-guided botulinum toxin injection into the pyloric sphincter for the treatment of gastroparesis. Endosc Ultrasound 2019;8(5):350–1.

51. Desprez C, Melchior C, Wuestenberghs F, et al. Pyloric distensibility measurement predicts symptomatic response to intrapyloric botulinum toxin injection. Gastrointest Endosc 2019;90(5):754–760 e1.

52. Gilsdorf D, Volckmann E, Brickley A, et al. Pyloroplasty Offers Relief of Postfundoplication Gastroparesis in Patients Who Improved After Botulinum Toxin Injection. J Laparoendosc Adv Surg Tech A 2017;27(11):1180–4.

53. Hirsch S, Nurko S, Mitchell P, et al. Botulinum toxin as a treatment for feeding difficulties in young children. J Pediatr 2020;226:228–35.

54. Mercier C, Ley D, Aumar M, et al. Comparison of symptom control in pediatric gastroparesis using endoscopic pyloric botulinum toxin injection and dilatation. J Pediatr Gastroenterol Nutr 2021;73(3):314–8.

55. Wellington J, Scott B, Kundu S, et al. Effect of endoscopic pyloric therapies for patients with nausea and vomiting and functional obstructive gastroparesis. Auton Neurosci 2017;202:56–61.

56. Soliman H, Oiknine E, Cohen-Sors B, et al. Efficacy and safety of endoscopic pyloric balloon dilation in patients with refractory gastroparesis. Surg Endosc 2022; 36(11):8012–20.

57. Jehangir A, Malik Z, Petrov RV, et al. EndoFLIP and pyloric dilation for gastroparesis symptoms refractory to pyloromyotomy/pyloroplasty. Dig Dis Sci 2021;66(8): 2682–90.

58. Israel DM, Mahdi G, Hassall E. Pyloric balloon dilation for delayed gastric emptying in children. Can J Gastroenterol 2001;15(11):723–7.

59. Santucci NR, Kemme S, El-Chammas KI, et al. Outcomes of combined pyloric botulinum toxin injection and balloon dilation in dyspepsia with and without delayed gastric emptying. Saudi J Gastroenterol 2022;28(4):268–75.

60. Kim SH, Keum B, Choi HS, et al. Self-expandable metal stents in patients with postoperative delayed gastric emptying after distal gastrectomy. World J Gastroenterol 2018;24(40):4578–85.

61. Maetani I, Ukita T, Tada T, et al. Gastric emptying in patients with palliative stenting for malignant gastric outlet obstruction. Hepatogastroenterology 2008;55(81): 298–302.

62. Clarke JO, Sharaiha RZ, Kord Valeshabad A, et al. Through-the-scope transpyloric stent placement improves symptoms and gastric emptying in patients with gastroparesis. Endoscopy 2013;45(Suppl 2 UCTN):E189–90.

63. Khashab MA, Besharati S, Ngamruengphong S, et al. Refractory gastroparesis can be successfully managed with endoscopic transpyloric stent placement and fixation (with video). Gastrointest Endosc 2015;82(6):1106–9.

64. Khashab MA, Stein E, Clarke JO, et al. Gastric peroral endoscopic myotomy for refractory gastroparesis: first human endoscopic pyloromyotomy (with video). Gastrointest Endosc 2013;78(5):764–8.

65. Kamal F, Khan MA, Lee-Smith W, et al. Systematic review with meta-analysis: one-year outcomes of gastric peroral endoscopic myotomy for refractory gastroparesis. Aliment Pharmacol Ther 2022;55(2):168–77.

66. Landreneau JP, Strong AT, Ponsky JL, et al. Enhanced recovery outcomes following per-oral pyloromyotomy (POP): a comparison of safety and cost with same-day discharge versus inpatient recovery. Surg Endosc 2020;34(7): 3153–62.

67. Ayinala S, Batista O, Goyal A, et al. Temporary gastric electrical stimulation with orally or PEG-placed electrodes in patients with drug refractory gastroparesis. Gastrointest Endosc 2005;61(3):455–61.

68. Kim SH, Kim HB, Chun HJ, et al. Minimally invasive gastric electrical stimulation using a newly developed wireless gastrostimulator: a pilot animal study. J Neurogastroenterol Motil 2020;26(3):410–6.

69. Islam S, Vick LR, Runnels MJ, et al. Gastric electrical stimulation for children with intractable nausea and gastroparesis. J Pediatr Surg 2008;43(3):437–42.

70. Islam S, McLaughlin J, Pierson J, et al. Long-term outcomes of gastric electrical stimulation in children with gastroparesis. J Pediatr Surg 2016;51(1):67–71.

71. Cook IJ, Talley NJ, Benninga MA, et al. Chronic constipation: overview and challenges. Neurogastroenterol Motil 2009;21(Suppl 2):1–8.

72. McCrea GL, Miaskowski C, Stotts NA, et al. A review of the literature on gender and age differences in the prevalence and characteristics of constipation in North America. J Pain Symptom Manage 2009;37(4):737–45.

73. Cash BD, Acosta RD, Chandrasekhara V, et al, ASGE Standards of Practice Committee. The role of endoscopy in the management of constipation. Gastrointest Endosc 2014;80(4):563–5.

74. Truong S, Willis S, Schumpelick V. Endoscopic therapy of benign anastomotic strictures of the colorectum by electroincision and balloon dilatation. Endoscopy 1997;29(9):845–9.

75. Virgilio C, Cosentino S, Favara C, et al. Endoscopic treatment of postoperative colonic strictures using an achalasia dilator: short-term and long-term results. Endoscopy 1995;27(3):219–22.

76. Di Lorenzo C, Flores AF, Reddy SN, et al. Colonic manometry in children with chronic intestinal pseudo-obstruction. Gut 1993;34(6):803–7.

77. Di Lorenzo C, Hillemeier C, Hyman P, et al. Manometry studies in children: minimum standards for procedures. Neurogastroenterol Motil 2002;14(4):411–20.

78. Rodriguez L, Sood M, Di Lorenzo C, et al. An ANMS-NASPGHAN consensus document on anorectal and colonic manometry in children. Neurogastroenterol Motil 2017;29(1).

79. van den Berg MM, Hogan M, Mousa HM, et al. Colonic manometry catheter placement with primary fluoroscopic guidance. Dig Dis Sci 2007;52(9):2282–6.
80. Rao SS, Singh S, Sadeghi P. Is endoscopic mucosal clipping useful for preventing colonic manometry probe displacement? J Clin Gastroenterol 2010;44(9): 620–4.
81. Rodriguez L, Flores A, Gilchrist BF, et al. Laparoscopic-assisted percutaneous endoscopic cecostomy in children with defecation disorders (with video). Gastrointest Endosc 2011;73(1):98–102.
82. Graham CD, Rodriguez L, Flores A, et al. Primary placement of a skin-level cecostomy tube for antegrade colonic enema administration using a modification of the laparoscopic-assisted percutaneous endoscopic cecostomy (LAPEC). J Pediatr Surg 2019;54(3):486–90.
83. Koyfman S, Swartz K, Goldstein AM, et al. Laparoscopic-assisted percutaneous endoscopic cecostomy (LAPEC) in children and young adults. J Gastrointest Surg 2017;21(4):676–83.
84. Colinet S, Rebeuh J, Gottrand F, et al. Presentation and endoscopic management of sigmoid volvulus in children. Eur J Pediatr 2015;174(7):965–9.
85. Parolini F, Orizio P, Bulotta AL, et al. Endoscopic management of sigmoid volvulus in children. World J Gastrointest Endosc 2016;8(12):439–43.
86. Atamanalp SS, Atamanalp RS. The role of sigmoidoscopy in thediagnosis and treatment of sigmoid volvulus. Pak J Med Sci 2016;32(1):244–8.
87. Atamanalp SS. Treatment of sigmoid volvulus: a single-center experience of 952 patients over 46.5 years. Tech Coloproctol 2013;17(5):561–9.
88. Osiro SB, Cunningham D, Shoja MM, et al. The twisted colon: a review of sigmoid volvulus. Am Surg 2012;78(3):271–9.
89. Patel RV, Njere I, Campbell A, et al. Sigmoid volvulus in an adolescent girl: staged management with emergency colonoscopic reduction and decompression followed by elective sigmoid colectomy. BMJ Case Rep 2014;2014. bcr2014206003.
90. Gershman G, Marvin A. Pediatric Colonoscopy. In: Gershman G, Marvin A, editors. Practical Pediatric Gastrointestinal Endoscopy. Malden: Blackwell Publishing Ltd Blackwell Publishing Inc; 2007. p. 272–341.
91. Raveenthiran V, Madiba TE, Atamanalp SS, et al. Volvulus of the sigmoid colon. Colorectal Dis 2010;12(7 Online):e1–17.
92. Choi D, Carter R. Endoscopic sigmoidopexy: a safer way to treat sigmoid volvulus? J R Coll Surg Edinb 1998;43(1):64.
93. Zeng M, Amodio J, Schwarz S, et al. Hirschsprung disease presenting as sigmoid volvulus: a case report and review of the literature. J Pediatr Surg 2013; 48(1):243–6.
94. Tsai MS, Lin MT, Chang KJ, et al. Optimal interval from decompression to semielective operation in sigmoid volvulus. Hepatogastroenterology 2006;53(69): 354–6.
95. Lacy BE, Crowell MD, Schettler-Duncan A, et al. The treatment of diabetic gastroparesis with botulinum toxin injection of the pylorus. Diabetes Care 2004;27(10): 2341–7.
96. Coleski R, Anderson MA, Hasler WL. Factors associated with symptom response to pyloric injection of botulinum toxin in a large series of gastroparesis patients. Dig Dis Sci 2009;54(12):2634–42.

Gastrointestinal Bleeding in Children

Current Management, Controversies, and Advances

Inna Novak, MD[a],*, Lee M. Bass, MD[b]

KEYWORDS

- Upper gastrointestinal bleeding • Hemoclips • Ulcer • Pediatric endoscopy
- Epinephrine • Portal hypertension • Esophageal varices • Transfusion

KEY POINTS

- Pediatric patients with complex comorbidities are at a higher risk for upper gastrointestinal bleeding (UGIB) and have higher mortality rates if bleeding occurs.
- Patients with gastrointestinal hemorrhage require immediate stabilization with the protection of the airway and fluid resuscitation to preserve tissue perfusion.
- Many endoscopic modalities, such as injection, mechanical, and thermal therapies are currently available for the treatment of UGIB in children.
- All patients with suspected gastrointestinal bleeding secondary to portal hypertension should be started on vasoactive therapy as soon as possible with endoscopy to perform band ligation or sclerotherapy within 24 h.
- Pre-endoscopic proton pump inhibitor therapy can significantly reduce the prevalence of high-risk endoscopic stigmata in patients with peptic ulcers and reduce the need for endoscopic intervention.

INTRODUCTION

Gastrointestinal (GI) bleeding in a child is not a rare event. There is a long list of potential etiologies that are based on age, location of bleeding, and severity of blood loss. Some bleeding may be mild and require little or no intervention, whereas some may be rapid and life-threatening. A systematic approach is necessary for both proper

I. Novak and L.M. Bass contributed equally to this work.
[a] Department of Pediatrics, Division of Pediatric Gastroenterology, Hepatology and Nutrition, Children's Hospital at Montefiore, Albert Einstein College of Medicine, 3415 Bainbridge Avenue, Bronx, NY 10467, USA; [b] Division of Gastroenterology, Hepatology and Nutrition, Ann & Robert H. Lurie Children's Hospital of Chicago, Northwestern University Feinberg School of Medicine, 225 E Chicago Avenue, Chicago, IL 60611, USA
* Corresponding author.
E-mail address: inovak@montefiore.org

Gastrointest Endoscopy Clin N Am 33 (2023) 401–421
https://doi.org/10.1016/j.giec.2022.11.003
1052-5157/23/© 2022 Elsevier Inc. All rights reserved.

diagnosis and treatment. This state-of-the-art review will discuss diagnosis and treatment of variceal and non-variceal GI bleeding and will focus on the current advances in the treatment of severe upper gastrointestinal bleeding (UGIB).

UPPER GASTROINTESTINAL BLEEDING

UGIB is defined as bleeding from the GI tract proximal to the ligament of Treitz. Pediatric studies on UGIB are mainly retrospective. The severity of UGIB varies significantly, and most children presenting to the emergency department require no intervention.[1] In more severe cases, patients are at risk for longer hospital stays and increased mortality. A recent study found that the overall mortality from UGIB was 2%, with 0.37% mortality in children with a primary diagnosis of UGIB and 2.96% mortality in those with UGIB as a secondary diagnosis, highlighting that mortality was significantly more likely in patients with multiple complex comorbidities. Endoscopy during admission was found to be protective.[2]

Presentation of UGIB can vary. A retrospective study found that 73% of children with UGIB present with hematemesis, 21% with melena, and 6% with coffee ground emesis. Other symptoms include abdominal pain or tenderness, and dizziness.[3] The rate and severity of UGIB is dependent on the etiology of the bleed (**Table 1**). UGIB should be suspected in any patient presenting with unexplained anemia. Although iron deficiency anemia is common, it is important to exclude GI blood loss in any child presenting with severe iron deficiency anemia. Nasopharyngeal bleeding can present similarly, and a thorough history and examination should be performed to differentiate it from bleeding originating in the upper GI tract.

Epidemiology

There are limited data on the incidence of UGIB in the pediatric population due to a lack of large multi-centered studies, especially because it can be difficult to distinguish from lower GI bleeding. It has been estimated that UGIB in children is three times more common than lower GI bleeding, and its incidence has increased over time, with a reported incidence of 6.4%.[4] Overall, 0.5% of all pediatric hospitalizations and 0.4% of critical care admissions are due to UGIB. The reported median age ranges from 9.3 to 11 years.[4] It remains unclear if there is a gender predisposition. Many children with UGIB have chronic medical problems, and other risk factors including trauma, coagulopathy, pneumonia, shock, organ failure, surgical procedures lasting more than 3 h, positive pressure ventilation, high pediatric risk of mortality (PRISM) score, multiple comorbidities, and prolonged nonsteroidal anti-inflammatory drugs use.

Etiology

There are many known causes of UGIB, and its prevalence varies by age. In general, bleeding is more likely to originate from the esophagus or the stomach than the small bowel. Common findings include diffuse inflammation, varices, and ulcerations. The age of the patient is an important factor in the differential diagnosis of UGIB (**Table 2**). For any critically ill child with UGIB, a stress ulcer should be considered; the etiology is unclear but presumed due to ischemia, especially in the fundus. Any significant stress on the body such as septic shock, organ failure, trauma (including burns), and cardiorespiratory collapse requiring extracorporeal membrane oxygenation can lead to the development of stress ulcers.

Comorbid conditions play a major role in understanding and treating UGIB in children. For example, patients with sickle cell disease can develop duodenal ulcers that can be a cause of frank or occult bleeding and lead to worsening anemia. These

Table 1		
Rate of upper gastrointestinal bleeding by etiology		
Low Bleeding Rate	High Bleeding Rate	Variable Bleeding Rate
• Reflux esophagitis	• Varices	• Esophagitis
• Vitamin K deficiency	• Ulcers	• Gastritis
• Mallory–Weiss tears	• Vascular malformations	
	• Dieulafoy lesions	
	• Hemobilia	

ulcers are often refractory to therapy with acid suppression but respond to treatment of underlying disease.[5] Children with previous UGIB, organ transplant recipients, and children with at least three comorbidities are also at increased risk. Medications may also contribute to UGIB by interfering with coagulation, increasing risk of mucosal ulcerations, or by causing direct mucosal damage, such as in pill esophagitis (**Table 3**). Oncology patients are particularly vulnerable to UGIB, as chemotherapy regiments often include high-dose steroids, non-steroidal anti-inflammatory drugs, and many other medications that may cause coagulopathy, mucositis, or other ulcerations of the GI tract. Angiogenesis inhibitors, which are now used in the treatment of various cancers, act by blocking growth of blood vessels to the tumor and can cause both bleeding and thrombosis.[6] Interestingly, angiogenic and anti-angiogenic therapy might also show promise in the treatment of GI ulcers.[7] In addition, cancer patients can be at risk for variceal bleeding caused by portal hypertension that develops as a result of diffuse liver infiltration with tumor, or portal or hepatic vein thrombosis.

Presentation by Age

Many common causes of UGIB depend on patient's age; however, there are many overlaps, as they can present at different ages (see **Table 2**).[8] Even congenital conditions are often not discovered until later in life. Intestinal duplications and malrotation can present with acute UGIB. Rare vascular lesions such as Dieulafoy lesion, hemangiomas, telangiectasias, and arteriovenous malformations are also on the differential for acute and chronic UGIB. Patients with the following syndromes have an increased risk of GI bleeding hereditary hemorrhagic telangiectasia or Rendu–Osler–Weber syndrome, Klippel–Trénaunay syndrome, blue rubber bleb nevus syndrome. Patients with polyposis syndromes are also at increased risk. *Helicobacter pylori* is a common cause of peptic ulcer disease, UGIB or anemia in older children, but has also been seen in toddlers and younger kids, especially in areas of high prevalence. Foreign body ingestion occurs frequently in the pediatric population, often accidental in younger children and non-accidental in adolescents. Button batteries and caustic ingestions have a high rate of complications, including UGIB. Portal hypertension secondary to liver disease can also present at any age. A thorough history and evaluation should be performed to help elucidate a potential etiology and exclude these causes.

Neonates and infants

UGIB is not common in the first few months of life; however, this symptom should be taken seriously as it can be the first presentation of a serious congenital anomaly. Swallowed maternal blood is the most common cause of UGIB in the newborn period and an Apt test can be used to differentiate maternal from fetal blood. Other considerations include coagulopathy due to vitamin K deficiency, especially if a baby was

Table 2
Common causes of upper gastrointestinal bleeding in pediatric patients

Neonatal (Birth— 1 Months)	Infancy (1 mo to 2 years)	Preschool (2 to 5 Years)	School Age (>5 Years)	All Ages
• Swallowed maternal blood • Necrotizing enterocolitis • Gastrointestinal (GI) malformations such as duodenal web, antral web, GI duplications, malrotation • Hemorrhagic disease of newborn • Cow's milk protein allergy	• Cow's milk protein allergy • GI malformations	• Esophageal varices • Foreign body/bezoar • Caustic ingestion • Mallory-Weiss tear • Henoch Schönlein purpura	• Esophageal varices • Foreign body ingestion • Mallory-Weiss tear • Inflammatory bowel disease	• Peptic ulcer disease (except infants), especially H. pylori gastritis • Esophagitis/gastritis/duodenitis (infectious, allergic, or inflammatory) • Caustic/foreign body ingestion • Medications • Coagulopathy (liver disease or coagulation disorders) • Vascular malformations • Polyps • Anastomotic ulcers

Data from Owensby S, Taylor K, Wilkins T. Diagnosis and management of upper gastrointestinal bleeding in children. J Am Board Fam Med 2015;28:134-145.

Table 3	
Medications causing gastrointestinal bleeding	
Medications Causing Pill Esophagitis	**Medications that Increase Bleeding Risk**
• Acetaminophen	• Vascular endothelial growth factor inhibitors
• Doxycycline	• Antiplatelet medications
• Bisphosphonates	• Anticoagulants
• Ascorbic acid	• Selective serotonin reuptake inhibitors
• Ferrous sulfate	
• Potassium chloride	

born outside of the hospital and was not supplemented, or due to infectious or hematologic disorders. Protein allergy can present with gastritis and UGIB, although allergic colitis is a more common presentation.

Older children and adolescents

For older children, causes are often similar to adults. Mallory-Weiss tears, gastritis, esophagitis, duodenitis (infectious, IBD related or other), peptic ulcers, and polyps are on the differential as well as medications, drug toxicities, and trauma.

Stabilization and Initial Management

The patient with severe GI hemorrhage requires immediate stabilization. The airway must be protected, and intubation may be required to protect the airway and prevent aspiration pneumonia. The goal of fluid resuscitation is to preserve tissue perfusion. Intravenous lines must be placed rapidly and volume resuscitation with either colloid, crystalloid or blood products must be initiated to restore and maintain hemodynamic stability. Persistent tachycardia may be a sign of compensated shock, whereas central venous oxygen saturation and venous lactate can be indicators of adequate tissue perfusion.[9]

Transfusions

Care should be taken to avoid volume overload, particularly in variceal hemorrhage, as this might increase portal pressure, potentially causing further bleeding. Blood transfusion with packed red blood cells (PRBCs) should be performed with the goals of maintaining hemodynamic stability and a hemoglobin of approximately 7 to 8 g/dL.[9] Compared with a more liberal transfusion strategy (goal Hgb 9 g/dL), a transfusion policy designed to transfuse only when Hgb drops below 7 g/dL in adults with GI bleeding showed fewer patients receiving blood products, fewer patients with continued bleeding and a higher probability of survival in patients with cirrhosis.[10] Prothrombin time with an internationalized normalized ratio (INR) should be measured and in children with elevation of these values, vitamin K should be administered to correct for possible deficiency.[9,11] As UGIB leads to whole blood loss with depletion of clotting factors, administration of fresh frozen plasma (FFP) may be of value. However, it should be noted that coagulation status is difficult to measure and although prothrombin time gives some indication of status, simply correcting this measurement with exogenous factor supplementation may not decrease the bleeding risk.[12] Administration of platelets should be considered if marked thrombocytopenia (less than 20,000/μL) is present.[9]

Nasogastric tube and lavage

Nasogastric tube (NGT) aspiration and lavage were previously recommended to assess UGIB; however, more recent studies show that NGT aspiration does not help predict presence of high-risk lesions.[13,14] In the setting of a suspected variceal bleed, an NGT should be placed to monitor ongoing bleed and remove blood from the GI tract, which can predispose patients with cirrhosis to encephalopathy. All patients with suspected bleeding secondary to portal hypertension should have vasoactive drug therapy initiated as soon as possible.[9,15] For likely non-variceal bleeding, a review concluded that NGT aspiration does not differentiate upper from lower GI bleeding in patients with melena. Moreover, a randomized, single-blind, noninferiority study comparing NGT placement (with aspiration and lavage) to no NGT placement (140 patients in each arm), failed to show that NGT aspiration could accurately predict the presence of a high-risk lesion requiring endoscopic therapy (39% vs 38%, respectively). In addition, adverse events (pain, nasal bleeding, or failure of NGT placement) occurred in 34% and there were no observed differences in rebleeding rates or mortality.[14]

Acid suppression

It is reasonable to start high-dose proton pump inhibitor (PPI) for any patient presenting with significant UGIB until etiology is identified and treated. There is evidence that pre-endoscopic PPI administration can significantly reduce the prevalence of high-risk endoscopic stigmata in patients with hemorrhage due to peptic ulcers, which in turn reduces the need for endoscopic intervention.[16] No pediatric data is available at this time; however, in adult patients there is no evidence that pre-endoscopic PPI therapy has an impact on patient outcomes including mortality, need for surgery, or recurrent hemorrhage. Nevertheless, importance of pre-endoscopic PPI therapy should not be undervalued because reduced need for endoscopic intervention can be particularly important when there is a delay in treatment due to lack of endoscopic facility or expertise in the treatment of UGIB in a pediatric patient. PPI administration should, however, never delay early endoscopy. Occasionally patient presenting with rapid UGIB can present without hematemesis or melena; therefore, pre-endoscopic PPI therapy can be considered in patients with clinically severe or ongoing hematochezia until a bleeding source is identified.[17] Sucralfate should not be used before endoscopy because it can obscure visualization. Post-endoscopic acid suppression is recommended for patients needing endoscopic hemostasis. Current adult guidelines all recommend 3 days of high-dose continuous or intermittent intravenous PPI, and most recommend twice daily PPI for the following 2 weeks.[18]

Prokinetics

Good endoscopic visualization is extremely important in diagnosis and treatment of UGIB. Endoscopic evaluation is adversely affected by presence of blood, clots, and fluids in the stomach. Administration of erythromycin enhances emptying of the stomach and may improve visualization on endoscopy.[19–22] A meta-analysis showed that visualization of gastric mucosa was greatly improved by administration of erythromycin before endoscopy.[23] The most common dosing reported, was either 250 mg or 3 mg/kg/dose, with medication administered most commonly 30 min before endoscopy (30 to 120 min). In addition, erythromycin administration significantly improved need for second-look endoscopy and decreased the length of hospital stay. The study did not show any effect on duration of procedure, need for surgical intervention, or units of blood transfused. No pediatric data are available.

Lactulose

Lactulose therapy may be considered, either orally or via enema, to reduce ammonia absorption.[24] Bacterial infection, either present before the bleed or acquired secondary to bacterial translocation during GI bleeding in patients with cirrhosis, is associated with both failure to control bleeding from esophageal varices and early re-bleeding.[25,26]

Antibiotics

Many studies have documented the benefit of antibiotics in adult cirrhotic patients who have had a variceal bleed and recent practice guidelines recommend the use of prophylactic antibiotics, generally intravenous ceftriaxone, following acute esophageal variceal hemorrhage in children.[9,27,28]

Vasoactive therapy

All patients with suspected bleeding secondary to portal hypertension should have vasoactive drug therapy initiated as soon as possible.[9,15] In the United States, octreotide is the primary vasoactive drug used in response to acute GI bleeding. Octreotide can be given as a bolus (1 μg/kg) and followed by continuous infusion (1 to 5 μg/kg/h). Use of octreotide to slow GI bleeding has been shown to be safe in children with varices.[29] Use of somatostatin or octreotide is not recommended in non-variceal bleeding.

Anticoagulants

Adult guidelines suggest that for patients with an acute UGIB receiving anti-coagulants, coagulopathy should be treated as necessary, but endoscopy should not be delayed.[30] Adult studies analyzing patients on anticoagulants, show that undertaking endoscopic therapy in a patient with an INR less than 2.5 appears to be safe.[31] For patients on anti-thrombotic medications or anti-coagulants before their bleeding event, halting the medication is associated with an increased risk of thromboembolic events when the medication is halted. The risk of re-bleeding may increase if the patient takes the anti-thrombotic agent again; however, it is important to take into account the overall risk to the patient of not being on the agents.[32]

Endoscopy

Scales that evaluate the clinical profile of a patient presenting with UGIB can be useful at stratifying risk and planning for the potential need for endoscopic intervention. The Glasgow Blatchford score is commonly used in adult studies and uses parameters, including blood urea nitrogen, hemoglobin, blood pressure, heart rate, the presence of melena, syncope, and co-morbidities such as hepatic disease and cardiac failure.[18] Thomson and colleagues created the Sheffield scoring system to identify pediatric patients who are likely to require endoscopic intervention. A history of co-existing medical co-morbidities, a history of large volume hematemesis, melena, heart rate greater than 20 bpm from the mean heart rate for age, prolonged capillary refill, hemoglobin drop of more than 2 g/dL, and need for fluid or blood resuscitation are all components of the score. This scoring system has shown a 91.18% positive predictive value and a negative predictive value of 88.57% in identifying patients with a need for intervention.[33]

The recommendation of the American College of Gastroenterology and European Society of Gastrointestinal Endoscopy (ESGE) guidelines is to undergo an endoscopy within 24 h of presentation for patients who require transfusions due to an acute drop of hemoglobin by 2 g/dL or a drop to a hemoglobin below 8 g/dL.[34] In patients who require ongoing circulatory support, endoscopy should be performed more urgently. A patient with UGIB should be placed nil per os immediately when they present for evaluation. Urgent endoscopy (in less than 6 h) is not recommended except in cases of button battery ingestion. A recent adult study found that urgent endoscopy was not associated with improvement in mortality in patients who were at high risk for further bleeding or death compared with those who underwent early endoscopy.[35] It is worth-while noting that there may be practical factors, such as availability of resources, that may influence the timing of endoscopy, and in a stable patient, timing can be altered to secure all the resources needed to ensure a successful procedure.[18,36]

Preparation of the endoscopy suite or operating room is also vital to the success of treating UGIB (**Box 1**). The patient should have a secure airway for the procedure. Blood or other blood products for transfusion should be present if needed. A water pump or irrigation method should be set up. Additional external suction tubing should be available and able to be used in the event of large clots. Medical therapies, such as epinephrine or sclerotherapy medications, should be available in the room. Other coagulation therapies, including hemostatic clips, argon plasma coagulation (APC), bipolar cautery, variceal band ligators, and hemospray should all be present and in working order. A back-up endoscope should be in the room in case there is a malfunction or clog in the scope you are using and finally, a consideration of a surgical or interventional radiology consultation should be made in the event that the bleeding is not amenable to endoscopic treatment.

NON-VARICEAL BLEEDING

A thorough endoscopic evaluation is likely to reveal the source of bleeding in the majority of cases. The Forrest classification developed almost 50 years ago continues to be useful in identifying features of peptic ulcers which are associated with an increased risk of continuous bleeding and rebleeding (**Table 4**).[37] Recent studies using Doppler endoscopic probes classified lesions as "high risk" (1a, 2a, and 2b), "medium risk" (1b and 2c) and low risk.[3] Other endoscopic features have been found to correlate with outcomes such as large ulcer size (greater than 2 cm), large non-bleeding vessel, ulcer location on the posterior duodenal wall or proximal lesser curvature of the stomach (see **Table 4**). Endoscopic ultrasound and through the scope Doppler probes have been used as a more objective alternative to endoscopic stigmata to identify a vascular bleeding source and assess the need for endoscopic therapy. Research has shown that use of Doppler probes is more cost-effective than visual assessment and standard therapy for non-variceal bleeding.[30]

Box 1
Preparation for endoscopic intervention

- Airway secured
- Blood for transfusion present
- Water pump/irrigation method
- Suction tubing
- Band ligator
- Sclerotherapy needle/sclerosant
- Epinephrine
- Bipolar cautery and argon plasma coagulation with equipment in working order
- Over the scope and through the scope hemoclips
- Hemospray
- Back up endoscope
- ± Surgical and/or interventional radiology consult back-up

Table 4
Forrest classification

Forrest Classification	Stigmata	Risk of Rebleeding Without Intervention
1a	Spurting active bleeding	100%
1b	Oozing active	30%
2a	Non-bleeding visible vessel	50%
2b	Adherent clot	30%
2c	Flat spot	<8%
3	Clean base	<3%

Treatment Modalities

There are many treatment modalities available to the endoscopist today. Choice of modality should depend on the type and location of the lesion, the expertise of the endoscopist with these devices, and their availability on the unit. A variety of devices should be available and prepared for use before the start of the procedure. A pediatric endoscopist is often aware of limitations of scope size and patient size when performing therapeutic procedures. The minimum channel size needed for use of the devices should be reviewed before the start of the procedure. Injection needles, APC, and electrocautery probes are available in sizes small enough to pass through a 2.0 mm channel and can be used when a child is too small for a standard scope and an infant endoscope is used.

Injectables

Epinephrine 1:10,000 dilution was used for injection around the bleeding lesion. It is usually injected in 4 quadrants around the lesion in 0.5 to 2 mL aliquots, with maximum volume of 10 mL recommended for pediatric patients.[38] In adults, volume up to 20 mL are used. Epinephrine injections work by vasoconstriction, mechanical tamponade, and platelet aggregation. Many recommend epinephrine injection before clot removal when an adherent clot is present. However, vasoconstrictive effects are not long lasting. The latest ESGE guidelines do not recommend epinephrine injection as monotherapy, but do recommend combination therapy with second endoscopic thermal or mechanical hemostasis modality.[34]

Mechanical

Endoclips achieve hemostasis by applying mechanical pressure to the bleeding site. Clips are passed through the endoscope channel and are available in variety of opening widths and jaw lengths. Many can be rotated, opened and closed and, therefore, repositioned to optimally target the bleeding lesion. They are likely to remain in place for days to weeks but will slough off eventually after placement. Many endoclips used for hemostasis are not considered magnetic resonance imaging (MRI) safe. An X-ray confirming clip passage might be necessary before proceeding with MRI, if required.[39]

Over-the-scope clips (OTSC) are a relatively novel device used for hemostasis, fistula closure or perforation. Their benefits include increased grasping strength and large diameter. They have been used successfully in adult patients for the treatment of peptic ulcer bleeding. OTSC devices are mounted on a cap similar to a band ligator

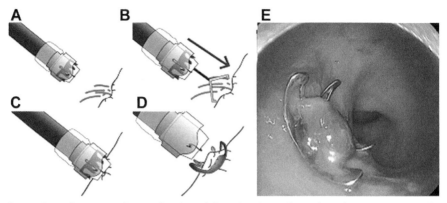

Fig. 1. Over-the-scope clip application: (*A*) Lesion is evaluated, and scope position for application of the clip determined; (*B*) the applicator is positioned over the lesion with help of grasper or forceps if needed; (*C*) the applicator is brought into close contact with mucosa and clip is deployed; and (*D*) the endoscope is withdrawn, lesion and clip position evaluated. (*E*) Endoscopic image of and ever-the-scope clip in situ. (*From* Kirschniak A, Kratt T, Stüker D, et al. A new endoscopic over-the-scope clip system for treatment of lesions and bleeding in the GI tract: first clinical experiences. Gastrointest Endosc. 2007;66(1):162-167).

and are deployed directly onto the bleeding site (**Fig. 1**). They typically slough off weeks after placement. Although devices can be removed with a special cutter they cannot be reopened once deployed. Good tissue opposition is important for proper deployment, making placement difficult in some anatomic locations. These devices come in a variety of sizes but all increase intubation diameter. The smallest have a diameter of 8.5 to 9.8 mm, resulting in an intubation diameter of 14.6 mm, which is an issue in younger children. A recent study outlined successful use of OTSC in the treatment of nonvariceal bleeding in pediatric patients.[40]

Thermal therapies

There are two types of thermal modalities that are currently available: contact and non-contact. Contact thermal probes are applied directly to the tissue and some pressure is applied during treatment. The probe should be pulled away gently to avoid dislodging a newly created clot. There are heater probes that generate heat directly and multipoloar/bioplar probes that use electric current to produce heat. Heat generated by these devices causes edema, coagulation, and vasoconstriction which lead to hemostasis (**Fig. 2**).

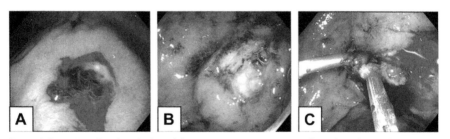

Fig. 2. (*A*) Oozing duodenal ulcer, (*B*) status post treatment with multipolar probe; and (*C*) post application of endoclips.

APC uses electron flow through a stream of ionized argon gas to cause coagulation of mucosa without direct contact of the probe with the area being treated (**Fig. 3**). To achieve coagulation, the APC probe is held few millimeters away from the tissue, the pulse setting is used, and area is "painted" by the endoscopist by gently moving the

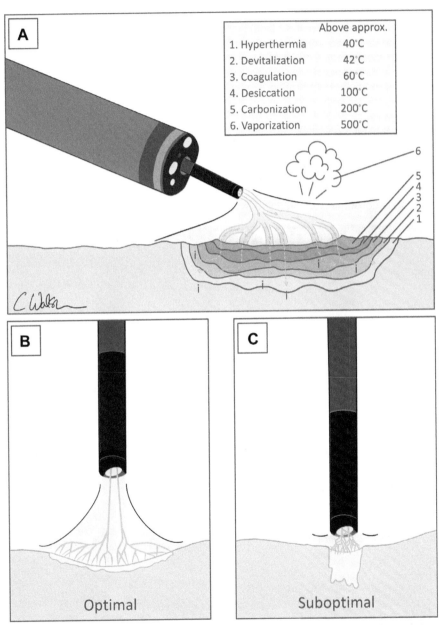

Fig. 3. (*A*) Energy is transferred between argon plasma coagulation (APC) probe and tissue without contact creating temperature dependent tissue effects (*arrows* labeled "i" represent current flow). (*B*) A distance less than 1 to 2 mm can lead to submucosal emphysema and undesirable tissue effect. (*C*) A distance of more than 1 to 2 mm is recommended for even distribution of current and optimal coagulation effect. (Courtesy of Catharine M. Walsh MD, MEd, PhD, Toronto, ON, Canada)

probe over the tissues until the desired effect is achieved. This therapy is usually reserved for coagulation of superficial lesions as the depth of penetration is only a few millimeters. Visible vessels are better treated with contact thermal probes, whereas superficial lesions (eg, telangiectasias) and large continuous lesions (eg, gastric antral vascular ectasia) respond well to APC techniques.[41]

Monopolar hemostatic forceps (MHS) is a new contact thermal endoscopic device that has been used to control bleeding during endoscopic mucosal dissection. One recent study showed improved hemostasis when comparing MHF and hemoclips for peptic ulcer bleeding.[42] When compared with other thermal therapies, MHF with soft coagulation works at a lower voltage than other coagulation devices, theoretically decreasing the risk of perforation by having decreased depth of tissue penetration.

Topical agents

Topical hemostatic powders are another therapeutic modality available to endoscopists treating actively bleeding lesions. Hemospray (TC-325) is an absorptive powder that can be sprayed onto the mucosal surface through a catheter, when it comes into contact with fluid it causes desiccation and has a rapid procoagulant effect (**Fig. 4**). It was available in many countries since 2011 and was approved by the Food and Drug Administration (FDA) in the United States in 2018.

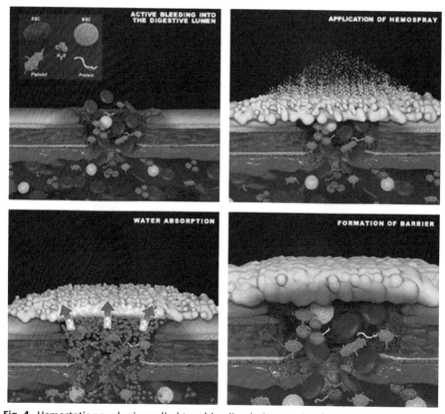

Fig. 4. Hemostatic powder is applied to a bleeding lesion causing formation of an adhesive layer when it comes into contact with fluid and/or blood. It provides a mechanical barrier and promotes hemostasis. (*From* Hookey L, Barkun A, Sultanian R, Bailey R. Successful hemostasis of active lower GI bleeding using a hemostatic powder as monotherapy, combination therapy, or rescue therapy. Gastrointest Endosc. 2019;89(4):865-871).

EndoClot, spray, consisting of absorbable modified polymers, was approved by FDA in 2021. There are other topical agents currently available in countries other than the United States. Currently, topical agents are mostly used as salvage therapy when other endoscopic modalities have failed or when there is diffuse mucosal bleeding. In recent meta-analysis, the pooled immediate hemostasis rate was 93%, with rebleeding occurring in 14.4%. In patients with variceal bleeding, immediate hemostasis was achieved in 92.3%, with rebleeding rate of 3.1% of patients.[43] A recent study showed that addition of Hemospray appears to improve immediate success rates but does not decrease re-bleeding or mortality.[44] Hemospray is easy to use and can lead to immediate successful hemostasis but might only act as a bridge to more definitive therapy as re-bleeding rates are relatively high.

Radiologic studies

Workup of UGIB starts with endoscopy as it can provide both diagnosis and treatment options for various etiologies. However, challenges such as a large amount of blood obscuring the location of bleed, comorbid conditions, post-surgical anatomy, and difficult locations can contribute to failure of endoscopic management. Computed tomography angiography (CTA) can detect bleeding rates as low as 0.3 mL/min and is helpful in identifying variant vascular anatomy. If the patient is hemodynamically stable, CTA can be useful. If the patient is hemodynamically unstable catheter angiography should be the procedure of choice as it allows for diagnosis and treatment of bleeding at the same time. CTA might not be helpful if bleeding is intermittent. Winzelberg and colleagues[45] described use of technetium 99m labeled red blood cells (RBCs) to identify GI bleeds in 1979. Although there are some changes to the method, the concept behind tagged RBC scan is that RBCs are labeled and injected into the body followed by dynamic acquisition which allows visualization of extravascular deposition of the tracer. RBC scans are time-consuming but not invasive and can be used in patients with limited renal function and contrast allergies, can detect bleeding of 0.05 to 0.1 mL/min, and can be used to identify intermittent bleeding as images can be acquired for up to 24 h.

GASTROINTESTINAL BLEEDING SECONDARY TO VARICEAL HEMORRHAGE

GI bleeding secondary to esophageal or gastric varices, presenting as hematemesis and melena, may be the initial manifestation of portal hypertension. Variceal bleeding is associated with a hepatic venous pressure gradient of more than 12 mm Hg. There are several grading systems looking at the size of varices; however, few of them have been validated for inter-observer reliability (**Fig. 5**).[9,46] Gastric varices are typically supplied by the short gastric veins. Gastric varices in continuity with esophageal varices may regress following treatment of esophageal varices. In addition, varices may be noted in the small intestine,[47] gall bladder,[48] or may present as symptomatic hemorrhoids in the rectum.[49]

Portal hypertensive gastropathy (PHG) is characterized by dilation of the mucosal and submucosal vessels of the stomach, and visually appears as discrete cherry-red spots in a lacy mosaic pattern. Bleeding from PHG is usually chronic and should be suspected in cirrhotic patients with persistent iron-deficiency anemia. A high rate of PHG has been shown in pediatric patients with end-stage liver disease.[50] In addition, patients with portal hypertension are at increased risk of bleeding from other lesions not secondary to portal hypertension, such as gastric or duodenal ulcers and gastritis.

The incidence of gastroesophageal varices in children is disease dependent, as is the risk of bleeding. Large varices, elevated prothrombin time, ascites, increased total

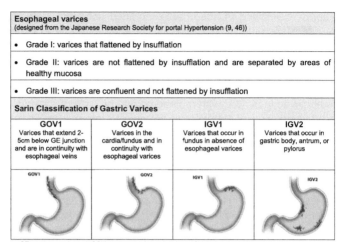

Esophageal varices (designed from the Japanese Research Society for portal Hypertension (9, 46))			
• Grade I: varices that flattened by insufflation			
• Grade II: varices are not flattened by insufflation and are separated by areas of healthy mucosa			
• Grade III: varices are confluent and not flattened by insufflation			
Sarin Classification of Gastric Varices			
GOV1	GOV2	IGV1	IGV2
Varices that extend 2-5cm below GE junction and are in continuity with esophageal veins	Varices in the cardia/fundus and in continuity with esophageal varices	Varices that occur in fundus in absence of esophageal varices	Varices that occur in gastric body, antrum, or pylorus

GE: gastro-esophageal; GOV: gastro-esophageal varices; IGV: isolated gastric varices

Fig. 5. Classification of esophageal and gastric varices. GE, gastro-esophageal; GOV, gastro-esophageal varices; IGV, isolated gastric varices. (*From* Henry Z, Patel K, Patton H, Saad W. AGA Clinical Practice Update on Management of Bleeding Gastric Varices: Expert Review. Clin Gastroenterol Hepatol. 2021;19(6):1098-1107.e1).

bilirubin, the presence of variceal red markings, and the presence of gastric varices are associated with an increased risk of bleeding.[51,52] In a recent multicenter study of variceal hemorrhage in biliary atresia, the overall incidence of variceal hemorrhage was 8 to 9.4% over 5 years, with 2.5% mortality in those who bled.[53] For patients with alpha-1 antitrypsin deficiency, 35% of patients presented with liver failure with variceal bleeding in a single-center study.[54] A majority of patients with cystic fibrosis-related liver disease (CFLD) have splenomegaly and varices[55] and 10 year cumulative variceal bleeding has been shown to be 6.6%.[56] Age at bleeding is also dependent on the underlying cause of cirrhosis, with patients who have surgically corrected but progressive biliary atresia bleeding for the first time at a mean age of 3 years and those with cystic fibrosis at a mean age of 11.5 years.[57]

Prophylaxis of Variceal Hemorrhage

Prevention of variceal hemorrhage is categorized by strategy. *Primary prophylaxis* refers to approaches to prevent the first episode of bleeding from established varices and *secondary prophylaxis* targets varices that have already bled.

Primary prophylaxis

In adults with cirrhosis and esophageal varices, the 1-year risk of a variceal hemorrhage is approximately 12%,[58] and primary prophylaxis to prevent bleeding is recommended. Although there are no clear pediatric guidelines, endoscopic surveillance of varices may identify children with cirrhosis and portal hypertension who have an increased risk of bleeding.

In children, both endoscopic variceal ligation (EVL) and sclerotherapy have been studied for primary prophylaxis. Duche and colleagues[59] used both techniques for primary prophylaxis in children with biliary atresia and major endoscopic risk factors for variceal bleeding and found that 11% of patients went on to have a GI bleed. Approaches for primary prophylaxis of gastric varices in both adults and children are based on bleeding risk, and surgical options or transjugular intrahepatic portosystemic shunt (TIPS) should be considered.[24]

Secondary prophylaxis. Owing to the high recurrence rate of variceal hemorrhage, once a first bleed has occurred, secondary prophylaxis is indicated.[9] In children, esophageal variceal obliteration by either EVL or sclerotherapy is recommended to decrease the risk of rebleeding. Treatment sessions should occur every 2 to 4 weeks until varices are eradicated.[60]

Therapy of Acute Variceal Hemorrhage

GI bleeding is a major cause of morbidity in patients with portal hypertension.[61] However, as previously discussed, the risk of mortality has decreased over the last few decades with improved medical management,[58,62] and mortality rates in children are lower than in adults.[53]

The treatment for a patient with portal hypertension and an acute GI hemorrhage is summarized in **Box 2**. The first steps to be taken include protecting the airway, assuring that the patient is breathing, and maintaining circulation. An NGT should be placed to monitor ongoing bleed and remove blood from the GI tract, which can predispose patients with cirrhosis to encephalopathy. Prophylactic antibiotics are recommended in the setting of acute esophageal variceal hemorrhage, and all patients should have vasoactive drug therapy, such as octreotide, initiated as soon as possible.[9,15] These drugs work by decreasing splanchnic blood flow, reducing portal venous inflow, and reducing portal pressure. Octreotide can be given as a bolus (1 μg/kg) followed by continuous infusion (1 to 5 μg/kg/h) or as subcutaneous injections three times daily and has been shown to safely slow the rate of GI bleeding in children with varices.[29]

Endoscopy should be performed as soon as possible once the patient is stable to determine the source of bleeding. Patients failing to respond to fluids, vasoactive medications and correction of coagulopathy may require emergent endoscopy, and rarely placement of a balloon tamponade device, emergent surgical intervention, or TIPS.[9] EVL has largely supplanted endoscopic sclerotherapy for the treatment of esophageal varices in both adults and children with good success.[59,63] In pediatrics, sclerotherapy is currently used only in infants and small children (under 10 kg) in whom the band ligation device is too large to pass through the upper esophageal sphincter. When sclerotherapy is performed, injections may be either intra-variceal, inducing thrombus formation within the vessel, or para-variceal, causing local inflammation

---

Box 2
Therapy of acute variceal hemorrhage

- Secure the airway
- Intravenous line placement with volume resuscitation with blood, crystalloid and/or colloid to achieve hemodynamic stability
- Nasogastric tube placement to evaluate ongoing bleed and remove blood from the stomach
- Blood–transfuse to a goal of approximately 7 to 8 g/dL
- Octreotide 1 mcg/kg bolus plus 1 mcg/kg/hr infusion
- Measurement of platelets and prothrombin time international normalized ratio
- Vitamin K administration
- Antibiotics–ceftriaxone or norfloxacin
- Consider urgent/emergent endoscopy if ongoing bleeding or hemodynamic instability
- Urgent elective endoscopy if controlled with octreotide and volume expansion[9]

that compresses the vessel. Sclerotherapy is effective in the treatment of variceal bleeding but is associated with a higher rate of complications than EVL, including aspiration pneumonia and esophageal stricture.[64] EVL causes thrombosis of the varix and the band and varix subsequently slough off together in approximately 5 to 7 days. Long-term administration of PPIs should be considered to reduce the risk of treatment failure after EVL.[65]

The approach to bleeding gastric varices is similar to that of esophageal varices, including initiation of medical therapy with vasoactive agents. Some gastric varices may regress the following thrombosis of associated esophageal varices. Injection of varices with tissue adhesives such as n-butyl-2-cyanoacrylate has been successful in halting gastric variceal bleeding in children,[66,67] but complications including pyrexia and abdominal pain have been described.[68] Balloon-occluded retrograde transvenous obliteration (BRTO) is an interventional radiology technique that obliterates gastric fundal varices,[69] and has been used safely in children.[70] Although both BRTO and cyanoacrylate injection may be considered in children with gastric varices, TIPS or portosystemic shunting may be associated with better long-term resolution and outcome.[9]

Surgical Therapy and Transjugular Intrahepatic Portosystemic Shunt

In patients who fail endoscopic therapy, or in whom there are additional problems such as refractory ascites, shunt surgery or TIPS may be considered. In many cases, children with progressive liver disease who fail endoscopic therapies are best treated with liver transplantation. In patients with stable liver disease who are not likely to progress to transplantation soon, surgical shunting may be an excellent option.

Surgical shunting is used to treat complications resulting from non-cirrhotic portal hypertension, including idiopathic portal hypertension, congenital hepatic fibrosis, and extra-hepatic portal vein obstruction (EHPVO). In the long term, surgical shunts control bleeding from esophageal or gastric varices in more than 90% of patients[71] and overall outcomes are very good.[72–74] The type of shunt selected depends on the underlying pathology and the vascular anatomy. Meso rex shunt is the recommended option for patients with EHPVO,[75] but requires normal liver architecture to ensure long-term patency. The distal splenorenal shunt selectively decompresses esophageal and gastric varices through the splenic vein to the left renal vein.

Creation of a TIPS effectively reduces portal pressure by creating a communication between the hepatic and portal vein. The shunt can be placed by an interventional radiologist and is technically feasible in children.[76] Indications for TIPS in pediatric patients with portal hypertension include recurrent variceal bleeding not responsive to more conservative therapy, hypersplenism, refractory ascites, hepatorenal syndrome, and hepatopulmonary syndrome.[77] Complications include portal vein leakage, encephalopathy, perforation, hemolysis, infection, and restenosis, but overall mortality from the procedure is low.[78] Studies of children with severe portal hypertensive and refractory variceal bleeding or ascites show a high degree of resolution of symptoms with TIPS.[79,80]

FUTURE ADVANCES

There are advances in use of artificial intelligence (AI) for the diagnosis and management of GI diseases.[81] Risk stratification in GI bleeding is an area of interest for many researchers in AI because identifying high-risk patients can guide both clinical decision-making and resource allocation.[82] Current prognostic models can predict rebleeding rates and need for endoscopic or surgical therapy, and many of these perform better than standard clinical scales available today, such as Glasgow-

Blatchford, Rockall, and others.[18] All the current research is being done in adult patient populations and more advances are anticipated. We hope that pediatric patients will benefit from these advances in the future.

SUMMARY

UGIB is a relatively common presentation to the pediatric gastroenterologist or pediatric emergency room. A careful history and evaluation must be performed to properly diagnose and treat UGIB in children and etiologies and treatments are very diverse. There continue to be many advances in both endoscopic techniques and equipment; however, the extant pediatric literature is limited, and much research is needed, as most data are extrapolated from adult studies and experiences.

CLINICS CARE POINTS

- Proper preparation of the endoscopy room to ensure availability of irrigation and suction, a selection of endoscopic hemostatic devices, a back-up endoscope, medications, and blood products (if required), is vital to successful treatment of upper gastrointestinal bleeding (UGIB).
- The recommended threshold level for transfusion in children with gastrointestinal bleeding is a hemoglobin of less than 7 g/dL with a post-transfusion target of 7 to 8 g/dL.
- Consider use of transjugular intrahepatic portosystemic shunt in patients with ongoing bleeding secondary to portal hypertension.
- Epinephrine injection should not be used as monotherapy in the treatment of UGIB

DISCLOSURE

The authors have nothing to disclose.

REFERENCES

1. Pant C, Sankararaman S, Deshpande A, et al. Gastrointestinal bleeding in hospitalized children in the United States. Curr Med Res Opin 2014;30:1065–9.
2. Attard TM, Miller M, Pant C, et al. Mortality associated with gastrointestinal bleeding in children: a retrospective cohort study. World J Gastroenterol 2017; 23:1608–17.
3. Cleveland K, Ahmad N, Bishop P, et al. Upper gastrointestinal bleeding in children: an 11-year retrospective endoscopic investigation. World J Pediatr 2012; 8:123–8.
4. Romano C, Oliva S, Martellossi S, et al. Pediatric gastrointestinal bleeding: Perspectives from the Italian Society of Pediatric Gastroenterology. World J Gastroenterol 2017;23:1328–37.
5. Rao S, Royal JE, Conrad HA Jr, et al. Duodenal ulcer in sickle cell anemia. J Pediatr Gastroenterol Nutr 1990;10:117–20.
6. Tol J, Cats A, Mol L, et al. Gastrointestinal ulceration as a possible side effect of bevacizumab which may herald perforation. Invest New Drugs 2008;26:393–7.
7. Szabo S, Deng X, Tolstanova G, et al. Angiogenic and anti-angiogenic therapy for gastrointestinal ulcers: new challenges for rational therapeutic predictions and drug design. Curr Pharm Des 2011;17:1633–42.
8. Owensby S, Taylor K, Wilkins T. Diagnosis and management of upper gastrointestinal bleeding in children. J Am Board Fam Med 2015;28:134–45.

9. Shneider BL, Bosch J, de Franchis R, et al. Portal hypertension in children: expert pediatric opinion on the report of the Baveno v Consensus Workshop on Methodology of Diagnosis and Therapy in Portal Hypertension. Pediatr Transplant 2012; 16:426–37.

10. Villanueva C, Colomo A, Bosch A, et al. Transfusion strategies for acute upper gastrointestinal bleeding. N Engl J Med 2013;368:11–21.

11. Ling SC. Advances in the evaluation and management of children with portal hypertension. Semin Liver Dis 2012;32:288–97.

12. Tripodi A, Mannucci PM. The coagulopathy of chronic liver disease. N Engl J Med 2011;365:147–56.

13. Machlab S, García-Iglesias P, Martínez-Bauer E, et al. Diagnostic utility of nasogastric tube aspiration and the ratio of blood urea nitrogen to creatinine for distinguishing upper and lower gastrointestinal tract bleeding. Emergencias 2018; 30:419–23.

14. Rockey DC, Ahn C, de Melo SW Jr. Randomized pragmatic trial of nasogastric tube placement in patients with upper gastrointestinal tract bleeding. J Investig Med 2017;65:759–64.

15. de Franchis R. Revising consensus in portal hypertension: report of the Baveno V consensus workshop on methodology of diagnosis and therapy in portal hypertension. J Hepatol 2010;53:762–8.

16. Sreedharan A, Martin J, Leontiadis GI, et al. Proton pump inhibitor treatment initiated prior to endoscopic diagnosis in upper gastrointestinal bleeding. Cochrane Database Syst Rev 2010;2010:Cd005415.

17. Wilcox CM, Alexander LN, Cotsonis G. A prospective characterization of upper gastrointestinal hemorrhage presenting with hematochezia. Am J Gastroenterol 1997;92:231–5.

18. Laine L, Barkun AN, Saltzman JR, et al. ACG Clinical Guideline: Upper Gastrointestinal and Ulcer Bleeding. Am J Gastroenterol 2021;116:899–917.

19. Altraif I, Handoo FA, Aljumah A, et al. Effect of erythromycin before endoscopy in patients presenting with variceal bleeding: a prospective, randomized, double-blind, placebo-controlled trial. Gastrointest Endosc 2011;73:245–50.

20. Barkun AN, Bardou M, Martel M, et al. Prokinetics in acute upper GI bleeding: a meta-analysis. Gastrointest Endosc 2010;72:1138–45.

21. Carbonell N, Pauwels A, Serfaty L, et al. Erythromycin infusion prior to endoscopy for acute upper gastrointestinal bleeding: a randomized, controlled, double-blind trial. Am J Gastroenterol 2006;101:1211–5.

22. Osman D, Djibre M, Da Silva D, et al. Management by the intensivist of gastrointestinal bleeding in adults and children. Ann Intensive Care 2012;2:46.

23. Rahman R, Nguyen DL, Sohail U, et al. Pre-endoscopic erythromycin administration in upper gastrointestinal bleeding: an updated meta-analysis and systematic review. Ann Gastroenterol 2016;29:312–7.

24. Maruyama HS. A: portal hypertension: non-surgical and surgical management. In: Maddrey WS, Eugene R, Sorrell MF, editors. Schiff's diseases of the liver. 11 edition. Hoboken (NJ): Wiley; 2011.

25. Goulis J, Armonis A, Patch D, et al. Bacterial infection is independently associated with failure to control bleeding in cirrhotic patients with gastrointestinal hemorrhage. Hepatology 1998;27:1207–12.

26. Vivas S, Rodriguez M, Palacio MA, et al. Presence of bacterial infection in bleeding cirrhotic patients is independently associated with early mortality and failure to control bleeding. Dig Dis Sci 2001;46:2752–7.

27. Garcia-Tsao G, Sanyal AJ, Grace ND, et al. Prevention and management of gastroesophageal varices and variceal hemorrhage in cirrhosis. Am J Gastroenterol 2007;102:2086–102.

28. Fernandez J, Ruiz del Arbol L, Gomez C, et al. Norfloxacin vs ceftriaxone in the prophylaxis of infections in patients with advanced cirrhosis and hemorrhage. Gastroenterology 2006;131:1049–56 [quiz: 1285].

29. Eroglu Y, Emerick KM, Whitingon PF, et al. Octreotide therapy for control of acute gastrointestinal bleeding in children. J Pediatr Gastroenterol Nutr 2004;38:41–7.

30. Barkun AN, Almadi M, Kuipers EJ, et al. Management of Nonvariceal Upper Gastrointestinal Bleeding: Guideline Recommendations From the International Consensus Group. Ann Intern Med 2019;171:805–22.

31. Chaudhary S, Stanley AJ. Optimal timing of endoscopy in patients with acute upper gastrointestinal bleeding. Best Pract Res Clin Gastroenterol 2019;42-43:101618.

32. Kim JS, Kim BW, Kim DH, et al. Guidelines for Nonvariceal Upper Gastrointestinal Bleeding. Gut Liver 2020;14:560–70.

33. Thomson MA, Leton N, Belsha D. Acute upper gastrointestinal bleeding in childhood: development of the Sheffield scoring system to predict need for endoscopic therapy. J Pediatr Gastroenterol Nutr 2015;60:632–6.

34. Tringali A, Thomson M, Dumonceau JM, et al. Pediatric gastrointestinal endoscopy: European Society of Gastrointestinal Endoscopy (ESGE) and European Society for Paediatric Gastroenterology Hepatology and Nutrition (ESPGHAN) Guideline Executive summary. Endoscopy 2017;49:83–91.

35. Lau JYW, Yu Y, Tang RSY, et al. Timing of Endoscopy for Acute Upper Gastrointestinal Bleeding. N Engl J Med 2020;382:1299–308.

36. Thomson M, Tringali A, Dumonceau JM, et al. Paediatric Gastrointestinal Endoscopy: European Society for Paediatric Gastroenterology Hepatology and Nutrition and European Society of Gastrointestinal Endoscopy Guidelines. J Pediatr Gastroenterol Nutr 2017;64:133–53.

37. Forrest JA, Finlayson ND, Shearman DJ. Endoscopy in gastrointestinal bleeding. Lancet 1974;2:394–7.

38. Kay MBN, Wyllie R. Esophagogastroduodenoscopy and related techniques. In: Kay RWJHM, editor. Pediatric gastrointestinal and liver disease. Philadelphia: Elsevier; 2021.

39. Sung JJ, Tsoi KK, Lai LH, et al. Endoscopic clipping versus injection and thermocoagulation in the treatment of non-variceal upper gastrointestinal bleeding: a meta-analysis. Gut 2007;56:1364–73.

40. Tran P, Carroll J, Barth BA, et al. Over the scope clips for treatment of acute non-variceal gastrointestinal bleeding in children are safe and effective. J Pediatr Gastroenterol Nutr 2018;67:458–63.

41. Yeh PJ, Le PH, Chen CC, et al. Application of argon plasma coagulation for gastrointestinal angiodysplasia in children- experience from a tertiary center. Front Pediatr 2022;10:867632.

42. Toka B, Eminler AT, Karacaer C, et al. Comparison of monopolar hemostatic forceps with soft coagulation versus hemoclip for peptic ulcer bleeding: a randomized trial (with video). Gastrointest Endosc 2019;89:792–802.

43. Mutneja H, Bhurwal A, Go A, et al. Efficacy of hemospray in upper gastrointestinal bleeding: a systematic review and meta-analysis. J Gastrointestin Liver Dis 2020;29:69–76.

44. Chahal D, Sidhu H, Zhao B, et al. Efficacy of Hemospray (TC-325) in the Treatment of Gastrointestinal Bleeding: An Updated Systematic Review and Meta-analysis. J Clin Gastroenterol 2021;55:492–8.

45. Winzelberg GG, McKusick KA, Strauss HW, et al. Evaluation of gastrointestinal bleeding by red blood cells labeled in vivo with technetium-99m. J Nucl Med 1979;20:1080–6.

46. Beppu K, Inokuchi K, Koyanagi N, et al. Prediction of variceal hemorrhage by esophageal endoscopy. Gastrointest Endosc 1981;27:213–8.

47. Bass LM, Kim S, Superina R, et al. Jejunal varices diagnosed by capsule endoscopy in patients with post-liver transplant portal hypertension. Pediatr Transplant 2017;21.

48. Yamada RM, Hessel G. Ultrasonographic assessment of the gallbladder in 21 children with portal vein thrombosis. Pediatr Radiol 2005;35:290–4.

49. Heaton ND, Davenport M, Howard ER. Symptomatic hemorrhoids and anorectal varices in children with portal hypertension. J Pediatr Surg 1992;27:833–5.

50. Ng NB, Karthik SV, Aw MM, et al. Endoscopic Evaluation in Children With End-Stage Liver Disease-Associated Portal Hypertension Awaiting Liver Transplant. J Pediatr Gastroenterol Nutr 2016;63:365–9.

51. Duche M, Ducot B, Tournay E, et al. Prognostic value of endoscopy in children with biliary atresia at risk for early development of varices and bleeding. Gastroenterology 2010;139:1952–60.

52. Duche M, Ducot B, Ackermann O, et al. Portal hypertension in children: High-risk varices, primary prophylaxis and consequences of bleeding. J Hepatol 2017;66: 320–7.

53. Bass LM, Ye W, Hawthorne K, et al. Risk of variceal hemorrhage and pretransplant mortality in children with biliary atresia. Hepatology 2022;76(3):712–26.

54. Bakula A, Pawlowska J, Niewiadomska O, et al. Liver transplantation in polish children with alpha1-antitrypsin deficiency: a single-center experience. Transplant Proc 2016;48:3323–7.

55. Stonebraker JR, Ooi CY, Pace RG, et al. Features of severe liver disease with portal hypertension in patients with cystic fibrosis. Clin Gastroenterol Hepatol 2016; 14:1207–15.e3.

56. Ye W, Narkewicz MR, Leung DH, et al. Variceal hemorrhage and adverse liver outcomes in patients with cystic fibrosis cirrhosis. J Pediatr Gastroenterol Nutr 2018; 66(1):122–7.

57. Debray D, Lykavieris P, Gauthier F, et al. Outcome of cystic fibrosis-associated liver cirrhosis: management of portal hypertension. J Hepatol 1999;31:77–83.

58. Garcia-Tsao G, Bosch J. Management of varices and variceal hemorrhage in cirrhosis. N Engl J Med 2010;362:823–32.

59. Duche M, Ducot B, Ackermann O, et al. Experience with endoscopic management of high-risk gastroesophageal varices, with and without bleeding, in children with biliary atresia. Gastroenterology 2013;145:801–7.

60. D'Antiga L. Medical management of esophageal varices and portal hypertension in children. Semin Pediatr Surg 2012;21:211–8.

61. Carneiro de Moura M, Chen S, Kamath BM, et al. Acute variceal bleeding causes significant morbidity. J Pediatr Gastroenterol Nutr 2018;67:371–6.

62. Carbonell N, Pauwels A, Serfaty L, et al. Improved survival after variceal bleeding in patients with cirrhosis over the past two decades. Hepatology 2004;40:652–9.

63. dos Santos JM, Ferreira AR, Fagundes ED, et al. Endoscopic and pharmacological secondary prophylaxis in children and adolescents with esophageal varices. J Pediatr Gastroenterol Nutr 2013;56:93–8.

64. Abd El-Hamid N, Taylor RM, Marinello D, et al. Aetiology and management of extrahepatic portal vein obstruction in children: King's College Hospital experience. J Pediatr Gastroenterol Nutr 2008;47:630–4.
65. Hidaka H, Nakazawa T, Wang G, et al. Long-term administration of PPI reduces treatment failures after esophageal variceal band ligation: a randomized, controlled trial. J Gastroenterol 2012;47:118–26.
66. Rivet C, Robles-Medranda C, Dumortier J, et al. Endoscopic treatment of gastroesophageal varices in young infants with cyanoacrylate glue: a pilot study. Gastrointest Endosc 2009;69:1034–8.
67. Fuster S, Costaguta A, Tobacco O. Treatment of bleeding gastric varices with tissue adhesive (Histoacryl) in children. Endoscopy 1998;30:S39–40.
68. Turler A, Wolff M, Dorlars D, et al. Embolic and septic complications after sclerotherapy of fundic varices with cyanoacrylate. Gastrointest Endosc 2001;53:228–30.
69. Kumamoto M, Toyonaga A, Inoue H, et al. Long-term results of balloon-occluded retrograde transvenous obliteration for gastric fundal varices: hepatic deterioration links to portosystemic shunt syndrome. J Gastroenterol Hepatol 2010;25:1129–35.
70. Hisamatsu C, Kawasaki R, Yasufuku M, et al. Efficacy and safety of balloon-occluded retrograde transvenous obliteration for gastric fundal varices in children. Pediatr Surg Int 2008;24:1141–4.
71. de Ville de Goyet J, D'Ambrosio G, Grimaldi C. Surgical management of portal hypertension in children. Semin Pediatr Surg 2012;21:219–32.
72. Emre S, Dugan C, Frankenberg T, et al. Surgical portosystemic shunts and the Rex bypass in children: a single-centre experience. HPB (Oxford) 2009;11:252–7.
73. Lillegard JB, Hanna AM, McKenzie TJ, et al. A single-institution review of portosystemic shunts in children: an ongoing discussion. HPB Surg 2010;2010:964597.
74. Scholz S, Sharif K. Surgery for portal hypertension in children. Curr Gastroenterol Rep 2011;13:279–85.
75. Shneider BL, de Ville de Goyet J, Leung DH, et al. Primary prophylaxis of variceal bleeding in children and the role of MesoRex Bypass: Summary of the Baveno VI Pediatric Satellite Symposium. Hepatology 2016;63:1368–80.
76. Lorenz JM. Placement of transjugular intrahepatic portosystemic shunts in children. Tech Vasc Interv Radiol 2008;11:235–40.
77. Paramesh AS, Husain SZ, Shneider B, et al. Improvement of hepatopulmonary syndrome after transjugular intrahepatic portasystemic shunting: case report and review of literature. Pediatr Transplant 2003;7:157–62.
78. Gazzera C, Righi D, Doriguzzi Breatta A, et al. Emergency transjugular intrahepatic portosystemic shunt (TIPS): results, complications and predictors of mortality in the first month of follow-up. Radiol Med 2012;117:46–53.
79. Di Giorgio A, Agazzi R, Alberti D, et al. Feasibility and efficacy of transjugular intrahepatic portosystemic shunt (TIPS) in children. J Pediatr Gastroenterol Nutr 2012;54:594–600.
80. Heyman MB, LaBerge JM, Somberg KA, et al. Transjugular intrahepatic portosystemic shunts (TIPS) in children. J Pediatr 1997;131:914–9.
81. Dhaliwal J, Walsh CM. Artificial intelligence in pediatric endoscopy: current status and future applications. Gastrointest Endosc Clin N Am 2023;33(2):305–22.
82. Kröner PT, Engels MM, Glicksberg BS, et al. Artificial intelligence in gastroenterology: A state-of-the-art review. World J Gastroenterol 2021;27:6794–824.

The Role of Endoscopy in the Diagnosis and Management of Small Bowel Pathology in Children

Amornluck Krasaelap, MD[a],*, Diana G. Lerner, MD[b], Salvatore Oliva, MD, PhD[c]

KEYWORDS

- Capsule endoscopy • Enteroscopy • Device-assisted enteroscopy • Small bowel
- Small bowel bleeding

KEY POINTS

- Capsule endoscopy provides a reliable and noninvasive method for small bowel evaluation.
- Device-assisted enteroscopy is crucial for diagnosing and treating a wide range of small bowel pathology that is not achievable by conventional endoscopy.
- Various small bowel imaging modalities can be used to accurately diagnose small bowel pathology and localize the site of small bowel bleeding.

INTRODUCTION

Capsule endoscopy (CE) has revolutionized small bowel (SB) imaging by providing a reliable and noninvasive method for complete visualization and assessment of the mucosal surface. Given the increased detection of SB disease by CE, innovations in device-assisted enteroscopy (DAE) have been crucial for histopathological confirmation, enabling endoscopic therapy in selected cases and thus avoiding surgery for a broad range of SB pathology.

[a] Division of Pediatric Gastroenterology, Hepatology and Nutrition, Children's Mercy Hospital, 2401 Gillham Road, Kansas City, MO 64108, USA; [b] Division of Pediatric Gastroenterology, Department of Pediatrics, Hepatology and Nutrition, Medical College of Wisconsin, 8701 Watertown Plank Road, Milwaukee, WI 53226, USA; [c] Maternal and Child Health Department, Pediatric Gastroenterology and Liver Unit, Sapienza - University of Rome, Piazzale Aldo Moro, 5 00185, Roma, RM, Italy
* Corresponding author.
E-mail address: akrasaelap@cmh.edu

Gastrointest Endoscopy Clin N Am 33 (2023) 423–445
https://doi.org/10.1016/j.giec.2022.11.007
1052-5157/23/© 2022 Elsevier Inc. All rights reserved.

The purpose of this review is to provide a comprehensive overview of the indications, techniques, and clinical applications of CE, DAE, and imaging studies for SB evaluation in children.

INDICATIONS FOR SMALL BOWEL EVALUATION

Multiple indications warrant SB evaluation with either CE and DAE.[1–3] In adults, the most common indications for SB endoscopy are SB bleeding (66%), pain, diarrhea, and/or weight loss (11%) and evaluation of Crohn's disease (10%).[1] In older children, suspected or known inflammatory bowel disease (IBD) is the most common reason for SB endoscopy, whereas in younger children, suspected SB bleeding is the most common indication.[4] **Box 1** summarizes common pediatric indications of SB endoscopy.

CAPSULE ENDOSCOPY

Capsule endoscopy (CE) is a noninvasive, accurate diagnostic technique for viewing intestinal mucosa, invented in the 1990s by Israeli engineer Gavriel Iddan. After the Food and Drug Administration's approval in 2001, CE was recognized as the first-choice diagnostic tool for SB lesions (**Fig. 1**). In the United States, its use was approved for children aged 10 years and up in 2004 and children aged 2 years and up in 2009. However, CE has been done safely in children as young as 8 months and 7.9 kg.[5,6] Younger children may have difficulty swallowing the capsule, necessitating endoscopic placement under sedation or general anesthesia with endotracheal intubation.[7]

The main characteristics of several capsule devices that are now available are summarized in **Table 1**. A capsule endoscope, a sensing system attached to the patient that includes either a sensing array or a sensing belt, a data recorder, a battery pack, and software for image review and interpretation are typically included in these systems. Upgrading CE's technical aspects (dual or rotational cameras, wider field of vision, longer battery life) and the software (dynamic imaging speed, real-time viewing)

Box 1
Indications of small bowel endoscopy in children

- Small bowel Crohn's disease
- Small bowel bleeding
- Iron deficiency anemia
- Small bowel polyps
- Familial and other polyposis syndromes
- Malabsorption and protein-losing enteropathies
- Celiac disease
- Eosinophilic and food-allergic enteropathies
- Intestinal lymphangiectasia
- Chronic abdominal pain
- Small bowel tumors
- Transplantation
- Intestinal graft versus host disease

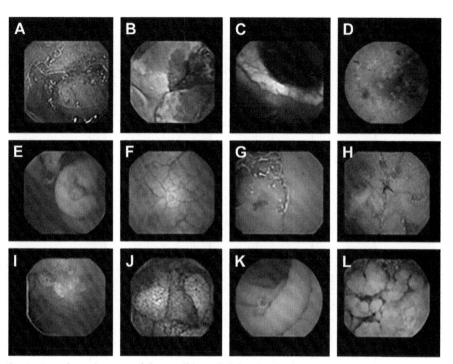

Fig. 1. Capsule endoscopy of the small bowel. (*A*) Polyp in the jejunum; (*B*) Crohn's disease, with ulceration and stenosis; (*C*) Crohn's disease small bowel stricture; (*D*) ulceration in the jejunum in inflammatory bowel disease; (*E*) small bowel intussusception; (*F*) aphthous ulcers in the colon; (*G*) arteriovenous malformation; (*H*) vascular malformation; (*I*) patchy lymphangiectasia; (*J*) extensive lymphangiectasia; (*K*) scalloping mucosa in celiac disease; and (*L*) lymphoid hyperplasia. (*Adapted from* Cohen SA, Oliva S. Capsule Endoscopy in Children. Front Pediatr. 2021;9:664722.)

and better bowel cleansing have improved diagnostic accuracy. However, these features differ across currently available CE systems.

CE is continuing to evolve. A slightly larger colon capsule (Medtronic) and a pan-enteric capsule (dubbed the Crohn's capsule, Medtronic, USA) to evaluate the SB and colon in the same procedure are already available in Europe. The colon capsule endoscopy (PillCam COLON 2, Medtronic, Minneapolis, USA) has also been proposed as a useful "one-step," noninvasive method in monitoring pediatric patients with IBD, considering its reported high accuracy in evaluating both the SB and the colon (sensitivity and specificity of 89% and 92%, respectively).[8] The pan-enteric capsule has shown promising results in the adult population.[9,10]

Despite advances in technology, CE has some limitations. First, the battery life may not be long enough to evaluate the entire intestine depending on the SB transit time; however, battery life is continuing to improve. Second, neither biopsies nor therapeutic interventions can be completed during the procedure. Third, the lack of steerability and limited view may lead to suboptimal visualization. Studies have shown that CE can miss about 30% of discrete lesions, particularly in the proximal SB where capsules are rapidly propelled by gut motility.[11–14] In addition, lesions appearing on a single frame may be challenging to interpret. Finally, there is a risk of capsule retention. A recent meta-analysis found that retention risk varies by procedure indication, with lower rates

Table 1
Capsule endoscopy

	PillCam				EndoCapsule EC-S10	MiroCam MC1600, MC2000	OMOM	CapsoCam Plus
	UGI	SB3	CROHN'S	COLON2				
Manufacturer	Medtronic, Minneapolis, MN, USA				Olympus, Tokyo, Japan	IntroMedic, Seoul, Korea	Jinshan Science and Technology, Chongqing, China	CapsoVision, Saratoga, CA, USA
Dimensions, mm	11.6 × 32.3	11.4 × 26.2	11.6 × 32.3	11.6 × 32.3	11 × 26	11 × 24.5	11 × 25.4	11 × 31
Weight, g	3	3	3	3	3.3	3.25–4.7	3	4
Frame rate, fps	18–35	2–6	4–35	4–35	2	3, 6	2–10	20 max
Operating time	1.5 h	≥8 h	≥10 h	≥10 h	≥12 h	11 h	12 h	15 h
Imaging heads	2	1	2	2	1	1, 2	1	4
Field of view, °	172 × 2	156	168 × 2	172 × 2	160	170 (× 2)	172	360
MDO, mm	>0.1	>0.07	>0.1	>0.1	ns	ns	ns	ns
Transmission mode	RF	RF	RF	RF	RF	EFP	RF	USB
Features	—	—	—	3D Track		MiroCam Navi can be controlled by magnetic force		Capsule retrieval, no external receiver equipment

Abbreviations: EFP, electric field propagation; fps, frames per second; MDO, minimum detectable object; ns, not specified; RF, radiofrequency; USB, universal serial bus.

among children than adults (1.64 vs 3.49%).[15] Nevertheless, CE is an evolving technology undergoing continual improvements aimed at overcoming many of these limitations.

Patency Capsule

The patency capsule (PC) was designed to prevent capsule retention in high-risk patients. Despite being identical to a CE in size and shape, a PC is filled with lactose and protected by a plug with a hole that allows the influx of intestinal fluid, causing it to dissolve the lactose in approximately 30 to 40 hours. PCs also have a transmitter that allows them to be detected by a hand-held scanner placed near the abdominal wall or on a radiograph. The Agile PC (Given Imaging, Yoqneam, Israel) has dissolvable plugs at both ends that implode after 30 hours to improve its noninvasive use in assessing the functional patency of intestinal strictures.[16]

In a meta-analysis of 35 papers involving 4219 adult and pediatric patients with Crohn's disease, 3.32% had retention. Patients with known Crohn's disease had a higher retention risk (4.63%) than suspected Crohn's disease (2.35%). Retention rates were 3.49% in adults and 1.64% in those younger than 18 years. In adults, the retention risk was 3.4 times higher in individuals with established Crohn's disease compared with suspected disease, but there was no difference in children. In established Crohn's disease, retention risk decreased if a PC or magnetic resonance/computed tomography enterography (MRE/CTE) was performed ahead of the procedure to evaluate for potential luminal narrowing.[17]

In a retrospective analysis, CE was performed successfully in all but 1 of 19 children where patency was established.[18] A prospective trial of children aged 10 to 16 years showed that most children excreted an intact PC within a mean of 34.5 hours, and no PC retentions or side effects were noted.[19] Crohn's disease was eventually diagnosed in all patients with a PC transit time of more than 40 hours and in 9 of 12 patients who passed the PC in 40 hours or less. Thus, the PC can be a useful guide and reduce the risk of CE retention, especially in children with known Crohn's disease.

Bowel Cleansing

Debris, bubbles, bile, and blood in the distal SB can limit CE's diagnostic ability.[20] Because of the inability to flush or suction fluids or gas during CE, adequate bowel cleaning is essential. Various cleansing regimens have been tested in adults.[21,22] The only pediatric prospective study to evaluate bowel preparation for CE showed that polyethylene glycol solution at a dose of 1.75 g/25 mL per kg (up to 70 g/1000 mL) the night before the procedure with 20 mL (376 mg) of oral simethicone given 30 min was most successful, lessening discomfort and improving visualization in the distal ileum, the portion most often impaired by debris.[23] Domperidone, metoclopramide, or sodium phosphate can be used to promote the transit of CE with a 95% completion rate and 84% excretion rate.[8,24] The Korea-Canada score has been validated to evaluate SB cleansing for CE in adults and has nearly perfect interrater and intrarater reliability.[25]

Contraindications

The only absolute contraindication to CE is luminal gastrointestinal tract obstruction or significant narrowing. Because safety data are unavailable, CE should be limited to urgent cases in pregnant individuals. In addition, manufacturers still advise against CE for people with implanted cardioassistive devices, although CE is theoretically safe. Although CEs are not proved safe with MRI, patients who have incidentally undergone MRI have been reported, showing susceptibility artifacts but no clinical harm.[17]

DEVICE-ASSISTED ENTEROSCOPY

The development of DAE has revolutionized SB evaluation in children and adults. Current options for DAE include balloon-assisted enteroscopy (BAE, ie, single-balloon enteroscopy [SBE] and double-balloon enteroscopy [DBE]), and spiral enteroscopy (SE). Enteroscope systems are further described in **Table 2**.[26,27]

DAE was first developed in 2001 by Yamamoto, who described DBE (Fujifilm, Tokyo, Japan).[28] This system includes an enteroscope with a distal mounted balloon, an overtube with a balloon, and a pump system; this was followed by the SBE (Olympus Medical Systems Corporation, Tokyo, Japan) in 2007. The main difference with SBE is the lack of a balloon on the enteroscope. It still includes an overtube with an inflatable balloon and a pump. Spiral enteroscopy (Endo-Ease Discovery SB, Spirus Medical, Stoughton, MA, USA) came to market in 2008. This technology involves an overtube fitted over a standard flexible enteroscope. Active rotation leads to pulling the intestine onto the scope.[28] BAE (SMART Medical Systems Ltd, Ra'anana, Israel) is an on-demand enteroscopy. It is easy to add to any ongoing procedure, as this device can be used with a standard endoscope/colonoscope in the SB. Motorized Spiral Enteroscopy (Olympus Medical Systems Corporation, Tokyo, Japan) is currently under investigation. It has high-definition imaging, enhanced optics, narrow-band imaging, a 3.2-mm accessory channel, and a separate channel for irrigation. It involves the endoscopist using an electric motor in the handle, which facilitates the rotation of the overtube. A foot pedal activates the rotation, and a light-emitting diode monitor gives feedback on tissue pressure to prevent damage to the SB.[27] Surgery-assisted intraoperative enteroscopy is accomplished sterilely with the enteroscope introduced directly into the SB via an enterotomy or the mouth. Still, it is advanced with the assistance of laparoscopy or laparotomy.

DAE enables direct visualization of SB lesions (**Fig. 2**) and a safe and effective means to treat SB pathology. Although diagnostic yields among SBE, DBE, and SE are similar, DBE has the deepest insertion capabilities and the longest procedure time.[26] BAE is commonly performed and well tolerated in children. The procedure is more challenging in smaller children, but it can be performed safely in children 3 years of age and older and weighing more than 14 kg.[29,30]

Diagnostic indications for enteroscopy include evaluation of abnormal findings detected on CE or imaging as well as those summarized in **Box 1**. Therapeutic enteroscopy allows for control of SB bleeding, dilation of SB stenosis, removal of polyps and foreign bodies, tattooing of lesions, placement of jejunal feeding tubes, SB stenting, SB intussusception, and access to the hepatobiliary tree in altered anatomy.[31]

Preprocedure Preparation

For both anterograde and retrograde approaches, abstaining from food for 8 to 12 hours and liquid for 4 to 6 hours ahead of the procedure is recommended. Colonoscopy preparation is also needed for the retrograde approach. If a slower transit is expected due to patient-specific factors, a longer NPO duration may be necessary.

Intraprocedural Technique

Lubricants such as olive or vegetable oil, antifoam solution, and irrigation system can improve procedural efficiency. An irrigation valve (BioShield irrigator; US Endoscopy, Mentor, Ohio, USA) is available for immediate, direct irrigation even with a device in the channel. It is common to have backflow of intestinal secretions from the overtube during the procedure. Personal protective equipment should include foot covers, mask and eye protection, hair covers, and a water-resistant gown.[32]

Table 2
Enteroscopy systems

Manufacturer	Model	Scope Diameter (mm)	Overtube Diameter (mm)	Working Channel (mm)	Working Length (mm)	Diagnostic Yield %	Advantages	Disadvantages
Fujinon (double-balloon enteroscopy)	EI-580BT	9.4	13.2	3.2	1550	40–88	Depth of insertion	2 operators
	EN-580T	9.4	13.2	3.2	2000		Smaller overtube available	Complex
	EN-580XP	7.5	11.6	2.2	2000			Longer procedure
Olympus (single-balloon enteroscopy)	SIF-Q180	9.2	13.2	2.8	2000	41–65	Shorter procedure time	Lower depth of insertion
	SIF-H290S	9.2	13.2	3.2	1520		Easier to master	
	SIF-H190	9.2	13.2	3.2	2000			
Olympus (motorized spiral enteroscopy)	PSF-1	11.3	18.1	3.2	1680	65–80	Short procedure Easy to use	Large insertion diameter May require esophageal dilation
Smart Medical Systems	NaviAid	N/A				45–59	Device used with existing scopes	Limited data
Spirus Medical	Endo-Ease Discover SB, Endo-Ease Vista Retrograde	N/A	14.5 mm	N/A		30–65	Shorter procedure	2 operators

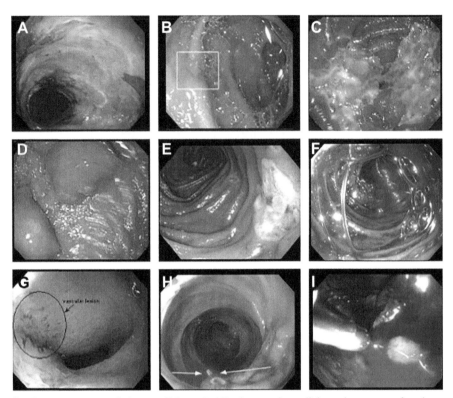

Fig. 2. Enteroscopy of the small bowel. (*A*) abnormal small bowel mucosa after bone marrow transplant; (*B*) Crohn's disease ulcer (*Yellow box*); (*C*) mid-small bowel stricture; (*D*) jejunal polyps; (*E*) postpolypectomy site in the jejunum; (*F*) active bleeding in the distal jejunum; (*G*) vascular lesion in the small bowel; (*H*) dieulafoy lesion in mid jejunum (*Yellow arrows*); and (*I*) single balloon enteroscopy for control of bleeding, with a clip applied to the area of active bleeding.

The average duration of DAE is 90 to 120 minutes.[31] Sedation is critical for maximizing diagnostic yield and patient comfort. Although retrospective adult studies suggest that conscious sedation is safe, with an adverse anesthesia event rate of 0% to 0.5%,[2] the authors recommend general anesthesia with endotracheal intubation in pediatrics based on expert opinion.

A dedicated team familiar with preprocedural and intraprocedural assistance will help facilitate the most effective, efficient, and safe DAE. Carbon dioxide, versus air insufflation, increases insertion depth and patient comfort.[2] Fluoroscopy was routinely used during the early stages of DAE, but it is now used based on endoscopist preference. There is no evidence to suggest that using fluoroscopy increases yield.

The antegrade route is preferred in the setting of massive overt bleeding or if the area of interest is unknown or seen on CE before 75% of the total time from ingestion to the cecum or 60% of the time from pylorus to the cecum.[33,34] A retrograde approach, although more technically difficult, is preferred when evaluating Crohn's disease or neuroendocrine tumors.

SB insertion depth should be estimated by counting the net advancement of the DAE during the insertion phase, with confirmation of this estimate during withdrawal.

A thorough evaluation of lesions generally takes place during the withdrawal portion of the procedure to limit overinflation. It is recommended that a tattoo be placed to mark the identified lesion and/or the deepest point of insertion. It is not advisable to combine retrograde and anterograde approaches on the same day.[2]

BAE involves advancing and retracting motions that allow the bowel to be plicated onto the endoscope using balloons to stabilize it during retraction (**Figs. 3** and **4**).[35]

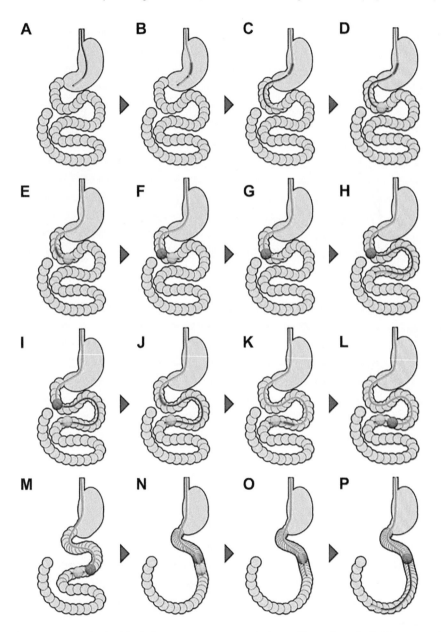

Fig. 3. Antegrade double-balloon enteroscopy technique. (*From* Sunada K, Yamamoto H. Double Balloon Enteroscopy: Techniques. Techniques in Gastrointestinal Endoscopy. 2008;(10)2:46-53; with permission.)

Because of the length and repetition of this procedure, proper ergonomics can help prevent strain and injury. It is best to position the patient in the left lateral position. The monitor should be at eye level in front of the endoscopist. There should be enough space behind the endoscopist to allow the assistant to hold the overtube and extend

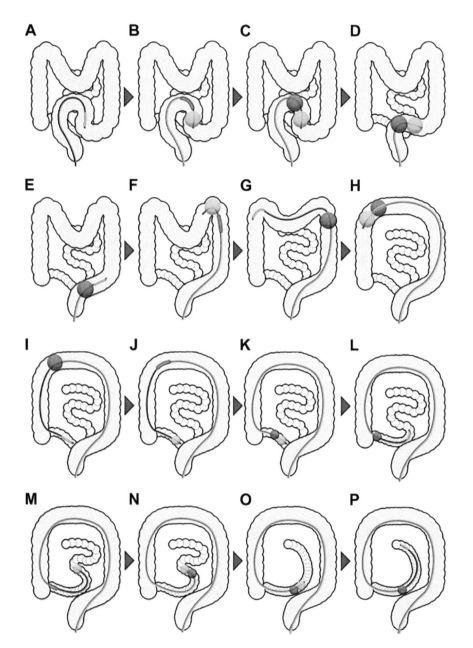

Fig. 4. Retrograde double-balloon enteroscopy technique. *From* Sunada K, Yamamoto H. Double Balloon Enteroscopy: Techniques. Techniques in Gastrointestinal Endoscopy. 2008;(10)2:46-53; with permission.

the enteroscope fully.[32] The assistant should be seated at the patient's mouth, facing the legs, with an arm board to rest both elbows while holding the overtube straight. Helpful images of proper room setup are described by Lo and colleagues.[32]

To avoid balloon pressure on the ampulla, the endoscope with the overtube must reach the jejunum before inflating the balloon. To avoid looping, place the patient supine and apply pressure to the left/epigastric region for an anterograde approach and the right/midline region for a retrograde approach. A small amount of oil in the channel can make passage easier.

Newer DAEs have 3.2 mm channels to aid in therapeutics.[36] Given the thin wall of the SB, therapeutic interventions should be performed with caution. Keeping the voltage to minimally effective settings is recommended for therapy for vascular and bleeding lesions. Injection of 1 to 2 mL of a lifting agent (1 in 100,000 epinephrine or adrenaline in normal saline) and placing the snare close to the stalk head can decrease the risk of perforation during polypectomy. Prior imaging should be used to plan stricture dilation and possibly intraoperative fluoroscopy. Favorable strictures for SB dilation include straight, short (<5 cm), and those without active inflammation.[2] Through-the-scope balloons with a soft tip wire are preferred if the narrowing cannot be traversed by the enteroscope.

Postprocedure

Most diagnostic procedures are outpatient procedures unless the patient is at high risk for complications. Most patients can resume eating within 1 to 2 hours. Postprocedural care following therapeutic DAE should be individualized. Pancreatitis after DAE is rare, so routine pancreatic enzyme testing is not recommended.

Training

Enteroscopy training can be considered when both diagnostic and therapeutic upper and lower endoscopy procedures have been mastered. Proctoring at least 10–15 anterograde DBE or SBE, 5 SE, and 30–35 retrograde procedures is suggested, though the exact number depends on the individual.[37] No formal training guidelines or competency assessment tools exist for pediatric endoscopy.

Adverse Events

Overall, DAE is safe and effective. The reported adverse event rate for diagnostic procedures is approximately 1% in adults.[38] For therapeutic enteroscopy, the reported rate increases up to 10% in adults,[38] with the highest risk in patients with altered anatomy and for intraoperative enteroscopy. Severe adverse events include perforation, pancreatitis, bleeding, and death.[26] Other adverse events include mucosal stripping, cardiovascular events, and parotid gland swelling.

A large retrospective study of 257 DBE procedures in children found an overall complication rate of 5.4%, with a rate of 10.4% in patients younger than 10 years.[39] All of the complications occurred during therapeutic procedures, such as endoscopic polypectomy, endoscopic bile-duct dilation, and removal of intrahepatic biliary stones.[39]

IMAGING MODALITIES OF THE SMALL BOWEL

Because of its length, anatomic complexity, and relative mobility, radiological examination of the SB remains challenging, particularly in children.

Small Bowel Ultrasound

In Central Europe and Canada, SB ultrasonography (SBUS) is widely used.[40] SBUS is comparable to MRE in detecting Crohn's disease, assessing SB thickness and the size of mesenteric lymph nodes.[41] SBUS has the advantages of not emitting ionizing radiation, being inexpensive, and being widely available. However, ultrasound can be limited in the presence of intestinal gas. In addition, quality is operator dependent. Contrast-enhanced ultrasonography is a recent approach that is as or more accurate than MRE in assessing Crohn's disease activity.[42,43]

Computed Tomography

Computed tomography (CT) is the primary imaging modality for SB evaluation in the acute setting, with good sensitivity in detecting blockage and ischemia. CT is also useful in detecting extraintestinal diseases such as malignancies and adhesions.

CTE uses a neutral oral contrast agent to distend the SB and thin-slice image acquisition to improve visualization of the SB wall thickness and enhancement characteristics. With a sensitivity of 33% and a specificity of nearly 90%, multiphase CTE can help identify the cause of occult gastrointestinal bleeding in hemodynamically stable adult patients.[44] The overall diagnostic yield of CTE for suspected SB bleeding is higher in overt or occult SB bleeding with heme-positive stool than in occult SB bleeding with iron-deficiency anemia only.[45]

Although CT and CTE are quite safe, there is a concern about ionizing radiation exposure. New reconstruction approaches enable significant radiation dose reductions while enhancing image quality and maintaining diagnostic accuracy.

Magnetic Resonance Enterography

MRE is the modality of first choice for diagnosing and monitoring the course of IBD in children. In evaluating Crohn's disease in children, MRE has demonstrated good agreement with CE.[46] The key advantage of MRE is its lack of ionizing radiation and superior contrast resolution compared with any other radiographic modality. However, its drawbacks include a long acquisition time, a higher cost, requirement for anesthesia, and susceptibility to artifacts.

Fluoroscopic Angiography

Fluoroscopic angiography can help diagnose gastrointestinal bleeding (**Fig. 5**), although its sensitivity varies depending on many factors, including the location and rate of bleeding.[47] A bleeding rate of at least 0.5 mL/min is required to be detected on fluoroscopic angiography.[48]

An advantage of angiography is the ability to perform transarterial embolization at the time of diagnosis by selectively occluding bleeding vessels while preserving collateral blood flow to lessen the risk of bowel infarction.[49] Common embolic agents include Gelfoam and polyvinyl alcohol particles. Because of its ability to evaluate and treat bleeding promptly, fluoroscopic angiography has become critical in patients suspected of having rapid active bleeding and those who do not respond to resuscitation.

Computed Tomography Angiography

CT angiography (CTA) has emerged as a promising modality for use in the emergency setting, as it can quickly identify the presence and the source of active bleeding (see **Fig. 5**). Using timed intravenous contrast, CTA can visualize the extravasation of contrast material into the gastrointestinal lumen in the presence of bleeding. CTA

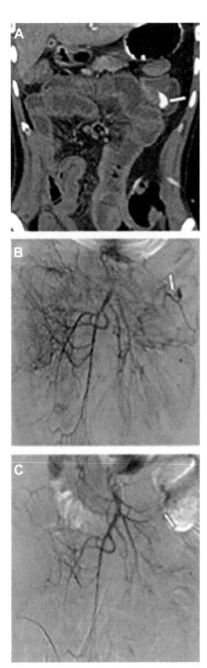

Fig. 5. (*A*) An enhanced CT scan shows active bleeding (*arrow*) from the jejunal loop. (*B*) Superior mesenteric angiography shows contrast extravasation (*arrow*) from the jejunal loop and multiple scattered, small aneurysms in the small bowel. (*C*) On postembolization angiography, the bleeding focus was embolized using gelatin sponge particles and 2 microcoils (*arrow*). (*From* Zheng L, Shin JH, Zhou WZ, Yoon HK. Transcatheter embolization of small bowel bleeding in a patient with polyarteritis nodosa. Gastrointestinal Intervention. 2015;4(1):65-67.)

can detect bleeding at a rate as slow as 0.3 mL/min.[49] CTA can also detect vascular malformations and masses, with limitations in assessing the bowel wall and intraluminal contents compared with CTE.

A meta-analysis of data from 672 adults with acute gastrointestinal bleeding revealed an overall sensitivity of 83% and a specificity of 92% for detecting the bleeding site.[50] The detection rates with CTA increase when patients have evidence of severe bleeding or hemodynamic instability.[47,51]

Scintigraphy

The most sensitive radiologic approach for detecting active bleeding is ^{99m}Tc-labeled red blood cell scintigraphy, or red blood cell (RBC) scan, which may detect bleeding at rates as low as 0.1 mL/min (**Fig. 6**). ^{99m}Tc-labeled RBCs stay in circulation for up to 24 hours, allowing for intermittent or delayed imaging.[47,49] When compared with CTA, the drawbacks of RBC scan include limited availability and the inability to identify the site of bleeding accurately. However, because of its great sensitivity and ability to detect intermittent bleeding, the RBC scan is an ideal tool for detecting slow, intermittent bleeding, that other methods have failed to detect.[47] A negative RBC scan predicts better outcomes and implies that the bleeding may stop without intervention.[52]

^{99m}Tc-pertechnetate scintigraphy, also known as a Meckel scan, detects ectopic gastric mucosa that secretes the radiotracer to diagnose Meckel diverticulum (**Fig. 7**). In children, sensitivities range from 50% to 90%, which can be enhanced by pretreatment with a histamine-2 blocker, proton pump inhibitor, or glucagon.[53]

Provocative Angiography

Provocative angiography involves using anticoagulants, vasodilators, or thrombolytic agents to induce bleeding when all other diagnostic techniques have been unrevealing.[49] Although provocative angiography can improve the identification of bleeding, it can potentially worsen bleeding complications. Early involvement of the surgical team is strongly advised.[54]

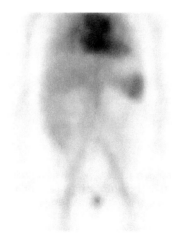

Fig. 6. Positive red blood cell scan showing active bleeding in the rectosigmoid colon. (*Courtesy of* Doug Rivard, MD, MO, USA.)

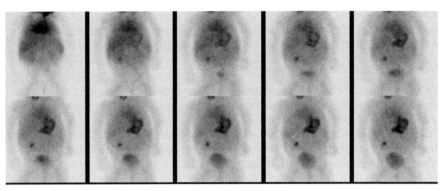

Fig. 7. Positive Meckel scan in the terminal ileum. *Courtesy of* Doug Rivard, MD, MO, USA.

SMALL BOWEL EVALUATION IN SPECIFIC POPULATIONS
Polyposis

Assessment of polyposis syndromes in the SB demonstrates positive findings in 80% of CE examinations in children, the highest diagnostic yield of any indication (see **Fig. 1A**).[55] CE is considered "feasible, safe, and accurate" for detecting SB polyps in Peutz-Jeghers and similar syndromes (eg, familial adenomatous polyposis, Gardner syndrome). The timing of screening, surveillance intervals, and the need for MRE versus DAE remain controversial.[56] Of note, SB screening in cases of juvenile polyposis has shown no benefit.[57]

Although the polyp detection rate has been shown to be comparable among DAE and CE,[58] DAE also allows polypectomy in the SB (see **Fig. 2D–E**).[59] DAE, however, should not be routinely recommended as a surveillance tool as it is technically challenging. Further details can be found in the "Polyps and Polyposis Syndromes in Children: Novel Endoscopic Considerations" manuscript in this volume.[60]

Inflammatory Bowel Disease

Because 70% of pediatric patients with Crohn's disease have SB involvement, and 40% have active disease exclusively in the SB, European and North American societies recommend a full gastrointestinal evaluation at the time of Crohn's disease diagnosis to assess the extent and severity of disease and to clarify a classification of indeterminate colitis.[61–63] Repeated studies have shown the superiority of CE to accomplish this task, especially in the initial evaluation of SB disease or more proximal SB disease, either alone or following an MRE, which can also detect strictures that would be a contraindication for CE (see **Fig. 1B–D**).[64]

In addition to its use in evaluating the extent of SB disease in IBD, several studies have demonstrated the feasibility of sequential CE as a minimally invasive method to evaluate mucosal response to treatment.[65,66] In addition, pan-enteric capsule endoscopy has been adapted to guide a treat-to-target therapeutic modifications strategy using a modified colon capsule to perform a pan-intestinal evaluation.[24]

DAE is recommended when conventional endoscopy, imaging, and CE have not yielded the desired results, and a histologic diagnosis and/or therapeutic procedure would alter disease management.[67] In the setting of established Crohn's disease, DAE is indicated when endoscopic visualization and biopsies of the SB beyond the reach of conventional endoscopy are necessary to exclude an alternative diagnosis (eg, lymphoma, tuberculosis, or carcinoma) or undertake a therapeutic procedure, including dilation of a stricture, removal of retained capsule, and treatment of bleeding lesions (see **Fig. 2**B).[68] Further details are outlined in the accompanying manuscript "Advances in Endoscopy for Pediatrics Inflammatory Bowel Disease" in this volume.[69]

Eosinophilic Gastrointestinal Disorders

Eosinophilic gastrointestinal disorders are characterized by gastrointestinal symptoms and dense mucosal eosinophilia. Eosinophilic enteritis is rare but can manifest with diarrhea, abdominal pain, protein-losing enteropathy, or gastrointestinal bleeding.[70] Salmon patches on CE in the setting of peripheral eosinophilia should raise suspicion for eosinophilic enteritis,[71] and mucosal biopsies by SB enteroscopy provided an important diagnostic approach.[72]

Celiac Disease

One of the gold standards for diagnosing celiac disease in children remains duodenal histology.[73] CE has a high sensitivity (89%) and specificity (95%) for diagnosing celiac disease.[74] CE can be helpful in patients who refuse gastroscopy,[75] have conflicting histology and celiac serology, or have refractory celiac disease.[76] Its wider angle of view, better magnification than conventional endoscopy, lack of insufflation, and underwater navigation make celiac disease features such as scalloping of folds, fissuring of the mucosa, villous atrophy, and mosaic appearance more prominent (see **Fig. 1**K). Suspicious abnormalities should be confirmed by histology, and DAE may be helpful in this regard.[77]

Small Bowel Bleeding

Bleeding from SB is uncommon and only accounts for 5% of all gastrointestinal bleeding. However, in both children and adults, SB bleeding is responsible for most gastrointestinal bleeding that persists or recurs without an obvious cause. In the past, "obscure" bleeding was defined as endoscopically unexplained. Recently, it has been proposed that the term "obscure" only be used if a source of bleeding has not been identified after a thorough examination of the gastrointestinal tract, including the SB.[78] The causes of SB bleeding in children are summarized in **Table 3**.

The evaluation and management of suspected SB bleeding should consider the patient's age, prior endoscopic results, bleeding severity, procedure availability, patient preferences, and physician expertise. Hemodynamic resuscitation is key for all

---

Table 3
Causes of small bowel bleeding[84]

Inflammation:	Bleeding Diathesis:
• Duodenitis	• Vitamin K deficiency
• Duodenal ulcers	• Coagulation disorders
• Nonsteroidal antiinflammatory drug enteropathy	Anatomic Abnormalities:
• Crohn's disease	• Duplication of bowel
Ingestions:	• Small bowel polyps
• Foreign bodies	• Meckel's diverticulum
• Caustic ingestions	• Aortoenteric fistula
Vascular Abnormalities:	• Small bowel intussusception
• Angioectasia	Ischemia:
• Dieulafoy lesion	• Midgut volvulus
• Arteriovenous malformation	• Necrotizing enterocolitis
• Blue rubber bleb nevus syndrome	Other:
• Osler-Weber-Rendu disease	• Small bowel tumors
• Small bowel varices	• Radiation enteropathy
	• Hemosuccus pancreaticus

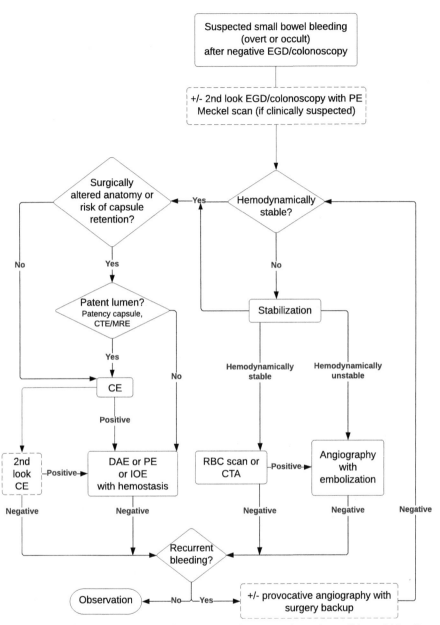

Fig. 8. Proposed diagnostic approach to suspected overt and occult small bowel bleeding. The approach may differ depending on the institution's expertise and availability, and multiple tests may be complementary. Positive test results should guide specific therapy. CE, capsule endoscopy; CTA, computed tomography angiography; CTE, computed tomography enterography; DAE, device-assisted enteroscopy; EGD, esophagogastroduodenoscopy; IOE, intraoperative enteroscopy; MRE, magnetic resonance enterography; PE, push enteroscopy; RBC, red blood cell.

gastrointestinal bleeding patients. A proposed diagnostic approach to suspected overt and occult SB bleeding is shown in **Fig. 8**. Enteroscopy is pivotal to the diagnosis and management of SB bleeding.[79] In children, the diagnostic yield of CE for SB bleeding is 42%,[80] and more with a second-look CE,[81] especially with a newer CE model that contain a double camera and a larger number of images per second.[82] DAE in children has been shown to have a high diagnostic yield for SB bleeding (70%–100%), and the yield considerably enhanced when lesions are previously identified by CE (see **Fig. 2**F–I).[82,83] If a patient remains hemodynamically unstable after resuscitation or has overt SB bleeding that cannot be managed endoscopically, interventional radiology and surgical consultation should be sought promptly.[79]

SUMMARY

CE, DAE, and SB imaging can provide an effective and safe means to evaluate the small intestine for pathology beyond the reach of conventional endoscopy. When used in combination, these tools can be complementary, offering more comprehensive answers and better-directed therapy for children.

CLINICS CARE POINTS

- In patients with Crohn's disease, a patency capsule or cross-sectional enterography reduces the risk of capsule endoscopy retention.
- Preparing the bowel with polyethylene glycol solution the night before and oral simethicone 30 minutes before CE can lessen patient discomfort and increase distal ileum visibility.
- CE is safe for children as young as 8 months or 8 kg, whereas DBE is safe for children older than 3 years and 14 kg.
- The antegrade approach of DAE is suggested in cases of massive gastrointestinal bleeding or if the area of interest is unknown or observed on capsule endoscopy before 75% of the total time from intake to the cecum or 60% of the time from pylorus to the cecum.
- For small intestinal bleeding, capsule endoscopy's diagnostic yield is close to 50% and greater with a second look. DAE has 70% to 100% diagnostic yield and is greater when lesions are previously identified by capsule endoscopy.

DISCLOSURE

A. Krasaelap and S. Oliva have nothing to disclose. D.G. Lerner is the founder of Lerner Media inc.

REFERENCES

1. Melson J, Trikudanathan G, Abu Dayyeh BK, et al. Video capsule endoscopy. Gastrointest Endosc 2021;93(4):784–96.
2. Rondonotti E, Spada C, Adler S, et al. Small-bowel capsule endoscopy and device-assisted enteroscopy for diagnosis and treatment of small-bowel disorders: European Society of Gastrointestinal Endoscopy (ESGE) Technical Review. Endosc 2018;50(4):423–46.
3. Friedlander JA, Liu QY, Sahn B, et al. NASPGHAN Capsule Endoscopy Clinical Report. J Pediatr Gastroenterol Nutr 2017;64(3):485–94.
4. Cohen SA, Klevens AI. Use of capsule endoscopy in diagnosis and management of pediatric patients, based on meta-analysis. Clin Gastroenterol Hepatol 2011; 9(6):490–6.

5. Nuutinen H, Kolho KL, Salminen P, et al. Capsule endoscopy in pediatric patients: technique and results in our first 100 consecutive children. Scand J Gastroenterol 2011;46(9):1138–43.
6. Oikawa-Kawamoto M, Sogo T, Yamaguchi T, et al. Safety and utility of capsule endoscopy for infants and young children. World J Gastroenterol 2013;19(45): 8342–8.
7. Cohen SA, Oliva S. Capsule endoscopy in children. Front Pediatr 2021;9:664722.
8. Oliva S, Cucchiara S, Civitelli F, et al. Colon capsule endoscopy compared with other modalities in the evaluation of pediatric Crohn's disease of the small bowel and colon. Gastrointest Endosc 2016;83(5):975–83.
9. Tamilarasan AG, Tran Y, Paramsothy S, et al. The Diagnostic Yield of Pan-enteric Capsule Endoscopy in Inflammatory Bowel Disease: A Systematic Review and Meta-analysis. J Gastroenterol Hepatol 2022;37(12):2207–16.
10. Brodersen JB, Knudsen T, Kjeldsen J, et al. Diagnostic accuracy of pan-enteric capsule endoscopy and magnetic resonance enterocolonography in suspected Crohn's disease. United European Gastroenterol J 2022;10(9):973–82.
11. Koulaouzidis A, Plevris JN. Detection of the ampulla of Vater in small bowel capsule endoscopy: experience with two different systems. J Dig Dis 2012; 13(12):621–7.
12. Selby WS, Prakoso E. The inability to visualize the ampulla of Vater is an inherent limitation of capsule endoscopy. Eur J Gastroenterol Hepatol 2011;23(1):101–3.
13. Clarke JO, Giday SA, Magno P, et al. How good is capsule endoscopy for detection of periampullary lesions? Results of a tertiary-referral center. Gastrointest Endosc 2008;68(2):267–72.
14. Kong H, Kim YS, Hyun JJ, et al. Limited ability of capsule endoscopy to detect normally positioned duodenal papilla. Gastrointest Endosc 2006;64(4):538–41.
15. Wang YC, Pan J, Liu YW, et al. Adverse events of video capsule endoscopy over the past two decades: a systematic review and proportion meta-analysis. BMC Gastroenterol 2020;20(1):364.
16. Wray N, Healy A, Thurston V, et al. Premature dissolution of the Agile patency device: implications for capsule endoscopy. Frontline Gastroenterol 2019;10(3): 217–21.
17. Pasha SF, Pennazio M, Rondonotti E, et al. Capsule Retention in Crohn's Disease: A Meta-analysis. Inflamm Bowel Dis 2020;26(1):33–42.
18. Cohen SA, Ephrath H, Lewis JD, et al. Pediatric capsule endoscopy: review of the small bowel and patency capsules. J Pediatr Gastroenterol Nutr 2012;54(3): 409–13.
19. Cohen SA, Gralnek IM, Ephrath H, et al. The Use of a Patency Capsule in Pediatric Crohn's Disease: A Prospective Evaluation. Dig Dis Sci 2011;56(3):860–5.
20. Niv Y. Efficiency of bowel preparation for capsule endoscopy examination: a meta-analysis. World J Gastroenterol 2008;14(9):1313–7.
21. Rokkas T, Papaxoinis K, Triantafyllou K, et al. Does purgative preparation influence the diagnostic yield of small bowel video capsule endoscopy?: A meta-analysis. Am J Gastroenterol 2009;104(1):219–27.
22. Chen HB, Huang Y, Chen SY, et al. Small bowel preparations for capsule endoscopy with mannitol and simethicone: a prospective, randomized, clinical trial. J Clin Gastroenterol 2011;45(4):337–41.
23. Oliva S, Cucchiara S, Spada C, et al. Small bowel cleansing for capsule endoscopy in paediatric patients: a prospective randomized single-blind study. Dig Liver Dis 2014;46(1):51–5.

24. Oliva S, Aloi M, Viola F, et al. A Treat to Target Strategy Using Panenteric Capsule Endoscopy in Pediatric Patients With Crohn's Disease. Clin Gastroenterol Hepatol 2019;17(10):2060–2067 e1.

25. Alageeli M, Yan B, Alshankiti S, et al. KODA score: an updated and validated bowel preparation scale for patients undergoing small bowel capsule endoscopy. Endosc Int Open 2020;8(8):E1011–7.

26. Schneider M, Hollerich J, Beyna T. Device-assisted enteroscopy: A review of available techniques and upcoming new technologies. World J Gastroenterol 2019;25(27):3538–45.

27. Nehme F, Goyal H, Perisetti A, et al. The Evolution of Device-Assisted Enteroscopy: From Sonde Enteroscopy to Motorized Spiral Enteroscopy. Front Med (Lausanne) 2021;8:792668.

28. Yamamoto H, Sekine Y, Sato Y, et al. Total enteroscopy with a nonsurgical steerable double-balloon method. Gastrointest Endosc 2001;53(2):216–20.

29. Nardo GD, Esposito G, Ziparo C, et al. Enteroscopy in children and adults with inflammatory bowel disease. World J Gastroenterol 2020;26(39):5944–58.

30. Barth BA. Enteroscopy in children. Curr Opin Pediatr 2011;23(5):530–4.

31. Committee AT, Chauhan SS, Manfredi MA, et al. Enteroscopy Gastrointest Endosc 2015;82(6):975–90.

32. Lo SK, Yamamoto H. How we do deep enteroscopy. Endosc 2021;53(9):943–6.

33. Tanaka S, Mitsui K, Tatsuguchi A, et al. Current status of double balloon endoscopy–indications, insertion route, sedation, complications, technical matters. Gastrointest Endosc 2007;66(3 Suppl):S30–3.

34. Gay G, Delvaux M, Fassler I. Outcome of capsule endoscopy in determining indication and route for push-and-pull enteroscopy. Endosc 2006;38(1):49–58.

35. Sunada K, Yamamoto H. Double Balloon Enteroscopy: Techniques. Tech Gastrointest Endosc 2008;10(2):46–53.

36. Kawashima H, Nakamura M, Ohno E, et al. Impact of instrument channel diameter on therapeutic endoscopic retrograde cholangiography using balloon-assisted enteroscopy. Dig Endosc 2014;26(Suppl 2):127–9.

37. Kim J. Training in Endoscopy: Enteroscopy. Clin Endosc 2017;50(4):328–33.

38. Pohl J, Delvaux M, Ell C, et al. European Society of Gastrointestinal Endoscopy (ESGE) Guidelines: flexible enteroscopy for diagnosis and treatment of small-bowel diseases. Endosc 2008;40(7):609–18.

39. Yokoyama K, Yano T, Kumagai H, et al. Double-balloon Enteroscopy for Pediatric Patients: Evaluation of Safety and Efficacy in 257 Cases. J Pediatr Gastroenterol Nutr 2016;63(1):34–40.

40. Okuhira T, Yoden A, Kaji E, et al. Usefulness of ultrasonography for small intestinal evaluations in pediatric Crohn's disease. Pediatr Int 2022;64(1):e15206.

41. Radford SJ, Clarke C, Shinkins B, et al. Clinical utility of small bowel ultrasound assessment of Crohn's disease in adults: a systematic scoping review. Frontline Gastroenterol 2022;13(4):280–6.

42. Mudambi K, Sandberg J, Bass D, et al. Contrast enhanced ultrasound: comparing a novel modality to MRI to assess for bowel disease in pediatric Crohn's patients. Transl Gastroenterol Hepatol 2020;5:13.

43. Gokli A, Dillman JR, Humphries PD, et al. Contrast-enhanced ultrasound of the pediatric bowel. Pediatr Radiol 2021;51(12):2214–28.

44. Hara AK, Walker FB, Silva AC, et al. Preliminary Estimate of Triphasic CT Enterography Performance in Hemodynamically Stable Patients With Suspected Gastrointestinal Bleeding. Am J Roentgenol 2009;193(5):1252–60.

45. Deepak P, Pundi KN, Bruining DH, et al. Multiphase Computed Tomographic Enterography: Diagnostic Yield and Efficacy in Patients With Suspected Small Bowel Bleeding. Mayo Clin Proc Innov Qual Outcomes 2019;3(4):438–47.
46. Hwang JY, Moon SW, Lee YJ, et al. Capsule Endoscopy versus Magnetic Resonance Enterography for Evaluation of Pediatric Small Bowel Crohn's Disease: Prospective Study. J Clin Med 2022;11(10):2760.
47. Wells ML, Hansel SL, Bruining DH, et al. CT for Evaluation of Acute Gastrointestinal Bleeding. Radiographics 2018;38(4):1089–107.
48. Choi C, Lim H, Kim MJ, et al. Relationship between angiography timing and angiographic visualization of extravasation in patients with acute non-variceal gastrointestinal bleeding. BMC Gastroenterol 2020;20(1):426.
49. Gerson LB, Fidler JL, Cave DR, et al. ACG Clinical Guideline: Diagnosis and Management of Small Bowel Bleeding. Am J Gastroenterol 2015;110(9):1265–87.
50. Garcia-Blazquez V, Vicente-Bartulos A, Olavarria-Delgado A, et al. Accuracy of CT angiography in the diagnosis of acute gastrointestinal bleeding: systematic review and meta-analysis. Eur Radiol 2013;23(5):1181–90.
51. García Crespo JM, Martín Pinto F, Domínguez Vallejo J. [Intestinal polyp of infrequent localization: presentation of 2 cases]. An Esp Pediatr 1984;21(9):855–7.
52. Dolezal J, Vizda J, Kopacova M. Single-photon emission computed tomography enhanced Tc-99m-pertechnetate disodium-labelled red blood cell scintigraphy in the localization of small intestine bleeding: a single-centre twelve-year study. Digestion 2011;84(3):207–11.
53. Spottswood SE, Pfluger T, Bartold SP, et al. SNMMI and EANM practice guideline for meckel diverticulum scintigraphy 2.0. J Nucl Med Technol 2014;42(3):163–9.
54. Murphy B, Winter DC, Kavanagh DO. Small Bowel Gastrointestinal Bleeding Diagnosis and Management-A Narrative Review. Front Surg 2019;6:25.
55. Latchford A, Cohen S, Auth M, et al. Management of Peutz-Jeghers Syndrome in Children and Adolescents: A Position Paper From the ESPGHAN Polyposis Working Group. J Pediatr Gastroenterol Nutr 2019;68(3):442–52.
56. Arguelles-Arias F, Donat E, Fernandez-Urien I, et al. Guideline for wireless capsule endoscopy in children and adolescents: A consensus document by the SEGHNP (Spanish Society for Pediatric Gastroenterology, Hepatology, and Nutrition) and the SEPD (Spanish Society for Digestive Diseases). Rev Esp Enferm Dig 2015;107(12):714–31.
57. Burke CA, Santisi J, Church J, et al. The utility of capsule endoscopy small bowel surveillance in patients with polyposis. Am J Gastroenterol 2005;100(7):1498–502.
58. Thomson M, Tringali A, Dumonceau JM, et al. Paediatric Gastrointestinal Endoscopy: European Society for Paediatric Gastroenterology Hepatology and Nutrition and European Society of Gastrointestinal Endoscopy Guidelines. J Pediatr Gastroenterol Nutr 2017;64(1):133–53.
59. Chong AK, Chin BW, Meredith CG. Clinically significant small-bowel pathology identified by double-balloon enteroscopy but missed by capsule endoscopy. Gastrointest Endosc 2006;64(3):445–9.
60. Attard T, Cohen S, Durno C. Polyps and polyposis syndromes in children: Novel endoscopic Considerations. GI Clinics of North America; 2022.
61. Levine A, Koletzko S, Turner D, et al. ESPGHAN revised porto criteria for the diagnosis of inflammatory bowel disease in children and adolescents. J Pediatr Gastroenterol Nutr 2014;58(6):795–806.
62. Oliva S, Thomson M, de Ridder L, et al. Endoscopy in Pediatric Inflammatory Bowel Disease: A Position Paper on Behalf of the Porto IBD Group of the

European Society for Pediatric Gastroenterology, Hepatology and Nutrition. J Pediatr Gastroenterol Nutr 2018;67(3):414–30.

63. Maaser C, Sturm A, Vavricka SR, et al. ECCO-ESGAR Guideline for Diagnostic Assessment in IBD Part 1: Initial diagnosis, monitoring of known IBD, detection of complications. J Crohn's Colitis 2019;13(2):144–64.

64. Kopylov U, Yung DE, Engel T, et al. Diagnostic yield of capsule endoscopy versus magnetic resonance enterography and small bowel contrast ultrasound in the evaluation of small bowel Crohn's disease: Systematic review and meta-analysis. Dig Liver Dis 2017;49(8):854–63.

65. Niv E, Fishman S, Kachman H, et al. Sequential capsule endoscopy of the small bowel for follow-up of patients with known Crohn's disease. J Crohn's Colitis 2014; 8(12):1616–23.

66. Hall BJ, Holleran GE, Smith SM, et al. A prospective 12-week mucosal healing assessment of small bowel Crohn's disease as detected by capsule endoscopy. Eur J Gastroenterol Hepatol 2014;26(11):1253–9.

67. Di Nardo G, Calabrese C, Conti Nibali R, et al. Enteroscopy in children. United Eur Gastroenterol J 2018;6(7):961–9.

68. Di Nardo G, de Ridder L, Oliva S, et al. Enteroscopy in paediatric Crohn's disease. Dig Liver Dis 2013;45(5):351–5.

69. Carman N, Picoraro JA. Advances in endoscopy for pediatric inflammatory bowel disease. GI Clinics of North America; 2022.

70. Nguyen N, Kramer RE, Friedlander JA. Videocapsule Endoscopy Identifies Small Bowel Lesions in Patients With Eosinophilic Enteritis. Clin Gastroenterol Hepatol 2018;16(6):e64–5.

71. Endo H, Hosono K, Inamori M, et al. Capsule endoscopic evaluation of eosinophilic enteritis before and after treatment. Digestion 2011;83(1–2):134–5.

72. Okuda K, Daimon Y, Iwase T, et al. Novel findings of capsule endoscopy and double-balloon enteroscopy in a case of eosinophilic gastroenteritis. Clin J Gastroenterol 2013;6(1):16–9.

73. Hill ID, Fasano A, Guandalini S, et al. NASPGHAN Clinical Report on the Diagnosis and Treatment of Gluten-related Disorders. J Pediatr Gastroenterol Nutr 2016;63(1):156–65.

74. Rokkas T, Niv Y. The role of video capsule endoscopy in the diagnosis of celiac disease: a meta-analysis. Eur J Gastroenterol Hepatol 2012;24(3):303–8.

75. Kurien M, Evans KE, Aziz I, et al. Capsule endoscopy in adult celiac disease: a potential role in equivocal cases of celiac disease? Gastrointest Endosc 2013; 77(2):227–32.

76. Atlas DS, Rubio-Tapia A, Van Dyke CT, et al. Capsule endoscopy in nonresponsive celiac disease. Gastrointest Endosc 2011;74(6):1315–22.

77. Green PHR, Paski S, Ko CW, et al. AGA Clinical Practice Update on Management of Refractory Celiac Disease: Expert Review. Gastroenterology 2022;163(5): 1461–9.

78. Raju GS, Gerson L, Das A, et al. American Gastroenterological Association (AGA) Institute technical review on obscure gastrointestinal bleeding. Gastroenterology 2007;133(5):1697–717.

79. Sorge A, Elli L, Rondonotti E, et al. Enteroscopy in diagnosis and treatment of small bowel bleeding: A Delphi expert consensus. Dig Liver Dis 2023;55(1): 29–39.

80. Cohen SA. The potential applications of capsule endoscopy in pediatric patients compared with adult patients. Gastroenterol Hepatol (N Y) 2013;9(2):92–7.

81. Viazis N, Papaxoinis K, Vlachogiannakos J, et al. Is there a role for second-look capsule endoscopy in patients with obscure GI bleeding after a nondiagnostic first test? Gastrointest Endosc 2009;69(4):850–6.
82. Oliva S, Pennazio M, Cohen SA, et al. Capsule endoscopy followed by single balloon enteroscopy in children with obscure gastrointestinal bleeding: a combined approach. Dig Liver Dis 2015;47(2):125–30.
83. Rondonotti E, Marmo R, Petracchini M, et al. The American Society for Gastrointestinal Endoscopy (ASGE) diagnostic algorithm for obscure gastrointestinal bleeding: eight burning questions from everyday clinical practice. Dig Liver Dis 2013;45(3):179–85.
84. Romano C, Oliva S, Martellossi S, et al. Pediatric gastrointestinal bleeding: Perspectives from the Italian Society of Pediatric Gastroenterology. World J Gastroenterol 2017;23(8):1328–37.

Advances in Endoscopy for Pediatric Inflammatory Bowel Disease

Nicholas Carman, MD[a,b,*], Joseph A. Picoraro, MD[c,d]

KEYWORDS

- Colonoscopy • Crohn disease • Endoscopy • Inflammatory bowel disease
- Stricture • Treatment target • Ulcerative colitis • Video capsule endoscopy

KEY POINTS

- Systematic and thorough endoscopic evaluation of the upper gastrointestinal tract, ileum, and colon is critical for accurate and meaningful phenotypic assessment of inflammatory bowel disease (IBD) in children and adolescents.
- Reliable and consistent communication of endoscopic findings using appropriate scoring tools and known descriptors is important to standardize assessment, to measure treatment response, and to undertake meaningful research.
- Video capsule endoscopy is a valuable adjunctive tool to evaluate the small bowel, especially in the setting of otherwise inconclusive findings.
- Application of therapeutic and interventional endoscopy in pediatric IBD is emerging

INTRODUCTION

Endoscopy in the field of inflammatory bowel disease (IBD) has remained the cornerstone of diagnostic assessment and disease monitoring for both adult and pediatric patients. As our therapeutic armamentarium increases and we enter the era of precision medicine with treatments targeted to individual phenotypic features, it is

Disclosure Statement: The authors have nothing to disclose.
[a] Division of Gastroenterology, Hepatology and Nutrition, Department of Paediatrics, CHEO Inflammatory Bowel Disease Centre, Children's Hospital of Eastern Ontario, University of Ottawa, Ontario, Canada; [b] Division of Gastroenterology, Hepatology and Nutrition, Department of Paediatrics, Sickkids Inflammatory Bowel Disease Centre, The Hospital for Sick Children, University of Toronto, 555 University Avenue, Toronto, Ontario M5G 1X8, Canada; [c] Division of Pediatric Gastroenterology, Hepatology and Nutrition, Columbia University Irving Medical Center, 622 West 168th Street, PH17-105, New York, NY 10032, USA; [d] NewYork-Presbyterian Morgan Stanley Children's Hospital, New York, NY 10032, USA
* Corresponding author. Division of Gastroenterology, Hepatology and Nutrition, Department of Paediatrics, Sickkids Inflammatory Bowel Disease Centre, The Hospital for Sick Children, University of Toronto, 555 University Avenue, Toronto, Ontario M5G 1X8, Canada.
E-mail address: nicholas.carman@sickkids.ca

Gastrointest Endoscopy Clin N Am 33 (2023) 447–461
https://doi.org/10.1016/j.giec.2022.10.002
giendo.theclinics.com

increasingly important that we accurately describe and standardize endoscopic assessment of children and adolescents with IBD. In addition, imaging technology and the clinical application of pediatric endoscopy in IBD continues to evolve, with innovative techniques allowing for novel ways to assess disease activity using endoscopy. This review summarizes the role of endoscopy in pediatric IBD, focusing on disease assessment techniques and tools, as well as evaluating newer, advanced endoscopic procedures that are being introduced into pediatric practice.

DIAGNOSIS, CHARACTERIZATION, AND DISEASE MONITORING
The First Endoscopy in Suspected Inflammatory Bowel Disease

Endoscopy remains the most important part of the diagnostic assessment in a child or adolescent with suspected IBD. The updated Porto group of ESPGHAN guidelines in 2018 recommends complete esophagogastroduodenoscopy (EGD) and ileocolonoscopy at the time of diagnosis, along with multiple biopsies ($\geq$2) from each segment, even in the absence of macroscopic inflammation.[1] A complete evaluation as described is of particular importance in pediatric patients, who are more likely to have upper tract disease and ileocolonic disease than adult patients.[2] Furthermore, recent pediatric endoscopy quality guidelines endorsed by the American Society for Gastrointestinal Endoscopy highlighted standard lower endoscopy in children is best characterized as ileocolonoscopy given that ileal intubation is integral to ensuring complete mucosal assessment in children.[3]

Performing the endoscopic assessment for a child or adolescent with suspected IBD extends beyond categorization into Crohn disease (CD) or ulcerative colitis (UC). At the time of diagnostic endoscopy, the endoscopist should describe the IBD type, location/extent, behavior, and severity (**Table 1**) as accurately and thoroughly as possible, because subsequent investigations will be impacted by treatment effect. Furthermore, it is important to describe visualized lesions in detail using common descriptors (eg, vascularity, erosions, ulcers) and to undergo training in endoscopic scoring tools to improve reporting consistency. Rigorous and consistent description of endoscopic findings allows for retrospective review and clear understanding among other IBD practitioners. This is especially important for transition of care and for surgical planning. In addition, appropriate classification of patients with IBD is essential for conducting rigorous clinical and epidemiologic research.[4]

At present, IBD in pediatric patients is characterized using the Paris modification of the Montreal classification system, based on the macroscopic appearance of endoscopy combined with small bowel imaging (see **Table 1**).[5] Occasionally, "atypical" features are seen at endoscopy and make disease classification difficult, leading to a label of inflammatory bowel disease unclassified (IBDU) (**Box 1**). In a recent large pediatric IBD inception cohort study in Canada, 8% were labeled IBDU and 44% of these patients retained this label after 12 months.[5,6] In pediatric patients with colonic disease, the rate of IBDU may be up to 30%.[7]

Macroscopic rectal sparing in UC is an uncommon finding in adult patients, and in general suggests a diagnosis of CD.[8] However, this phenomenon is seen in children and adolescents with a rate of 5% observed in a large cohort of pediatric patients with UC in Europe, with young age being a predictor of rectal sparing in multivariable analysis.[9]

Similarly, inflammation in the terminal ileum termed "backwash ileitis" does not necessarily denote a diagnosis of CD in patients with UC in the setting of pancolitis. The rate of children and adolescents with UC containing abnormalities in the terminal ileum may be up to 10%.[9] Features of backwash ileitis that are suggestive of CD

Table 1
Paris classification for pediatric inflammatory bowel disease

Crohn disease location	
L1	Distal one-third of the ileum ± limited cecal disease
L2	Isolated colonic disease
L3	Ileocolonic disease
L4a L4b	Additional/isolated upper tract disease: Proximal to the ligament of Treitz Distal to the ligament of Treitz
Perianal disease (p)	Presence of fistula and/or abscesses
Crohn disease behavior	
B1	Inflammatory (nonstricturing, nonpenetrating)
B2	Stricturing
B3	Internally penetrating
Ulcerative colitis	
E1	Limited to the rectum (proctitis)
E2	Inflammation to the splenic flexure
E3	Inflammation to the hepatic flexure
E4	Inflammation beyond the hepatic flexure

Adapted from Levine A, Griffiths A, Markowitz J, et al. Pediatric modification of the Montreal classification for inflammatory bowel disease: the Paris classification. Inflamm Bowel Dis. 2011;17(6):1314-1321.

include discrete ulceration, extensive/patchy ulceration, severity worse than the cecum, and strictures.[10]

Periappendiceal inflammation, or a "cecal patch," is also consistent with a diagnosis of UC, despite normal mucosa in between the inflamed segment and the cecal patch. It is a relatively common phenomenon, with rates as high as 75% in patients with distal UC.[11] There are conflicting data to suggest that a cecal patch may be associated with subsequent disease extension, but there is no association between the presence of a cecal patch and risk of acute severe colitis or colectomy.[12–14]

Upper gastrointestinal tract findings are an increasingly identified phenomenon, because clinicians recognize the importance of performing an EGD at the time of diagnostic ileocolonoscopy. In addition to the macroscopic appearance, the presence of histologic granuloma in the esophagus, stomach, or duodenum is helpful in establishing a diagnosis of CD. The presence of macroscopic inflammation in the stomach and duodenum can be consistent with UC and was found in 25% and 8% of pediatric patients with UC in Canada, respectively.[6] The presence of large or discrete ulcers, however, should prompt consideration of a diagnosis of CD.

Box 1
Common atypical endoscopic features of ulcerative colitis

Gastritis/duodenitis

Backwash ileitis

Periappendiceal inflammation (patch) in the absence of pancolitis

Rectal sparing

Endoscopic Characterization

Although the emerging delineation of molecular pathway-based IBD subphenotypes may begin to correlate with endoscopic phenotypes, characterizing disease severity and activity within our current categorizations of CD and UC are helpful in facilitating our treatment approach. For CD, the simple endoscopic score for Crohn disease (SES-CD) and the Crohn disease endoscopic index of severity (CDEIS) are validated and reproducible measures of luminal endoscopic activity. The CDEIS measures types of lesions (ulcers, stenosis), extent of involvement, and segments of bowel affected (TI, right colon, transverse, left, sigmoid, rectum).[15] The scoring is complicated, time-consuming, requires specific training, and is largely reserved for clinical trials. The SES-CD was developed as a more accessible scoring system based on the CDEIS, with a similar structure, including lesion type, extent of involvement, and segments affected (TI, right, transverse, left/sigmoid, rectum).[16] Neither the CDEIS nor the SES-CD is validated in children and adolescents. A scoring system that is further simplified and has the potential to provide an accurate measure of disease activity in clinical practice, the simplified endoscopic mucosal assessment for Crohn's disease (SEMA-CD) was developed with pediatric data and has now been validated in pediatric and adult patients.[17,18] The SEMA-CD has strong correlation with SES-CD and has the potential for widespread adoption given its ease of use and applicability to current goals in therapy.[19]

In UC, the endoscopic subscore of the Mayo scoring index (Mayo-ES) has become the most widely used measure in clinical trials and in clinical practice. The Mayo-ES ranges from 0 to 3, with the 4 discrete values assigned to the interpretation of the degree of erythema, friability, decreased vascular pattern, and presence/absence of erosions/ulcerations.[20] Given interobserver variation for the Mayo-ES, the ulcerative colitis endoscopic index of severity (UCEIS) was developed, but its use in clinical practice is variable.[21] The Mayo-ES and the UCEIS have been incompletely validated in children and adolescents; however, a recent Canadian pediatric study demonstrated excellent reliability and construct validity of both scoring tools.[22]

Despite advances in medical therapies, pediatric patients undergo surgery at estimated rates of 26% in CD[23] and 13% to 14% in UC.[24,25] The surgically altered bowel represents a unique physiologic state influenced by the underlying CD or UC. In CD, the site of anastomosis following resection is a frequent area of postoperative recurrence, and the Rutgeerts endoscopic score was developed to determine the successful control of disease following the presumptive removal of affected bowel from the body. The Rutgeerts score is a validated and predictive measure of disease recurrence, and a modified Rutgeerts delineates lesion location at the ileocolonic anastomosis from the neoterminal ileum.[26] In UC, the restorative surgical intervention of J pouch creation with ileal pouch-anal anastomosis following proctocolectomy (restorative proctocolectomy with ileal pouch-anal anastomosis [RPC-IPAA]) lends to a state of absent primary disease, but potential for complications, including inflammation of the ileal pouch. The pouchitis disease activity index, which attempts to capture the state of inflammation in the ileal pouch, has an endoscopic component, but it has limitations.[27] Research to determine clinically meaningful endoscopic characterization of the ileal pouch is underway (see later discussion).[28,29]

Endoscopic Treatment Targets

The current treatment paradigm in IBD focuses on mucosal healing as the most important target to promote long-term remission and reduce the risk of disease complications. As therapeutic options have improved over the past 25 years, it has been recognized that clinical remission is an insufficient treatment target and does not reflect the potential for disease progression. Treatment targets should be both achievable with available therapies and predictive of future disease. The improvement and resolution of endoscopic activity emerged as the target that most closely represents the broader goal of mucosal healing. Endoscopic characterization and classification are, therefore, critical to both diagnosis and assessment of treatment response.

Selecting Therapeutic Targets in Inflammatory Bowel Disease (STRIDE) provides the foremost consensus on the goals of care in IBD, and the recent STRIDE-II guidelines brought forth greater attention to pediatric patients.[30] These guidelines, however, are primarily based on research in adults, and the applicability within pediatrics deserves individualized consideration. Recognizing those limitations, endoscopic healing is a long-term target, corresponding to an SES-CD score less than 3 points for CD and Mayo-ES score of 0 for UC. Endoscopic improvement is agreed upon as a short-term goal, although what constitutes a lack of endoscopic improvement remains debated. However defined, failure to achieve endoscopic improvement in the short term and endoscopic healing in the long term should prompt consideration to re-evaluate therapy.

Endoscopic healing in CD[31–33] and UC[34] is associated with durable improved outcomes, including reduction of hospitalization, surgery, and steroid dependence. In pediatrics, although robust long-term data following endoscopic healing are limited, endoscopic appearance does impact treatment[35] and endoscopic healing is an accepted treatment target for CD.[1]

Histologic remission in UC, and to a lesser degree CD, continues to receive attention but is not yet a treatment target. In adults, recent evidence has shown that in UC the addition of a histologic assessment to Mayo-ES was not superior to the Mayo-ES alone.[36] Transmural assessment continues to evolve with further research necessary to evaluate the utility of imaging modalities (computed tomographic enterography [CTE], magnetic resonance enterography [MRE], intestinal bowel ultrasonography [IBUS]) and associated scoring systems.[37]

Ileal Pouch-Anal Anastomosis

Although the staged surgeries of RPC-IPAA have transformed the quality of life for patients with medically refractory UC, the ileal pouch may develop a variety of inflammatory (eg, pouchitis, de novo CD and Crohn-like disease of the pouch, ischemic pouchitis, and cuffitis), structural (eg, leak, stricture and fistula), and functional (eg, irritable pouch syndrome) disorders.[29] Because clinical symptoms may be indistinguishable, endoscopic evaluation is necessary to differentiate the underlying cause. With knowledge of ileal pouch anatomy, endoscopy should delineate the features of the mucosal appearance (eg, erythema, altered vascularity, erosion, ulceration, exudate) as well as the portion and pattern of the ileal pouch affected (**Fig. 1**). A classification system of distinct endoscopic phenotypes of the pouch has been proposed.[28] Accurate endoscopic characterization of the pouch will guide appropriate treatment and reassessment.[38] Structural pouch disorders, specifically, may benefit from endoscopic intervention with an experienced endoscopist.

Colorectal Cancer Screening in Pediatric Inflammatory Bowel Disease

At present, there are no established recommendations for screening for colorectal carcinoma (CRC) in pediatric patients with IBD, with population studies showing an extremely low rate of CRC developing during childhood even with long-standing disease, despite an overall increased risk of developing CRC during a patient's lifetime.[39] In the adult population, screening colonoscopy for CRC is currently recommended 8 to 10 years after initial IBD diagnosis, and several new technologies may enhance

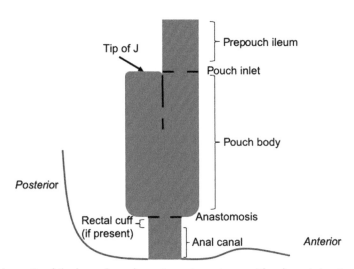

Fig. 1. Schematic of ileal-pouch anal anastomosis anatomy with relevant structures.

detection rate, including targeted biopsies with virtual or dye chromoendoscopy.[40] Surveillance colonoscopy is recommended every 1 to 5 years thereafter, depending on risk factors, and surveillance of the ileal pouch is recommended annually in high-risk patients. In pediatrics, endoscopy training rarely includes adequate exposure to CRC screening techniques. If surveillance is warranted, it should be performed by an appropriately trained endoscopist.

Central Reading and Video Reading

Owing to the poor correlation of subjective clinical tools with endoscopic disease activity in both adult[41] and pediatric patients,[42,43] it is now a requirement that endoscopic outcomes are included in registration trials by regulatory agencies. If endoscopic outcomes are to be interpreted meaningfully, reliable and consistent interpretation of endoscopic assessment is imperative. As with other imaging modalities, interpretation is subjective, and varies between observers, with potential for bias even among experienced clinicians. A recent study demonstrated relatively modest interrater agreement among experienced staff when interpreting endoscopic images for CD (kappa 0.37) and UC (kappa = 0.49).[44]

Variability in interpretation of endoscopy can be improved significantly by the use of "central reading," where endoscopic assessments are interpreted by an independent, experienced reader, who has been properly trained in regard to lesion definition and interpretation.[45] The use of centralized video review of endoscopic assessments has become a mainstay in adult clinical trials and has increasingly been applied outside of drug registration trials or clinical trial networks. In addition to trial outcomes, the use of centralized video review has allowed for validation research of existing endoscopic scoring indices, and for training in the use of scoring tools.

By using a formalized training program consisting of video clip presentations with a large pool of community gastroenterologists and internists involved in IBD clinics, interrater agreement in Mayo-ES and Rutgeerts scores were enhanced.[46] In pediatrics, the Canadian Children's Inflammatory Bowel Disease Network has used centralized video review to undertake validation studies of existing scoring tools in UC. This work has demonstrated that experienced, trained central readers can achieve excellent interrater and intrarater agreement using both a traditional and pan-colonic

UCEIS, and Mayo-ES, demonstrating the benefit of structured training in the scoring tools.[22] Last, the application of artificial intelligence to pediatric endoscopy has the potential to improve IBD characterization and scoring of disease activity.[47]

EMERGING TECHNIQUES AND TECHNOLOGIES
Endoscopic Ultrasonography

Disease evaluation beyond the superficial intestinal mucosa as measured by endoscopy has been of interest to clinicians, with increasing use of imaging techniques such as MRE and IBUS to evaluate depth of inflammation, and to determine presence of fibrosis and disease complications.

Endoscopic ultrasonography (EUS) is another imaging modality that allows real-time sonographic evaluation of the luminal wall and can be combined with EGD/ileocolonoscopy in the same procedural setting. Given the paucity of formal training programs in pediatric EUS, and ready availability of MRE and IBUS in most centers, experience with EUS in IBD is limited.

EUS in CD has largely been limited to the assessment of perianal fistula. In evaluating anatomy of perianal fistulae, EUS was found to be equivalent to examination under anesthesia (EUA) and MRI.[48] Although MRI remains a critical tool in evaluation of perianal fistula in pediatric CD, EUS does offer a potential adjunctive benefit in that it is possible to undertake a surgical EUA with real-time EUS guidance, ensuring that there is adequate drainage with or without seton placement.

In UC, there has been increasing recognition that inflammation is not only limited to the superficial mucosa but also extends to the deeper layers, with colectomy specimens demonstrating muscularis propriae thickening and submucosal fibrosis.[49,50] EUS is able to examine the deeper layers of the intestinal wall to evaluate for superficial and transmural inflammation. Experience with EUS in UC remains limited, and its potential role in the assessment of disease severity and/or as a prognostic tool remains undefined. Early studies were hindered by methodological issues and limited technology.[51–53] More recently, there have been several studies that demonstrate the potential of EUS to determine disease severity and prognosis.[54] Involvement of the muscularis propria layer or deeper, as identified by EUS, has been shown to be associated with an increased risk of colectomy.[50] Alternatively, in patients with quiescent disease, depth of disease activity, as specified by increased thickness of the first 3 layers of the bowel, may predict relapse.[55,56] EUS may also help evaluate and predict response to therapy. In a small study, patients with steroid-refractory severe UC who responded to cyclosporin demonstrated a reduction in wall thickness compared with nonresponders who had no significant sonographic change.[55]

Given the potential of EUS in UC, the operating properties of this technique using existing indices was examined, leading to the development of a new index of EUS activity in UC (EUS-UC) score.[52,54,57,58] The EUS-UC, which comprises 3 items (bowel wall thickening, depth of inflammation, and hyperemia),[54] was validated against defined pathologic features (**Table 2**). However, the operating characteristics of this new instrument have been incompletely evaluated. There are no data evaluating the use of EUS in children and adolescents. Because pediatric patients most commonly have moderate to severe disease with limited clinical predictors of severity and prognosis, the potential role of EUS as an additional measure of disease activity is compelling and requires further study.

Video Capsule Endoscopy

Video capsule endoscopy (VCE) has been used in adults since its approval in 2001 as a safe and effective method of assessing the small intestine, with FDA approval in children older than 2 years in 2009. VCE has emerged as an important adjunctive diagnostic imaging technique, especially in patients with suspected CD with inconclusive standard evaluation with EGD or ileocolonoscopy and MRE or in patients with isolated perianal fistulae.[59] VCE can also be used as a monitoring tool in patients with isolated small bowel disease. A recent meta-analysis demonstrated that the diagnostic yield of VCE was similar to that of MRE for detection of small bowel disease in both suspected and established CD odds ratio [OR], 1.17 (95% confidence interval [CI], 0.83–1.67) and was in fact superior to MRE in the detection of proximal small bowel lesions (OR, 2.79; 95% CI, 1.2–6.48).[60] VCE can thus evaluate for mucosal healing, especially in the setting of unexplained inflammatory marker elevation and for superficial small bowel inflammation in cases of IBDU, with rates of detection leading to change in diagnosis to CD ranging from 13.5% up to 50%.[61–63] Limitations in children and adolescents include risk of capsule retention in stricturing disease and the inability to swallow the capsule, thus requiring placement during EGD with anesthesia.

VCE scoring tools for IBD, namely, the Lewis score[64] and the capsule endoscopy CD activity index, have been developed with variable adoption and limited application in pediatrics.[65] Most recently, a novel pediatric VCE index (CE-CD score) has been developed to align with the more familiar and validated SES-CD.[66] It has not yet undergone validation in prospective studies.

Technology with VCE continues to evolve, with recent advances including the development of the pan-enteric capsule designed to examine the small and large bowel in one procedure and a beltless 360° capsule that can be performed remotely without an office visit. VCE has the potential for innovation with artificial intelligence and machine learning, and it is likely that we will see increased use of VCE in the evaluation of pediatric patients with IBD moving forward.

Deep Enteroscopy

Device-assisted enteroscopy, including single balloon enteroscopy, double balloon enteroscopy, and, more recently, through-the-scope balloon-assisted enteroscopy (TTS-BAE), allows for visualization, sampling, and intervention in the small bowel, and can be applied in both an antegrade and a retrograde fashion. For patients with IBD, the most common applications are the collection of histopathological specimens of suspicious lesions seen at VCE or MRE/CTE and for interventional techniques such as balloon dilatation of small bowel strictures. Data in pediatrics are sparse, because there are few pediatric gastroenterologists trained in this technique given the relative paucity of indications and the potential for complications in smaller patients.

TTS-BAE is a newer technique in which a novel single-use balloon is passed through the scope, with an inflation-deflation device that applies a set amount of pressure to the balloon, limiting potential for overinflation. This device may allow for broader uptake of the technique given the ability to use conventional colonoscopes and is a less technically challenging procedure. A recent prospective study has demonstrated feasibility and safety in the pediatric population.[67]

THERAPY AND INTERVENTIONS
Endoscopic Stricture Dilation

Primary strictures in IBD, predominantly in CD, are composed of inflammatory and fibrotic components. Early in CD, appropriate medical therapy may alter the development of medically refractory strictures.[68] However, the delineation of inflammatory and fibrotic components is challenging even with comprehensive imaging modalities such as MRE. Intestinal resection or surgical strictureplasty are the primary modalities

Table 2
Endoscopic ultrasonographic activity in ulcerative colitis score

Component	0	1	2	3
Component score				
Total wall thickening	Normal ($\leq$ 3.0 mm)	Mild (3.1–4.0 mm)	Moderate (4.1–6.0 mm)	Severe (>6.1 mm)
Depth of inflammation	Superficial (no disruption to the 5-layer echo pattern)	Subepithelial (disruption of the first 3 layers to the submucosa but not beyond)	Deep (disruption beyond the submucosa to the muscularis propria)	Transmural (disruption beyond the muscularis propria to the serosa or beyond)
Hyperemia	Normal absence of intramural vascular signal	Mild (intermittent signal)	Moderate (continuous signal)	Severe (presence of intramural anechoic vessel seen without power Doppler, with immediate continuous signal on power Doppler)
Total score (sum of 3 items) 0–9				

Adapted from Yan BM, Sey MSL, Belletrutti P, Brahm G, Guizzetti L, Jairath V. Reliability of the Endoscopic Ultrasound Ulcerative Colitis (EUS-UC) score for assessment of inflammation in patients with ulcerative colitis. Endosc Int Open. 2021;9(7):E1116-E1122.

to address medically refractory intestinal strictures. Anastomotic strictures are common postsurgery, where differentiating progressive IBD from postsurgical changes remains challenging. Disease activity commonly recurs at the site of anastomosis and adjacent areas, and endoscopic assessment plays a primary role in this differentiation. Stricture phenotyping, as suggested by pathologic delineation of constrictive and hypertrophic forms, may hold promise.[69] Despite current challenges in stricture phenotyping, interventional endoscopic techniques afford an opportunity to obviate or delay surgery.

Endoscopic balloon dilation (EBD) has been the mainstay of therapeutic intervention for strictures in the gastrointestinal tract. In IBD, it has been used as a temporizing measure for primary gastroduodenal, ileal, colonic and anorectal, and anastomotic strictures, including ileal pouch-anal and ileocolonic. The widespread use of EBD has been limited by its attendant risk of perforation and postprocedural bleeding. In children, the limited data in EBD has shown similar efficacy and safety to adults.[70,71] When performing EBD in IBD, patient selection is the most important step. Appropriate selection depends on the development of obstructive symptoms and dedicated imaging. MRE is the imaging modality that provides the most comprehensive characterization with fairly reliable capture of active disease, length, angulation, and delineation of associated fistulae or abscesses. Generally, EBD should not be attempted for strictures greater than 5 cm or for multiple strictures.[72] When fistulae or abscesses are present, EBD should generally be deferred due to increased risks. Barium defecography is most useful to characterize ileal pouch or anorectal strictures. Endoscopic characterization should include discernment of the degree of active inflammation. Minimal inflammation of characteristic postanastomotic areas is most amenable to successful EBD. Untreated or severe refractory inflammation at the stricture site may portend additional risk. Recurrent stricture is common with EBD, with the benefits of EBD typically providing extended time to surgery rather than avoidance of surgery altogether.

Electroincision Stricture Therapy

An advanced interventional technique that is gaining broader application in pediatrics, endoscopic electroincision therapy (EIT), has emerged in adult IBD. The technique entails directing electrocautery with an endoscopic needle knife or insulated tip knife to the intraluminal fibrotic tissue to expand and open the stricture from within the lumen. With endoscopic visualization, precise cuts can be made not only to target the most important areas but also to avoid areas at highest risk of complication, including surrounding anatomy. This is in contrast to EBD, in which the tear will preferentially occur at the weakest portion of the bowel wall. For example, in ileal pouch-anal anastomotic strictures, the knife is directed toward the posterior wall to avoid the risk of inciting rectovaginal fistula on the anterior wall. The use of EIT in this fashion achieves an endoscopic stricturotomy.[73] Depending on the depth of incision and complexity of the stricture, endoscopic clips may be applied to stent open the incisions and reduce the risk of bleeding, resulting in an endoscopic strictureplasty.[37] Both endoscopic stricturotomy and strictureplasty have shown promise in adult IBD with a lower rate of perforation when compared with EBD.[38,74–76]

Although EIT has been used in pediatric patients with esophageal and duodenal strictures, its use and description in children and adolescents with IBD is scant. EIT should be undertaken by experienced advanced endoscopists with expertise in IBD. The anastomotic stricture that is suspected to consist primarily of fibrosis is the best candidate. Further study of predictive radiographic and endoscopic characterization is needed.

SUMMARY

Endoscopy in pediatric IBD is the cornerstone of disease characterization, both during initial diagnostic evaluation and throughout monitoring of response to treatment and progression of disease. Although delineation of more precise phenotypes of IBD continues to evolve with advances in molecular characterization, endoscopic reporting should balance detailed individual description with standardized and validated assessment tools. The promise of advances in therapeutic intervention by endoscopy in pediatric IBD deserves further exploration.

CLINICS CARE POINTS

- Accurate endoscopic characterization of inflammatory bowel disease (IBD) in children and adolescents is required for disease characterization and to inform treatment decisions.
- Endoscopic reporting of IBD in the pediatric population requires attention to specific considerations, such as upper gastrointestinal tract disease and atypical features of colon-predominant disease.
- The use of validated scoring tools is beneficial in clinical practice, and when undertaking research, but requires training to ensure consistent and reliable application.
- Therapeutic endoscopy in pediatric patients with IBD is emerging but should be undertaken by experienced interventional endoscopists.

REFERENCES

1. Oliva S, Thomson M, de Ridder L, et al. Endoscopy in Pediatric Inflammatory Bowel Disease: A Position Paper on Behalf of the Porto IBD Group of the European Society for Pediatric Gastroenterology, Hepatology and Nutrition. J Pediatr Gastroenterol Nutr 2018;67(3):414–30.
2. Henderson P, Hansen R, Cameron FL, et al. Rising incidence of pediatric inflammatory bowel disease in Scotland. Inflamm Bowel Dis 2012;18(6):999–1005.
3. Walsh CM, Lightdale JR. Pediatric Endoscopy Quality Improvement Network (PEnQuIN) quality standards and indicators for pediatric endoscopy: an ASGE-endorsed guideline. Gastrointest Endosc 2022;96(4):593–602.
4. Bousvaros A, Antonioli DA, Colletti RB, et al. Differentiating ulcerative colitis from Crohn disease in children and young adults: report of a working group of the North American Society for Pediatric Gastroenterology, Hepatology, and Nutrition and the Crohn's and Colitis Foundation of America. J Pediatr Gastroenterol Nutr 2007;44(5):653–74.
5. Levine A, Griffiths A, Markowitz J, et al. Pediatric modification of the Montreal classification for inflammatory bowel disease: the Paris classification. Inflamm Bowel Dis 2011;17(6):1314–21.
6. Dhaliwal J, Walters TD, Mack DR, et al. Phenotypic Variation in Paediatric Inflammatory Bowel Disease by Age: A Multicentre Prospective Inception Cohort Study of the Canadian Children IBD Network. J Crohns Colitis 2020;14(4):445–54.
7. Carvalho RS, Abadom V, Dilworth HP, et al. Indeterminate colitis: a significant subgroup of pediatric IBD. Inflamm Bowel Dis 2006;12(4):258–62.
8. Shergill AK, Lightdale JR, Bruining DH, et al. The role of endoscopy in inflammatory bowel disease. Gastrointest Endosc 2015;81(5):1101–21, e1101-1113.
9. Levine A, de Bie CI, Turner D, et al. Atypical disease phenotypes in pediatric ulcerative colitis: 5-year analyses of the EUROKIDS Registry. Inflamm Bowel Dis 2013;19(2):370–7.

10. Haskell H, Andrews CW Jr, Reddy SI, et al. Pathologic features and clinical significance of "backwash" ileitis in ulcerative colitis. Am J Surg Pathol 2005;29(11): 1472–81.

11. D'Haens G, Geboes K, Peeters M, et al. Patchy cecal inflammation associated with distal ulcerative colitis: a prospective endoscopic study. Am J Gastroenterol 1997;92(8):1275–9.

12. Albayrak NE, Polydorides AD. Characteristics and Outcomes of Left-sided Ulcerative Colitis With a Cecal/Periappendiceal Patch of Inflammation. Am J Surg Pathol 2022;46(8):1116–25.

13. Bakman Y, Katz J, Shepela C. Clinical Significance of Isolated Peri-Appendiceal Lesions in Patients With Left Sided Ulcerative Colitis. Gastroenterol Res 2011; 4(2):58–63.

14. Anzai H, Hata K, Kishikawa J, et al. Appendiceal orifice inflammation is associated with proximal extension of disease in patients with ulcerative colitis. Colorectal Dis 2016;18(8):O278–82.

15. Mary JY, Modigliani R. Development and validation of an endoscopic index of the severity for Crohn's disease: a prospective multicentre study. Groupe d'Etudes Therapeutiques des Affections Inflammatoires du Tube Digestif (GETAID). Gut 1989;30(7):983–9.

16. Daperno M, D'Haens G, Van Assche G, et al. Development and validation of a new, simplified endoscopic activity score for Crohn's disease: the SES-CD. Gastrointest Endosc 2004;60(4):505–12.

17. Adler J, Eder SJ, Gebremariam A, et al. Development and Testing of a New Simplified Endoscopic Mucosal Assessment for Crohn's Disease: The SEMA-CD. Inflamm Bowel Dis 2021;27(10):1585–92.

18. Adler J, Colletti RB, Noonan L, et al. Validating the Simplified Endoscopic Mucosal Assessment for Crohn's Disease: A Novel Method for Assessing Disease Activity. Inflamm Bowel Dis 2022. [Epub ahead of print]. https://doi.org/10.1093/ibd/izac183.

19. Adler J, Eder SJ, Gebremariam A, et al. Quantification of Mucosal Activity from Colonoscopy Reports via the Simplified Endoscopic Mucosal Assessment for Crohn's Disease. Inflamm Bowel Dis 2022;28(10):1537–42.

20. Schroeder KW, Tremaine WJ, Ilstrup DM. Coated oral 5-aminosalicylic acid therapy for mildly to moderately active ulcerative colitis. A randomized study. New Engl J Med 1987;317(26):1625–9.

21. Travis SP, Schnell D, Krzeski P, et al. Reliability and initial validation of the ulcerative colitis endoscopic index of severity. Gastroenterology 2013;145(5):987–95.

22. Ricciuto A, Carman N, Benchimol EI, et al. Prospective Evaluation of Endoscopic and Histologic Indices in Pediatric Ulcerative Colitis Using Centralized Review. Am J Gastroenterol 2021;116(10):2052–9.

23. Kerur B, Machan JT, Shapiro JM, et al. Biologics Delay Progression of Crohn's Disease, but Not Early Surgery, in Children. Clin Gastroenterol Hepatol 2018; 16(9):1467–73.

24. Hyams JS, Brimacombe M, Haberman Y, et al. Clinical and Host Biological Factors Predict Colectomy Risk in Children Newly Diagnosed With Ulcerative Colitis. Inflamm Bowel Dis 2022;28(2):151–60.

25. Ihekweazu FD, Fofanova T, Palacios R, et al. Progression to colectomy in the era of biologics: A single center experience with pediatric ulcerative colitis. J Pediatr Surg 2020;55(9):1815–23.

26. Rutgeerts P, Geboes K, Vantrappen G, et al. Predictability of the postoperative course of Crohn's disease. Gastroenterology 1990;99(4):956–63.

27. Sandborn WJ. Pouchitis following ileal pouch-anal anastomosis: definition, pathogenesis, and treatment. Gastroenterology 1994;107(6):1856–60.
28. Akiyama S, Ollech JE, Rai V, et al. Endoscopic Phenotype of the J Pouch in Patients With Inflammatory Bowel Disease: A New Classification for Pouch Outcomes. Clin Gastroenterol Hepatol 2022;20(2):293–302 e299.
29. Shen B, Kochhar GS, Kariv R, et al. Diagnosis and classification of ileal pouch disorders: consensus guidelines from the International Ileal Pouch Consortium. Lancet Gastroenterol Hepatol 2021;6(10):826–49.
30. Turner D, Ricciuto A, Lewis A, et al. STRIDE-II: An Update on the Selecting Therapeutic Targets in Inflammatory Bowel Disease (STRIDE) Initiative of the International Organization for the Study of IBD (IOIBD): Determining Therapeutic Goals for Treat-to-Target strategies in IBD. Gastroenterology 2021;160(5):1570–83.
31. Ungaro RC, Yzet C, Bossuyt P, et al. Deep Remission at 1 Year Prevents Progression of Early Crohn's Disease. Gastroenterology 2020;159(1):139–47.
32. Baert F, Moortgat L, Van Assche G, et al. Mucosal healing predicts sustained clinical remission in patients with early-stage Crohn's disease. Gastroenterology 2010;138(2):463–8 [quiz: e410-461].
33. Yzet C, Diouf M, Le Mouel JP, et al. Complete Endoscopic Healing Associated With Better Outcomes Than Partial Endoscopic Healing in Patients With Crohn's Disease. Clin Gastroenterol Hepatol 2020;18(10):2256–61.
34. Shah SC, Colombel JF, Sands BE, et al. Mucosal Healing Is Associated With Improved Long-term Outcomes of Patients With Ulcerative Colitis: A Systematic Review and Meta-analysis. Clin Gastroenterol Hepatol 2016;14(9):1245–55.e8.
35. Thakkar K, Lucia CJ, Ferry GD, et al. Repeat endoscopy affects patient management in pediatric inflammatory bowel disease. Am J Gastroenterol 2009;104(3):722–7.
36. Nardone OM, Bazarova A, Bhandari P, et al. PICaSSO virtual electronic chromendoscopy accurately reflects combined endoscopic and histological assessment for prediction of clinical outcomes in ulcerative colitis. United Eur Gastroenterol J 2022;10(2):147–59.
37. Ordas I, Rimola J, Alfaro I, et al. Development and Validation of a Simplified Magnetic Resonance Index of Activity for Crohn's Disease. Gastroenterology 2019;157(2):432–9.e1.
38. Shen B, Kochhar GS, Rubin DT, et al. Treatment of pouchitis, Crohn's disease, cuffitis, and other inflammatory disorders of the pouch: consensus guidelines from the International Ileal Pouch Consortium. Lancet Gastroenterol Hepatol 2022;7(1):69–95.
39. Everhov ÅH, Ludvigsson JF, Järås J, et al. Colorectal Cancer in Childhood-onset Inflammatory Bowel Disease: A Scandinavian Register-based Cohort Study, 1969-2017. J Pediatr Gastroenterol Nutr 2022;75(4):480–4.
40. Murthy SK, Feuerstein JD, Nguyen GC, et al. AGA Clinical Practice Update on Endoscopic Surveillance and Management of Colorectal Dysplasia in Inflammatory Bowel Diseases: Expert Review. Gastroenterology 2021;161(3):1043–10451 e4.
41. Modigliani R, Mary JY, Simon JF, et al. Clinical, biological, and endoscopic picture of attacks of Crohn's disease. Evolution on prednisolone. Groupe d'Etude Therapeutique des Affections Inflammatoires Digestives. Gastroenterology 1990;98(4):811–8.
42. Carman N, Tomalty D, Church PC, et al. Clinical disease activity and endoscopic severity correlate poorly in children newly diagnosed with Crohn's disease. Gastrointest Endosc 2019;89(2):364–72.

43. Ricciuto A, Fish J, Carman N, et al. Symptoms Do Not Correlate With Findings From Colonoscopy in Children With Inflammatory Bowel Disease and Primary Sclerosing Cholangitis. Clin Gastroenterol Hepatol 2018;16(7):1098–105.e1.

44. Hart L, Chavannes M, Lakatos PL, et al. Do You See What I See? An Assessment of Endoscopic Lesions Recognition and Description by Gastroenterology Trainees and Staff Physicians. J Can Assoc Gastroenterol 2020;3(5):216–21.

45. Khanna R, Zou G, D'Haens G, et al. Reliability among central readers in the evaluation of endoscopic findings from patients with Crohn's disease. Gut 2016;65(7): 1119–25.

46. Daperno M, Comberlato M, Bossa F, et al. Training Programs on Endoscopic Scoring Systems for Inflammatory Bowel Disease Lead to a Significant Increase in Interobserver Agreement Among Community Gastroenterologists. J Crohns Colitis 2017;11(5):556–61.

47. Brooks-Warburton J, Ashton J, Dhar A, et al. Artificial intelligence and inflammatory bowel disease: practicalities and future prospects. Frontline Gastroenterol 2022;13(4):325–31.

48. Schwartz DA, Wiersema MJ, Dudiak KM, et al. A comparison of endoscopic ultrasound, magnetic resonance imaging, and exam under anesthesia for evaluation of Crohn's perianal fistulas. Gastroenterology 2001;121(5):1064–72.

49. Gordon IO, Agrawal N, Willis E, et al. Fibrosis in ulcerative colitis is directly linked to severity and chronicity of mucosal inflammation. Aliment Pharmacol Ther 2018; 47(7):922–39.

50. Yoshizawa S, Kobayashi K, Katsumata T, et al. Clinical usefulness of EUS for active ulcerative colitis. Gastrointest Endosc 2007;65(2):253–60.

51. Rasmussen SN, Riis P. Rectal wall thickness measured by ultrasound in chronic inflammatory diseases of the colon. Scand J Gastroenterol 1985;20(1):109–14.

52. Tsuga K, Haruma K, Fujimura J, et al. Evaluation of the colorectal wall in normal subjects and patients with ulcerative colitis using an ultrasonic catheter probe. Gastrointest Endosc 1998;48(5):477–84.

53. Hurlstone DP, Sanders DS, Lobo AJ, et al. Prospective evaluation of high-frequency mini-probe ultrasound colonoscopic imaging in ulcerative colitis: a valid tool for predicting clinical severity. Eur J Gastroenterol Hepatol 2005; 17(12):1325–31.

54. Yan B, Feagan B, Teriaky A, et al. Reliability of EUS indices to detect inflammation in ulcerative colitis. Gastrointest Endosc 2017;86(6):1079–87.

55. Higaki S, Nohara H, Saitoh Y, et al. Increased rectal wall thickness may predict relapse in ulcerative colitis: a pilot follow-up study by ultrasonographic colonoscopy. Endoscopy 2002;34(3):212–9.

56. Watanabe O, Ando T, El-Omar EM, et al. Role of endoscopic ultrasonography in predicting the response to cyclosporin A in ulcerative colitis refractory to steroids. Dig Liver Dis 2009;41(10):735–9.

57. Yan BM, Sey MSL, Belletrutti P, et al. Reliability of the Endoscopic Ultrasound Ulcerative Colitis (EUS-UC) score for assessment of inflammation in patients with ulcerative colitis. Endosc Int Open 2021;9(7):E1116–22.

58. Ruess L, Blask AR, Bulas DI, et al. Inflammatory bowel disease in children and young adults: correlation of sonographic and clinical parameters during treatment. AJR Am J Roentgenol 2000;175(1):79–84.

59. Maaser C, Sturm A, Vavricka SR, et al. ECCO-ESGAR Guideline for Diagnostic Assessment in IBD Part 1: Initial diagnosis, monitoring of known IBD, detection of complications. J Crohns Colitis 2019;13(2):144–64.

60. Kopylov U, Yung DE, Engel T, et al. Diagnostic yield of capsule endoscopy versus magnetic resonance enterography and small bowel contrast ultrasound in the evaluation of small bowel Crohn's disease: Systematic review and meta-analysis. Dig Liver Dis 2017;49(8):854–63.
61. Min SB, Le-Carlson M, Singh N, et al. Video capsule endoscopy impacts decision making in pediatric IBD: a single tertiary care center experience. Inflamm Bowel Dis 2013;19(10):2139–45.
62. Bokemeyer B, Luehr D, Helwig U, et al. Small bowel capsule endoscopy in ulcerative colitis: the capcolitis study: a prospective observational study. Eur J Gastroenterol Hepatol 2019;31(7):766–72.
63. Monteiro S, Boal Carvalho P, Dias de Castro F, et al. Capsule Endoscopy: Diagnostic Accuracy of Lewis Score in Patients with Suspected Crohn's Disease. Inflamm Bowel Dis 2015;21(10):2241–6.
64. Gralnek IM, Defranchis R, Seidman E, et al. Development of a capsule endoscopy scoring index for small bowel mucosal inflammatory change. Aliment Pharmacol Ther 2008;27(2):146–54.
65. Niv Y, Ilani S, Levi Z, et al. Validation of the Capsule Endoscopy Crohn's Disease Activity Index (CECDAI or Niv score): a multicenter prospective study. Endoscopy 2012;44(1):21–6.
66. Oliva S, Veraldi S, Cucchiara S, et al. Assessment of a new score for capsule endoscopy in pediatric Crohn's disease (CE-CD). Endosc Int Open 2021;9(10): E1480–90.
67. Broide E, Shalem T, Richter V, et al. The Safety and Feasibility of a New Through-the-scope Balloon-assisted Enteroscopy in Children. J Pediatr Gastroenterol Nutr 2020;71(1):e6–11.
68. Kugathasan S, Denson LA, Walters TD, et al. Prediction of complicated disease course for children newly diagnosed with Crohn's disease: a multicentre inception cohort study. Lancet 2017;389(10080):1710–8.
69. Liu Q, Zhang X, Ko HM, et al. Constrictive and Hypertrophic Strictures in Ileal Crohn's Disease. Clin Gastroenterol Hepatol 2022;20(6):e1292–304.
70. Foster EN, Quiros JA, Prindiville TP. Long-term follow-up of the endoscopic treatment of strictures in pediatric and adult patients with inflammatory bowel disease. J Clin Gastroenterol 2008;42(8):880–5.
71. McSorley B, Cina RA, Jump C, et al. Endoscopic balloon dilation for management of stricturing Crohn's disease in children. World J Gastrointest Endosc 2021; 13(9):382–90.
72. Shen B, Kochhar G, Navaneethan U, et al. Practical guidelines on endoscopic treatment for Crohn's disease strictures: a consensus statement from the Global Interventional Inflammatory Bowel Disease Group. Lancet Gastroenterol Hepatol 2020;5(4):393–405.
73. Shen B, Lian L, Kiran RP, et al. Efficacy and safety of endoscopic treatment of ileal pouch strictures. Inflamm Bowel Dis 2011;17(12):2527–35.
74. Lan N, Shen B. Endoscopic Stricturotomy Versus Balloon Dilation in the Treatment of Anastomotic Strictures in Crohn's Disease. Inflamm Bowel Dis 2018;24(4): 897–907.
75. Lan N, Shen B. Endoscopic Stricturotomy with Needle Knife in the Treatment of Strictures from Inflammatory Bowel Disease. Inflamm Bowel Dis 2017;23(4): 502–13.
76. Lan N, Stocchi L, Delaney CP, et al. Endoscopic stricturotomy versus ileocolonic resection in the treatment of ileocolonic anastomotic strictures in Crohn's disease. Gastrointest Endosc 2019;90(2):259–68.

Polyps and Polyposis Syndromes in Children
Novel Endoscopic Considerations

Thomas M. Attard, MD[a,b,]*, Shlomi Cohen, MD[c], Carol Durno, MSc, MD[d,e,f]

KEYWORDS

• Upper endoscopy • Colonoscopy • Polyposis syndromes • Cancer predisposition

KEY POINTS

• Polypectomy entails increased risk over routine endoscopy, and preprocedure preparation, an appreciation of high-risk patient and polyp attributes, and vigilance postprocedure can mitigate risk and limit adverse outcomes.

• Novel polypectomy techniques including cold snare polypectomy need to be tailored to pediatric polypectomy indications.

• Accurate identification of a hereditary polyposis syndrome rests on an understanding of the intestinal and extraintestinal clinical features including histology of resected polyps and a detailed family history. Whenever possible, it is supported by targeted genetic testing.

• The goals of endoscopic management are syndrome-specific and include polypectomy to limit symptoms, risk of obstruction, and malignant transformation.

INTRODUCTION

Polyps are frequently encountered in pediatric endoscopy during colonoscopy performed for painless hematochezia. Less frequently, syndromic polyps are encountered in the context of screening, or subsequent surveillance, in hereditary cancer predisposing syndromes. Multiple, potentially syndromic polyps may be encountered unexpectedly during endoscopy; their number, distribution, and histopathologic

[a] Division of Gastroenterology, Hepatology and Nutrition, Children's Mercy Hospital, 2401 Gillham Road, Kansas City, MO 64108, USA; [b] The University of Missouri in Kansas City School of Medicine, Kansas City, MO, USA; [c] Pediatric Gastroenterology Institute, Dana-Dwek Children's Hospital, Tel Aviv Sourasky Medical Center, Affiliated to the Sackler Faculty of Medicine, Tel Aviv University, Tel Aviv, Israel; [d] Division of Gastroenterology, Hepatology and Nutrition, The Hospital for Sick Children, 555 University Avenue, Toronto, Ontario M5G 1X8, Canada; [e] The Zane Cohen Centre for Digestive Diseases, 60 Murray Street, Toronto, Ontario M5T 3L9, Canada; [f] Mount Sinai Hospital, University of Toronto, Toronto, Ontario, Canada
* Corresponding author. Division of Gastroenterology, Hepatology and Nutrition, Children's Mercy Hospital, 2401 Gillham Road, Kansas City, MO 64108.
E-mail address: tmattard@cmh.edu

Gastrointest Endoscopy Clin N Am 33 (2023) 463–486
https://doi.org/10.1016/j.giec.2022.11.001
1052-5157/23/© 2022 Elsevier Inc. All rights reserved.

findings, along with a detailed family history (FH) will direct genetic testing and ultimately help to diagnose the particular polyposis syndrome and determine management strategies.

The management of polyposis syndromes includes endoscopy with polypectomy, focusing on treatment of bleeding, prevention of mechanical obstruction, and surveillance. The goals of surveillance include monitoring polyp burden, removing larger, potentially dysplastic lesions, and preventing progression to cancer. Gastrointestinal inherited polyposis syndromes may involve intergenerational trauma as multiple family members may be affected.[1] Compliance with endoscopy is crucial as lifelong surveillance in polyposis syndromes has been shown to improve long-term survival.[2]

Pediatric gastroenterologists play a key role in the multidisciplinary approach necessary to manage polyposis syndromes. Relatedly, they must be engaged in developing evidence-based guidelines focused on these disorders.[3] The objectives of these collaborative efforts encompass unique aspects of the pediatric population, including the age at first screening, screening modality, and timing of surgical intervention. This shared goal inspired the creation of the European Society of Pediatric, Gastroenterology, Hepatology and Nutrition (ESPGHAN) Working Group on Polyposis which spearheaded the creation of recently published position papers focused on the management of juvenile polyposis syndrome (JPS),[4] familial adenomatous polyposis (FAP),[5] and Peutz–Jeghers syndrome (PJS)[6] in children and adolescents. More recently the North American Society of Pediatric, Gastroenterology, Hepatology and Nutrition (NASPGHAN) Polyposis Special Interest Group convened with similar collaborative goals.

Polypectomy is the most common therapeutic intervention in pediatric endoscopy; as such it deserves attention in quality metrics toward detection and resection. The importance of the quality of endoscopy in children and adolescents has been a recent major focus of both NASPGHAN and ESPGHAN and has resulted in the development of the Pediatric Endoscopy Quality Improvement Network (PEnQuIN).[7]

This state-of-the-art review focuses on the accurate characterization of polyps, technical aspects of performing polypectomy and associated adverse events, goals of endoscopy in polyposis syndromes, cancer screening, and high-quality management of polyps and polyposis syndromes, including endoscopy quality standards.

CHARACTERIZING POLYPS

The distribution and visual assessment of intestinal polyps is central to their management as is photodocumentation. Isolated, usually pedunculated, lobular lesions characteristic of sporadic juvenile polyps are the most frequently encountered, especially in the distal colon. Gastric and small intestinal polyps are rare. Initial inspection determines shape and surface-mucosal characteristics that differentiate true polyps from extrinsic compression or suction blebs. A more detailed examination of the polyp surface can identify vascular and pit pattern characteristics that are suspect for a dysplastic or cancerous histology as opposed to a hyperplastic (inflammatory or hamartomatous) lesion. Chromoendoscopy may be useful to better define the surface characteristics. Optical diagnosis of pseudopolyps in the context of chronic inflammation and hematologic neoplastic lesions may prove challenging based on inspection alone, and biopsy confirmation may be required.

Chromoendoscopy and Virtual Chromoendoscopy

Several adjunct techniques have been adopted from adult gastroenterology practice toward enhanced polyp detection and intraprocedural histologic classification of polyps. Indigo carmine chromoendoscopy has been shown to increase colorectal neoplasia detection rate including diminutive adenomas in adults.[8] This may be relevant in pediatric practice toward establishing the diagnosis of FAP in at risk individuals, as well as more accurately determining polyp burden in established disease (particularly for detection of smaller duodenal polyps), and rectal surveillance following ileorectal anastomosis.

Virtual chromoendoscopy refers to electronic endoscopic imaging technologies, which use electronic image processing to enhance visualization of certain mucosal features. They provide enhanced visualization of tissues without the need for dyes, enabling endoscopists to differentiate polyps in real time. Several virtual chromoendoscopy technologies are available, including narrow-band imaging (NBI; Olympus Medical Systems, Tokyo, Japan), flexible spectral imaging color enhancement (Fujinon, Fujifilm Medical Co, Saitama, Japan), and i-SCAN (PENTAX Endoscopy, Tokyo, Japan).[9] Such optical imaging enhancing technologies require less training and time to implement than chromoendoscopy.

Polyp features that may indicate advanced dysplasia or malignancy are ulceration, surface bleeding, or adenoma diameter greater than 10 mm. Histologic characterization of lesions is based on the appraisal of both pit and vascular pattern in the lesion, and for which there are several well-established classifications, including the narrow-band imaging international colorectal endoscopic (NICE) classification (**Table 1**).[10]

Although more laborious and time-consuming, in FAP chromoendoscopy has been shown to be superior to NBI in detecting diminutive polyps and both were significantly better than traditional white light colonoscopy.[11] NBI can also be used to distinguish polyp histologic subtypes. In a pediatric study in patients with hamartomatous polyposis, Cheng and colleagues differentiated PJS and JPS polyps based on pit pattern and achieved a higher accuracy (93.9% compared with 84.1%) in the detection of adenomatous lesions.[12] Virtual chromoendoscopy can be further enhanced by underwater (**Fig. 1**)[13] or magnifying endoscopy.

TECHNICAL APPROACH TO POLYPECTOMY

Planning for polypectomy requires several technical considerations centered on the number, size, distribution, and anticipated histology of the polyps. In addition to the

Table 1
Narrow-band imaging international colorectal endoscopic classification

	Type 1	Type 2	Type 3
Color	Same/lighter than background	Brown relative to background	Brown/dark brown relative to background; patchy white areas
Vessels	None/isolated lacy	Brown vessels surrounding white structures	Areas of disrupted/missing vessels
Surface pattern	Dark or white spots, uniform size, homogenous pattern	Oval/tubular/branched white structures, brown vessels	Amorphous/absent surface pattern
Most likely pathology	Hyperplastic and sessile serrated adenoma	Adenoma	Deep submucosal invasive carcinoma

Adapted from Hamada Y, Tanaka K, Katsurahara M, et al. Utility of the narrow-band imaging international colorectal endoscopic classification for optical diagnosis of colorectal polyp histology in clinical practice: a retrospective study. BMC Gastroenterology 2021;21(1):336.

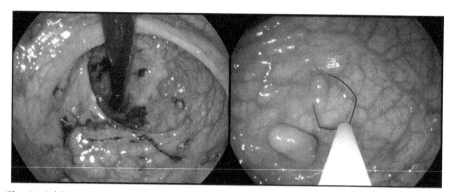

Fig. 1. Cold snare polypectomy for control of adenomatous polyp burden during surveillance proctoscopy after colectomy with ileorectal anastomosis in patient with familial adenomatous polyposis.

standard requirements for pediatric endoscopy, additional equipment needs should be anticipated. These include hot and cold polypectomy snares, endoclips, over-the-scope clips, lifting agents for flat lesions and the full complement of equipment related to the management of bleeding.

Preoperatively, the need for optimal bowel preparation underscores the importance of an unimpeded, thorough examination which, based on adenoma detection in adult patients, is best with good (eg, Boston Bowel Preparation Scale Score greater than 6–8), but paradoxically, not necessarily pristine (9), bowel preparation.[14,15] In addition, good bowel preparation is associated with lower morbidity following microperforation.[16] Planning may also include extra procedure time and provision for postprocedure admission if deemed necessary.

Operator specialization and experience is also a key to successful and safe polypectomy. There is robust evidence, in adults, correlating increased adverse events following polypectomy when performed by less specialized, lower volume endoscopists.[17] Parameters to determine level of experience and what constitutes a high-volume practice in pediatrics remain undefined. This is one of the goals of the PEn-QuIN moving forward.

Several patient and polyp characteristics factor in higher risk polypectomy (**Table 2**). The high-risk patient tends to be younger; Thakkar and colleagues[18] reported a threefold increased risk of bleeding in patients less than 10 years of age compared with older pediatric patients. In addition, Hispanic and medically frail pediatric patients with multiple chronic medical comorbidities are at a higher risk of admission following therapeutic procedures including polypectomy.[19]

The specific polypectomy technique (**Fig. 2**) is determined by polyp characteristics (**Table 3**) and operator experience. Complete excision and retrieval are important, especially in potentially dysplastic lesions. Retrieval of all polyps may be impracticable in children with polyposis syndromes with numerous, especially right-sided, lesions not amenable to suction retrieval through the scope. The use of an overtube during colonoscopy, although technically challenging, allows grasping, retrieval then reintubation to the same segment of the colon being examined.

Hot Snare Polypectomy

Hot snare polypectomy is currently the preferred technique in polyps greater than 10 mm in diameter. Sessile or flat polyps 6 to 10 mm are amenable to either hot or

Table 2
Characteristics associated with higher risk polypectomy

Characteristics	Comments
Patient	
Age ≤ 10	
Coagulopathy	• Increased risk of delayed bleeding
Multiple chronic comorbidities	• Including technology dependence
Polyp location	
Right colon and cecum	• Thin walled viscus, • Inverted appendix or ileocecal valve, may be misidentified as polyp • Visualization may be poor (fluid, bowel preparation)
Small intestinal	• Thin-walled viscera
Sigmoid colon	• Redundant (older children and adult)
Morphology	
Large polyps	• Sessile polyps 10–19 mm in size • Pedunculated polyps with head ≥ 20 mm/stalk ≥ 10 mm in diameter
Flat lesions serrated polyps	• May require endoscopic submucosal dissection (ESD)

cold snare polypectomy. For pedunculated polyps, hot snare is considered preferable as excision with simultaneous cautery will minimize bleeding from vasculature traversing the stalk. Epinephrine injection and/or prophylactic mechanical hemostasis (eg, clips or loop) may offer additional hemostasis and are

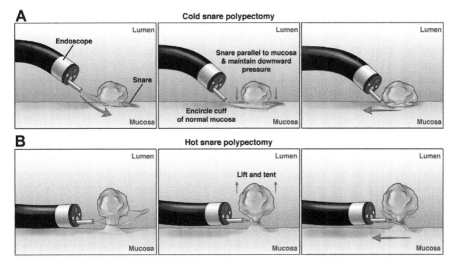

Fig. 2. Polypectomy technique. The approach to polypectomy illustrating key difference between hot snare polypectomy (*B*) with the snare lifting away from the mucosal surface to limit thermal injury, in contrast to cold snare polypectomy (*A*) with the snare pressing gently down on the mucosa, capturing a thin cuff of surrounding mucosa before excision. (*From Rutter MD, Jover R. Personalizing Polypectomy Techniques Based on Polyp Characteristics. Clin Gastroenterol Hepatol. 2020;18(13):2859-2867.*)

Table 3 Recommended approach to polypectomy technique		
Polyp Shape	**Polyp Size (mm)**	**Resection Method**
Sessile/Flat	≤3	Cold snare or cold biopsy forceps (en bloc)
	4–6	Cold snare (en bloc)
	7–10	Cold or hot snare polypectomy (en bloc)
	>10	Hot snare polypectomy (consider submucosal injection), EMR (en bloc preferred), ESD, or surgical resection depending on polyp site, size, morphology, and access
Pedunculated	Head < 20 mm and stalk width <10 mm	Hot snare polypectomy
	Head ≥20 mm or stalk width ≥10 mm	Hot snare polypectomy with bleeding prophylaxis (inject with adrenaline and/or prophylactic mechanical hemostasis [clips or loop] before polypectomy)

Abbreviations: EMR, endomucosal resection; ESD, endoscopic submucosal dissection.

recommended pre-polypectomy for larger pedunculated polyps. Given their characteristic smooth muscle core, polyps in PJS may require more forceful effort during resection.

The selection of an appropriately sized snare loop, orienting the polyp base to the 5 or 6 o'clock location and positioning of the endoscope directly above the polyp are universal recommendations for hot snare polypectomy. For non-adenomatous pedunculated polyps common in children, snaring the polyp stalk farther away from the bowel wall (but below the head) is advised. Residual polyp tissue is less likely to harbor malignancy in children compared with adults, and the availability of redundant stalk enables additional hemostatic measures, if needed, and minimizes the risk of thermal injury to the bowel wall.

Cold Snare Polypectomy

Cold snare polypectomy is superior to both cold and hot forceps polypectomy for diminutive lesions. Indeed, the use of hot forceps polypectomy is an outdated technique which carries an increased risk of diathermy-related deep thermal injury, inadequate histology, and incomplete excision.[20] Cold snare polypectomy is now established in the adult patient literature as the preferred modality to remove nonpedunculated lesions up to 10 mm in diameter (**Fig. 3**).[21–23] It renders better quality histopathologic material to ascertain complete resection, which is vital in the context of potentially malignant processes. A thin wire mini-snare (0.30 mm) seems superior to a thick wire snare in achieving complete histologic resection.[24] In addition, cold snare polypectomy obviates the possibility of thermal, electrocautery injury, post-polypectomy electrocautery syndrome (discussed below) and is associated with less delayed bleeding.[22] Underwater cold snare polypectomy is a promising permutation that allows for deeper resection of adenomata,[25,26] although the practical application in pediatric polyposis patients is as yet unclear.

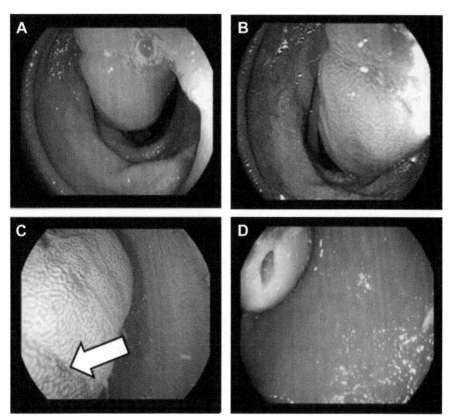

Fig. 3. Use of virtual chromoendoscopy with i-Scan to enhance surface morphology of large polyp (*A-B*) followed by water immersion to enhance buoyance and identify highest effective level (*arrow, C*) for hot snare resection in complex, obstructive small bowel hemolymphangioma (*D*).

Ischemic Polypectomy

Both cross-clip (clip) application and use of detachable snare (loop) will result in polyp strangulation and dehiscence, to obviate electrocautery in larger lesions, including small intestinal polyps in PJS.[27,28] This has been successfully implemented in adult patients, but caution needs to be exercised in that the strangulated lesion may preclude further advancing the endoscope and there is a theoretic risk that the detached, dehisced lesion may obstruct downstream if other large lesions are present.

Endoscopic Mucosal Resection

Endoscopic mucosal resection (EMR) is established as an effective and safe option in the management of adults with complex colon polyps and has considerably reduced the need for surgery in the adult population.[29] EMR has been reported in pediatric patients with intestinal polyposis, specifically in small and wide-based polyps, or piecemeal removal of larger polyps.[30] When reported, most polyps successfully removed by EMR in pediatric patients have been juvenile polyps in the rectum.[31] Indications for pediatric EMR need to be better defined and further investigation is needed.

POST-POLYPECTOMY ADVERSE EVENTS

Polypectomy is a higher risk endoscopic intervention, with associated early, delayed, and late adverse events (**Box 1**). In a single center, large cohort of patients who underwent therapeutic endoscopy including polypectomy, adverse events were reported in 11% of patients, with the majority (9% of total) requiring emergency room evaluation or admission.[32] The risk associated with polypectomy is therefore a key consideration in management and informed consent.

Post-Polypectomy Syndrome

Post-polypectomy electrocoagulation syndrome (PPECS) is a peritonitic reaction with systemic manifestations resulting from transmural thermal injury following hot snare polypectomy. Presentation is between 12 hours and 5 days postprocedure. The incidence of PPECS was 1.1% in a large pediatric study and the presentation included abdominal pain and fever, with leukocytosis and elevated C-reactive protein. Associated risk factors included younger age (<3 years), right-sided polyps, larger (>2.5 cm), broad-based lesions[33] with longer duration, and piecemeal polypectomy. Less than 10% of adult patients with PPECS evolve to florid perforation. Management includes hospitalization, bowel rest, fluid support, and broad-spectrum intravenous antibiotics.

Post-Polypectomy Bleeding

Techniques to reduce the risk of bleeding associated with polypectomy of larger (>1.5–2.5 cm), thick-stalked polyps include mechanical prophylaxis with endoclips[34] (**Fig. 4**) or detachable snares (ie, loops) at the base of the polyp and proximal to the planned resection plane. Evidence shows no clear advantages in adults with the use of routine endoclip application. Endoscopic loop-assisted polypectomy has been safely performed and reported in pediatric patients.[35]

POLYP SUBTYPES: SPORADIC AND SYNDROMIC
Sporadic (Non-Syndromic) Juvenile Polyps, Multiple (Non-Syndromic) Juvenile Polyps

Juvenile polyps are most often solitary and non-syndromic, they may also be reported as inflammatory or retention polyps due to their microscopic appearance. Solitary juvenile polyps will mostly appear in the left colon, but it may also appear proximal to the splenic flexure hence the need for complete colonoscopy with polypectomy. Patients with solitary JPs may have up to five polyps either at presentation or subsequently in follow-up. Although there are few reports of adenomatous changes, high-grade dysplasia is encountered rarely and only one report of adenocarcinoma in situ arising in a solitary JP.[36,37] Hence, if asymptomatic, no endoscopic follow-up is advised post-

---

Box 1
Post-polypectomy adverse events

Intraoperative/Early (<12 hours)
  Perforation
  Bleeding

Delayed (>12 hours) or Late (2–7 days)
  Bleeding
  Post-polypectomy electrocautery syndrome
  Post-polypectomy perforation

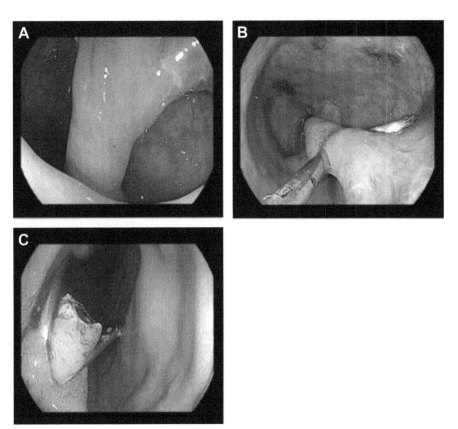

Fig. 4. Mechanical prophylaxis of post-polypectomy bleeding with large-stalked polyp (*A*). Cross-clip application before polypectomy (*B*) to limit bleeding following hot snare resection of a large juvenile (syndromic) colonic polyp (*C*).

polypectomy, unless there is concern of atypical features or suspicion of polyposis syndrome (ie, adenomatous changes in the polyps, polyposis syndrome in any member of the family, gastrointestinal cancer at early age or rebleeding).

Pediatric Polyposis Syndromes

Accurate diagnosis of polyposis is the keystone of effective management. This rests on a thorough clinical examination, detailed FH and characterization of the number, distribution, and histologic subtype of any polyps in the context of the patient's age (**Table 4**). The clinical diagnosis can be supplemented by targeted genetic testing. Clinical and endoscopic findings suspicious for a polyposis syndrome in the absence of a consistent FH may suggest de novo mutation. Conversely, the identification of a polyposis syndrome in a child may lead to recognition of presymptomatic disease in a parent. Thus, it is strongly recommended that genetic testing only be offered in collaboration with genetic counseling in order to determine the underlying specific genotype. Identification of a pathogenic variant allows cascade family genotyping, dissemination of important health information to multiple relatives, and the ability to make specific screening recommendations for the entire family. Relatedly, genotype–phenotype correlation in certain polyposis syndromes, notably FAP has

Table 4
Hereditary polyposis syndromes

	Familial Adenomatous Polyposis	Juvenile Polyposis Syndrome	Peutz–Jeghers Syndrome	PTEN-HS	Constitutional Mismatch Repair Defect
Incidence	1–3:10,000	1 in 100,000–160,000	1 in 200,000	1 in 200,000	Extremely rare
Inheritance pattern	Autosomal dominant	Autosomal dominant	Autosomal dominant	Autosomal dominant	Autosomal recessive
Genetic mutation	APC	SMAD4 or BMPR1A	STK11	PTEN (inactivation) WWP1 (gain-of-function)	MLH1, MSH2, MSH6, PMS2
Diagnostic criteria	Any number of colonic adenomas with positive known APC mutation OR positive FH	1. Five or more JPs of the colon or rectum 2. JPs in other parts of the GI tract 3. Any number of JPs and a positive FH	1. ≥2 histologically confirmed Peutz–Jeghers (PJ) polyps 2. Any number of PJ polyps OR characteristic mucocutaneous pigmentation in a person with an FH of PJS 4. Any number of PJ polyps in a person with the characteristic mucocutaneous pigmentation of PJS	Three or more major criteria including macrocephaly, Lhermitte–Duclos disease, or GI hamartomas OR Two major and three minor criteria	1. Child/young adult with a Lynch syndrome cancer 2. Child/young adult with colonic adenomatous polyposis not explained by a known polyposis syndrome mutation 3. Any child/young adult with cancer plus parental consanguinity, café-au-lait macules, or features of NF. 4. Any cancer with abnormal immunohistochemistry for the DNA-MMR proteins in normal and tumor tissue 5. History of brain cancer, lymphoma, or leukemia without history of radiation 6. Any child/adult with hypermutated tumor

Intestinal manifestation during childhood	• Mostly no symptoms • Abdominal pain • GI bleeding	• GI bleeding • Autoamputation of polyp	• GI bleeding • Intussusception	• GI polyps • Bleeding	• GI bleeding
Extraintestinal manifestations	• Osteomas • Exostoses • Dental abnormalities • Desmoid tumors • Fibroma • CHRPE • Glioblastoma • Thyroid mass/cancer • Hepatoblastoma	• *Cardiac* - mitral valve prolapse, VSD, PS, bicuspid AV • *Vascular/skin lesions;* telangiectasia, pigmented nevi, aneurysm, pulmonary AVM • *Cranial/skeletal;* macrocephaly, hydrocephalus, cleft palate, polydactyly, hypertelorism • *Thyroid disease* • *ADHD/autism* • *Epilepsy* • *Undescended testes* • *Ocular abnormalities*	• Mucocutaneous pigmented lesions	• Macrocephaly • Developmental delay • Hemangiomas • Lipomas	• Brain tumors • Leukemia • Lymphoma • Café-au-lait macules
Subtypes/Variants	• Attenuated FAP mutation at 3' or 5' end of APC • GAPPS - *Exon 1B APC* mutation	• Juvenile polyposis of infancy - Contiguous deletion of *BMPR1A* and *PTEN*		• Cowden syndrome • Bannayan-Riley-Ruvalcaba syndrome • PTEN-related Proteus syndrome • PTEN-PS like syndrome	

Abbreviations: ADHD, attention-deficit hyperactivity disorder; AV, aortic valve; CHRPE, congenital hypertrophy of the retinal pigment epithelium; DNA-MMR, DNA-mismatch repair; FH, family history; GAPPS, gastric adenocarcinoma and proximal polyposis of the stomach syndrome; GI, gastrointestinal; HHT, hereditary hemorrhagic telangiectasia; JP, juvenile polyps; NF, neurofibromatosis; PJ, Peutz–Jeghers; PJS, PJ syndrome; PS, pulmonary stenosis; VSD ventricular septal defect.

management implications, for example, the risk of desmoids factoring in surgical decision-making.

A key aspect of management of children with polyposis syndromes includes diagnosing premalignant conditions. The risk of developing malignant tumors in the gastrointestinal tract or in extraintestinal sites depends primarily on the underlying polyposis syndrome (**Table 5**).

The risk of malignancy is a major, albeit not the only driver of the current surveillance guidelines for childhood and adolescent hereditary polyposis syndromes[4–6] (**Table 6**). The timing of endoscopic surveillance is individualized and reflects multiple influencing factors including, age, symptoms, underlying gene mutation, and relatedly the disease expression in other family members. Although helpful, even within a particular kindred, genotype-phenotype correlation is imperfect and endoscopic assessment remains key. However, any surveillance strategy must factor the potential morbidity of colonoscopy and subsequent polypectomies.

ADENOMATOUS POLYPOSIS SYNDROMES
Familial Adenomatous Polyposis

FAP is the most common hereditary polyposis syndrome in childhood. The critical consideration in these patients is to eliminate the risk of colorectal cancer. The onus for management is therefore determining polyp burden and risk of dysplasia including polypectomy of larger lesions (>10 mm), or those with concerning appearance. Polypectomy of larger lesions is preferred over biopsy alone; the latter may fail to identify high grade dysplasia or carcinoma in situ. Polypectomy of adenomas is not intended to delay the inevitable colectomy; the goal of endoscopy is to optimize timing for colectomy and assist in the type of colectomy that can be offered (**Fig. 5**). Thus, the detailed documentation of polyp number, size, and distribution is a key consideration in FAP management.

Upper gastrointestinal tract involvement in FAP includes duodenal adenomata, which tend to cluster around the ampulla of Vater as well as fundic gland polyps in the stomach. Although reported, the incidence of advanced dysplastic or malignant lesions is believed to be very low and current pediatric guidelines do not support routine upper endoscopy unless the child is symptomatic.[38,39]

Lynch Syndrome and Constitutional Mismatch Repair Defect

Lynch syndrome is an autosomal dominant disorder, caused by the presence of a pathogenic mismatch repair (MMR) gene variant, with high risk for colorectal and other extraintestinal malignancies.[40,41] The risk of cancer varies according to the MMR gene mutation, gender, and other factors. As the mean age at the diagnosis of colorectal cancer is 44 to 61 years, current recommendations are to start colonoscopy surveillance at early adulthood (age 25–35 years), depending on the mutation type. If a first degree relative has early onset colorectal cancer the age to start surveillance would be modified.

In contrast, Biallelic/Constitutional Mismatch Repair Defect (BMMRD/CMMRD) is a rare, but much more aggressive cancer syndrome, originating from the biallelic/constitutional MMR gene mutations. This syndrome may include brain tumors, colonic polyposis, colorectal and small-bowel cancers, leukemia, and lymphoma. In these individuals, the lifetime risk of gastrointestinal cancer is the highest reported of all gastrointestinal cancer predisposition syndromes. Tumors are often diagnosed in the first decade of life.[42] Consequently, endoscopic surveillance is started early and is more intense. It is vital that the first-degree relatives of affected patients be screened for Lynch syndrome-associated cancers.[43]

Table 5
Risk of cancer in pediatric and adult patients with polyposis syndromes

	Familial Adenomatous Polyposis	Juvenile Polyposis Syndrome	Peutz–Jeghers Syndrome	PTEN Hamartoma Syndrome	Constitutional Mismatch Repair Deficiency		
					Site	*%*	*Age Range (years)*
Pediatric	CRC: 0.2% Upper GI: very rare Hepatoblastoma: 1.5% Brain tumor: 1% Thyroid cancer	GI: Rare (case reports)	GI: Rare (case reports) Testicular: 6% (age range 6–9 y)		CRC Small bowel	70 10	8–48 11–42
Adult	CRC: 100% (mean age 36 y) Gastric Small intestine: 4%–12% Pancreatic/ampullary cancer: 2% Desmoid tumor: 5% Thyroid cancer: 2%	CRC: 34% Gastric (*SMAD4* PV)	CRC: 39% Gastric: 29% Small intestine: 13% Breast: 32%–54% Other: 7%–36%	CRC: 9%–18% Thyroid: 3%–38% Uterus: 5%–28% Breast: 25%–85% Kidney: 15%–34%	Brain Hematological	40–50 20	2–40 0–30

Abbreviations: CRC, colorectal cancer; GI, gastrointestinal; PV, pathogenic variant.

Table 6
Screening and surveillance recommendations for hereditary polyposis syndromes in pediatric patients

	Familial Adenomatous Polyposis	Juvenile Polyposis Syndrome	Peutz–Jeghers Syndrome	Constitutional Mismatch Repair Defect
Age at first colonoscopy	12–14 year old	12–15 year old	8 year old	6 year old
Colonoscopy interval	Every 1–3 y	Every 1–5 y	Every 3 y If no polyps: at age 18	Annually
After colectomy surveillance	Every 6–12 mo			
Age at first EGD	Up to 25 year old	12–25 year old	8 year old	8 year old then annually
Age at first small bowel surveillance	—	—	8 year old	8 year old
Extraintestinal	Annual thyroid ultrasound	SMAD4 mutation evaluated for hereditary hemorrhagic telangiectasia	Annual testicular self-examination or ultrasound	Brain MRI every 6 mo beginning at 2 year old CBC every 6 mo beginning at 1 year old Urinalysis annually beginning at 10 year old

Abbreviations: CBC, complete blood count; EGD, esophagogastroduodenoscopy.

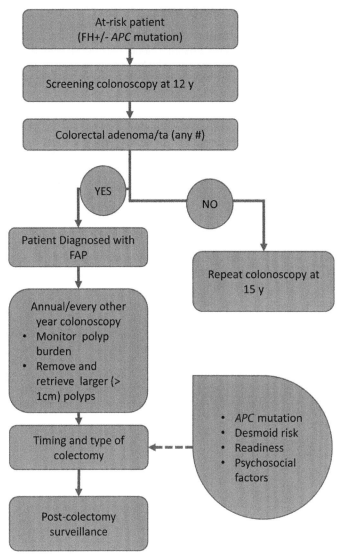

Fig. 5. **Colonoscopy management of familial adenomatous polyposis.** *FAP, familial adenomatous polyposis; FH, family history.* Children at risk of FAP should undergo predictive genetic testing following genetic counseling if a pathogenic variant is identified in the family. Earlier colonoscopy is justified in individuals with symptoms OR known aggressive pathogenic variant APC mutation OR family history of early (<20 years of age) CRC. Routine retroflexion in the rectum during colonoscopy may benefit detailed assessment of the rectum. Timing of colectomy factors polyp burden-based assessment of risk of CRC in next 12 months: (*A*) low burden—negligible risk → colonoscopy in 1 year; (*B*) increased adenoma size and/or number → surgery when convenient; (*C*) high-grade dysplasia or carpeting with adenomatous polyps → surgery soon. The type of surgery factors rectal polyp burden, desmoid risk, and available surgical expertise. Post-colectomy (rectal preserving) proctoscopy is needed every 6 to 12 months depending on polyp burden.

HAMARTOMATOUS POLYPOSIS SYNDROMES

Hamartomatous polyposis syndromes include JPS, PJS, and the PTEN hamartoma syndrome (PTEN-HS) which may present during childhood with rectal bleeding, abdominal pain, and/or extraintestinal manifestations. Endoscopic management of hamartomatous polyposis syndromes primarily focuses on polypectomy to prevent bleeding and mechanical obstruction, notably in PJS.

Juvenile Polyposis Syndrome

The clinical diagnosis of JPS is based on the number and distribution of polyps, and the presence of a FH[44] (see **Table 4**). A critical consideration in the management of these patients is determining the related gene mutation; the presence of a *SMAD4* pathogenic variant identifies a subgroup of patients with JPS at risk of vascular, including cerebral and pulmonary arteriovenous malformations related to hereditary hemorrhagic telangiectasia (HHT) and whose treatment is best coordinated through a specialized HHT referral center. The risk of HHT has implications for increased anesthetic risk so this is vital to communicate to the anesthetist well ahead when planning for endoscopy. Surveillance for colonic polyps starts at age 12 to 15 years (**Fig. 6**), although JPS patients with negative mutation generally have a milder phenotype that may require a different surveillance program.[45]

Peutz–Jeghers Syndrome

Gastroscopy and colonoscopy with polypectomy are a necessary surveillance tool in PJS with the goal of managing bleeding and anemia. Mitigating cancer risk is a central

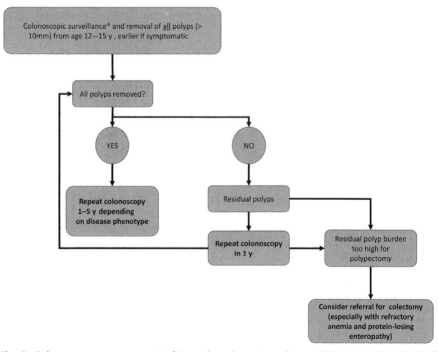

Fig. 6. Colonoscopy management of juvenile polyposis syndrome. [a]Alert anesthesiologist if SMAD4 pathogenic variant and expressing hereditary hemorrhagic telangiectasia phenotype.

consideration in PJS management in adults[3]; in children, however, monitoring and limiting the growth of small intestinal polyps through enteroscopy is the critical consideration. The early, presymptomatic identification and resection of small intestinal polyps in PJS has been shown to decrease the likelihood of intussusception, obstruction, and hence intestinal resection. There are diverse diagnostic and therapeutic options in surveillance for these children. (**Fig. 7**) shows the proposed algorithm that reflects the recommendations made in the pediatric guidelines.

PTEN Hamartoma Syndrome

PTEN-HS includes a variety of phenotypic variations caused by mutation in the *PTEN* gene. Because no cases of cancer during childhood were reported, colonoscopy surveillance in asymptomatic individuals is recommended starting at 35 years of age (or 10 years younger than the age of any relative with colorectal cancer) and repeated at intervals no greater than 5 years, depending on the burden of polyps. Children with PTEN-HS may present with a spectrum of gastrointestinal symptoms including weight loss and protein-losing enteropathy, therefore endoscopy is often required for diagnostic workup. The histology from polyps and non-polyp mucosa in these individuals may reflect prominent eosinophilic infiltrate of unclear significance.

POLYPOSIS SYNDROMES: SPECIAL CONSIDERATIONS
Promoting Compliance and Managing Anxiety Around Procedures

An important goal of the endoscopic experience for children and adolescents with a polyposis syndrome is to develop a positive culture and experience. A multidisciplinary approach is best suited for caring children and their families with polyposis

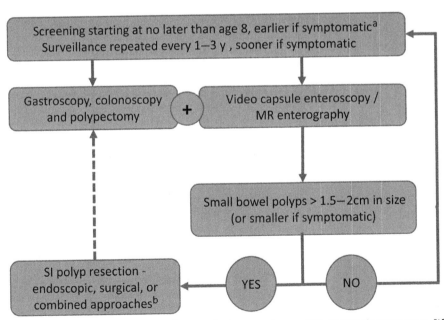

Fig. 7. Endoscopic management of Peutz–Jeghers syndrome. MR, magnetic resonance. [a]If no polyps are noted during initial examination, surveillance should be resumed by age 18 years. [b]The optimal modality for small bowel polypectomy is determined by polyp size, distribution, and available expertise.

syndromes. Team members typically include a pediatric gastroenterologist, primary care physician, genetic counselor, behavioral or mental health care providers, gastroenterology nurse, social worker, and surgeon.[46] Team members can work with the individual patient to encourage the child and/or adolescent to have age and developmentally appropriate control over certain decisions. The young person can decide when to have their annual scope. Some adolescents prefer to schedule procedures and surgery during summer vacation so not to interfere with sports and school. Siblings may decide to have their scopes booked on the same day, whereas others want their parent to be able to focus on them solely and stagger the endoscopy dates. Timing of colectomy for patients with FAP is an important decision, wherein the adolescent should be given a voice in the choice.[47]

Many young patients report significant fears and anxieties around imaging procedures and endoscopy. Specific concerns frequently include a fear of needles, fear of waking up during the procedure and being scared to be "put to sleep." Pre-endoscopy the most common concerns expressed by patients and parents are pain, procedure adverse events ("accidents related to the endoscopy"), and hunger.[48]

Some pediatric polyposis patients and families struggle with the potential, albeit low risk of discovering a malignant lesion. An honest, comprehensible discussion of the relatively low risk of malignancy, tailored to the patient and family's understanding is important to minimize distress and anxiety. Multimedia resources tailored to polyposis pre-endoscopy should be routinely used in this population.

Impact of Coronavirus Disease on Pediatric Endoscopy Patients

Currently, many pediatric gastroenterologists are reporting encountering more patients with polyps and polyposis syndromes (personal communication). This observation is not believed to be due to an increased prevalence but related to the coronavirus disease-19 pandemic. Patients with polyposis syndromes undergo regular surveillance which often is a schedule of annual colonoscopies. During the pandemic, many patients did not have surveillance due to the lack of access to endoscopy.[49,50] Currently, as the pandemic moves to an endemic, there is a catch-up occurring within this population. Patients with polyposis syndromes such as JPS have developed more polyps, which are often larger and more difficult to remove due to the delay in surveillance protocol. Secondly, more patients with rectal bleeding who were not able to access care for several reasons during the pandemic are now undergoing colonoscopy.

Inequity in Access to Care Including Endoscopic Management

There are several barriers to care that are unique or accentuated in the practice patterns prevalent in North America. Socialized care facilitates access to centralized centers of excellence, offering a more standardized and evidence-driven model of care, including endoscopic management. This is one of the factors that accounts for the impact of national and regional registries in the care of hereditary polyposis.[51] Disparities in care can also result from rural in comparison with urban residence,[52] income and race require a conscious collaborative approach including the active engagement of social work and financial assistance programs early in the care of these patients.[46]

QUALITY IMPROVEMENT AND TRAINING IN PEDIATRIC POLYPECTOMY

Quality metrics are increasingly prominent in pediatric endoscopy.[53,54] The NASP-GHAN and ESPGHAN endorsed PEnQuIN working group set out to standardize quality standards and indicators for pediatric gastrointestinal endoscopic procedures through a rigorous guideline consensus process.[7]

Competence in polypectomy can be categorized through measures of polyp detection and, independently, measures of safe, successful, and complete resection of the polyp. Measures of polyp detection and accurate classification, exemplified by the adenoma detection rate (ADR), are a key quality measure in adult practice but do not have a clear correlate in pediatric practice.[55] Successful resection entails an understanding of the polypectomy technique and specific factors related to size, localization, and patient characteristics as outlined above. Simulation-based and hands-on training sessions in tandem with formal didactic activities can be tailored for physicians in training and offer a necessary introduction before clinical exposure is allowed.[56] This is in line with the progressive acquisition of skills necessary to ensure competence to perform procedures independently on completion of a training program. Specific minimal targets on polyp resection are needed to ensure standardized care and quality benchmarking.

Finally, high-quality documentation of gastrointestinal procedures is another key aspect of quality improvement. This is especially relevant in polypectomy where determining polyp burden is a major factor in management. The inclusion of all key reporting elements is foundational to high-quality pediatric endoscopy.[57]

SUMMARY: CHALLENGES AND FUTURE DIRECTIONS

The technical repertoire available for polypectomy is ever expanding. Clearly, pediatric gastroenterology picks cues from adult gastroenterology in, among other aspects of care, polypectomy. However, the differences in patients, predisposing risk factors, and the implications of the different histologic types of lesions need to be considered. Missing diminutive lesions does not entail the same catastrophic sequelae in pediatric patients as in adults. This has bearing on the quality of bowel preparation needed, and the specific quality metrics (eg, ADR) that need to be emphasized in auditing procedure outcomes and the choice of polypectomy resection technique itself. Relatedly, the adoption of adjunct techniques, chromoendoscopy and virtual chromoendoscopy underwater resection, and EMR deserve more study to define their role, associated risk, and implications for training.

A key consideration in regard to children with polyposis syndromes is the heterogeneity and relative rarity of the syndromes that makes collaboration on a national and international level essential toward building capacity for observations and trials. An encouraging recent project is the ESPGHAN funded Polyposis Registry which brings together several European and North American Centers.

The very rationale for colonoscopy in FAP seems to be in de facto transition, as we witness a shift from the goal of establishing polyp burden needed to advocate for colectomy to a more interventional approach of decreasing polyp burden ostensibly toward delaying the need for colectomy. The risk benefit assessment of aggressive multiple polypectomies to delay colectomy needs to be qualified better before universal adoption. The need for upper endoscopy in FAP is similarly contentious as, relatedly, would be the aggressive treatment of periampullary changes in the pediatric population.[58,59]

There is considerable interest, by young patients and their parents, as well as by pharmaceutical companies in chemoprevention of polyposis. Current guidelines do not support routine treatment, although a spectrum of agents have been trialed. A critical challenge aside from identifying a suitable agent with a favorable adverse profile is to determine meaningful clinical endpoints to justify treatment.

There is a dire need for safe therapeutic options that impact small intestinal polyp growth, highlighted by the need for invasive enteroscopy with polypectomy in

Peutz–Jeghers patients.[60] Another meaningful therapeutic goal for which mTOR inhibitors, everolimus, and sirolimus have been proposed[61] is the reduction of polyp burden in juvenile polyposis of infancy, mitigating hypoalbuminemia and growth failure with the goal to delay colectomy.

Proficiency in routine polypectomy and awareness of the complexity and broader implications of polyposis syndromes are necessary competencies in pediatric gastroenterology. Novel polypectomy techniques need to be critically appraised, and close multidisciplinary collaboration, both with allied health care providers as well as basic and translational scientists, are the key components for future success.

CLINICS CARE POINTS

- Planning for polypectomy requires several technical considerations centered on the number, size, distribution, and anticipated histology of the polyps.
- Cold snare polypectomy is now established as the preferred modality to remove small (3–9 mm) nonpedunculated polyps.
- Simulation-based and hands-on training sessions in tandem, with formal didactic activities, can be tailored for physicians in training and organized to offer a necessary introduction before clinical exposure is allowed.

DISCLOSURE

The authors have nothing to disclose.

ACKNOWLEDGEMENT

The Zane Cohen Center donors, The Mullin Family and Friends.

REFERENCES

1. Silva E, Gomes P, Matos PM, et al. "I have always lived with the disease in the family": family adaptation to hereditary cancer-risk. BMC Prim Care 2022;23(1): 93. https://doi.org/10.1186/s12875-022-01704-z.
2. Durno C, Ercan AB, Bianchi V, et al. Survival Benefit for Individuals with Constitutional Mismatch Repair Deficiency Undergoing Surveillance. J Clin Oncol 2021; 39(25):2779–90.
3. Boland CR, Idos GE, Durno C, et al. Diagnosis and Management of Cancer Risk in the Gastrointestinal Hamartomatous Polyposis Syndromes: Recommendations from the US Multi-Society Task Force on Colorectal Cancer. Gastroenterology 2022;162(7):2063–85.
4. Cohen S, Hyer W, Mas E, et al. Management of juvenile polyposis syndrome in children and adolescents: A position paper from the ESPGHAN polyposis working group. J Pediatr Gastroenterol Nutr 2019;68(3):453–62. https://doi.org/10.1097/MPG.0000000000002246.
5. Hyer W, Cohen S, Attard T, et al. Management of Familial Adenomatous Polyposis in Children and Adolescents: Position Paper from the ESPGHAN polyposis working group. J Pediatr Gastroenterol Nutr 2019;68(3):428–41.
6. Latchford A, Cohen S, Auth M, et al. Management of peutz-jeghers syndrome in children and adolescents: a position paper from the ESPGHAN polyposis working group. J Pediatr Gastroenterol Nutr 2019;68(3):442–52.

7. Lightdale JR, Thomson MA, Walsh CM. The pediatric endoscopy quality improvement network joint NASPGHAN/ESPGHAN guidelines: a global path to quality for pediatric endoscopy. J Pediatr Gastroenterol Nutr 2022;74(S1 Suppl 1):S1–2.

8. Brooker JC, Saunders BP, Shah SG, et al. Total colonic dye-spray increases the detection of diminutive adenomas during routine colonoscopy: a randomized controlled trial. Gastrointest Endosc 2002;56(3):333–8.

9. Lerner DG, Mencin A, Novak I, et al. Advances in pediatric diagnostic endoscopy: a state-of-the-art review. JPGN Rep 2022;3(3):e224.

10. Hamada Y, Tanaka K, Katsurahara M, et al. Utility of the narrow-band imaging international colorectal endoscopic classification for optical diagnosis of colorectal polyp histology in clinical practice: a retrospective study. BMC Gastroenterol 2021;21(1):336. https://doi.org/10.1186/S12876-021-01898-Z.

11. Matsumoto T, Esaki M, Fujisawa R, et al. Chromoendoscopy, narrow-band imaging colonoscopy, and autofluorescence colonoscopy for detection of diminutive colorectal neoplasia in familial adenomatous polyposis. Dis Colon Rectum 2009;52(6):1160–5.

12. Cheng W, Liu H, Gu Z, et al. Narrow-band imaging endoscopy is advantageous over conventional white light endoscopy for the diagnosis and treatment of children with Peutz-Jeghers syndrome. Medicine (Baltimore) 2017;96(19):e6671. https://doi.org/10.1097/MD.0000000000006671.

13. Halma J, Attard T. Small Bowel Hemolymphangioma Treated by Polypectomy in a Pediatric Patient with Cystic Fibrosis. JPGN Rep 2021;2(2):e060.

14. Calderwood AH, Thompson KD, Schroy PC, et al. Good is better than excellent: Bowel preparation quality and adenoma detection rates. Gastrointest Endosc 2015;81(3):691.

15. Adike A, Buras MR, Gurudu SR, et al. Is the level of cleanliness using segmental Boston bowel preparation scale associated with a higher adenoma detection rate? Ann Gastroenterol 2018;31(2):217–23.

16. Christie JP, Marrazzo J. Mini-perforation" of the colon–not all postpolypectomy perforations require laparotomy. Dis Colon Rectum 1991;34(2):132–5.

17. Paszat LF, Sutradhar R, Luo J, et al. Perforation and post-polypectomy bleeding complicating colonoscopy in a population-based screening program. Endosc Int Open 2021;9(4):E637–45.

18. Thakkar K, El-Serag HB, Mattek N, et al. Complications of pediatric colonoscopy: a five-year multicenter experience. Clin Gastroenterol Hepatol 2008;6(5):515–20. Available at: http://doi.org/10.1016/j.cgh.2008.01.007.

19. Attard TM, Miller M, Walker AA, et al. Pediatric elective therapeutic procedure complications: A multicenter cohort analysis. J Gastroenterol Hepatol (Australia) 2019;34(9):1533–9. Available at: http://doi.org/10.1111/jgh.14626.

20. Metz AJ, Moss A, McLeod D, et al. A blinded comparison of the safety and efficacy of hot biopsy forceps electrocauterization and conventional snare polypectomy for diminutive colonic polypectomy in a porcine model. Gastrointest Endosc 2013;77(3):484–90.

21. Qu J, Jian H, Li L, et al. Effectiveness and safety of cold versus hot snare polypectomy: A meta-analysis. J Gastroenterol Hepatol 2019;34(1):49–58.

22. Arimoto J, Chiba H, Ashikari K, et al. Management of Less Than 10-mm-Sized Pedunculated (Ip) Polyps with Thin Stalk: Hot Snare Polypectomy Versus Cold Snare Polypectomy. Dig Dis Sci 2021;66(7):2353–61.

23. Willems P, Orkut S, Ditisheim S, et al. An international polypectomy practice survey. Scand J Gastroenterol 2020;55(4):497–502.

24. Din S, Ball AJ, Riley SA, et al. Cold snare polypectomy: does snare type influence outcomes? Dig Endosc 2015;27(5):603–8.

25. Maruoka D, Kishimoto T, Matsumura T, et al. Underwater cold snare polypectomy for colorectal adenomas. Dig Endosc 2019;31(6):662–71.

26. Myung YS, Kwon H, Han J, et al. Underwater versus conventional cold snare polypectomy of colorectal polyps 4-9 mm in diameter: a prospective randomized controlled trial. Surg Endosc 2022;36(9):6527–34.

27. Yano T, Shinozaki S, Yamamoto H. Crossed-clip strangulation for the management of small intestinal polyps in patients with Peutz-Jeghers syndrome. Dig Endosc 2018;30(5):677.

28. Khurelbaatar T, Sakamoto H, Yano T, et al. Endoscopic ischemic polypectomy for small-bowel polyps in patients with Peutz-Jeghers syndrome. Endoscopy 2021; 53(7):744–8.

29. Raju GS, Lum PJ, Ross WA, et al. Outcome of EMR as an alternative to surgery in patients with complex colon polyps. Gastrointest Endosc 2016;84(2):315–25.

30. Zhan Q, Jiang C. Chromoendoscopy Plus Mucosal Resection Versus Conventional Electrocoagulation for Intestinal Polyps in Children: Two Case Series. J Laparoendosc Adv Surg Tech A 2018;28(11):1403–7.

31. Vitale DS, Wang K, Jamil LH, et al. Endoscopic Mucosal Resection in Children. J Pediatr Gastroenterol Nutr 2022;74(1):20–4.

32. Kramer RE, Narkewicz MR. Adverse Events Following Gastrointestinal Endoscopy in Children: Classifications, Characterizations, and Implications. J Pediatr Gastroenterol Nutr 2016;62(6):828–33.

33. Wang YS, Zhang J, Li XQ, et al. [Clinical characteristics and risk factors of post polypectomy electrocoagulation syndrome in children]. Zhonghua Er Ke Za Zhi 2021;59(3):201–5.

34. Luigiano C, Ferrara F, Ghersi S, et al. Endoclip-assisted resection of large pedunculated colorectal polyps: Technical aspects and outcome. Dig Dis Sci 2010; 55(6):1726–31.

35. Lin YC, Chou JW, Chen AC, et al. Endoloop-Assisted Polypectomy for a Symptomatic Giant Colonic Polyp in a Pediatric Patient. Children (Basel) 2022;9(2): 222. Available at: http://doi.org/10.3390/CHILDREN9020222.

36. Gupta SK, Fitzgerald JF, Croffie JM, et al. Experience with juvenile polyps in North American children: the need for pancolonoscopy. Am J Gastroenterol 2001;96(6): 1695–7.

37. Fox VL, Perros S, Jiang H, et al. Juvenile polyps: recurrence in patients with multiple and solitary polyps. Clin Gastroenterol Hepatol 2010;8(9):795–9.

38. Attard TM, Cuffari C, Tajouri T, et al. Multicenter Experience with Upper Gastrointestinal Polyps in Pediatric Patients with Familial Adenomatous Polyposis. Am J Gastroenterol 2004;99(4). https://doi.org/10.1111/j.1572-0241.2004.04115.x.

39. Jagelman DG, Decosse JJ, Bussey HJR. Upper gastrointestinal cancer in familial adenomatous polyposis. Lancet 1988;1(8595):1149–51.

40. Giardiello FM, Allen JI, Axilbund JE, et al. Guidelines on genetic evaluation and management of Lynch syndrome: a consensus statement by the US Multi-Society Task Force on colorectal cancer. Gastroenterology 2014;147(2):502–26.

41. Seppälä TT, Latchford A, Negoi I, et al. European guidelines from the EHTG and ESCP for Lynch syndrome: an updated third edition of the Mallorca guidelines based on gene and gender. Br J Surg 2021;108(5):484–98.

42. Aronson M, Gallinger S, Cohen Z, et al. Gastrointestinal findings in the largest series of patients with hereditary biallelic mismatch repair deficiency syndrome:

Report from the international consortium. Am J Gastroenterol 2016;111(2): 275–84.

43. Durno C, Boland CR, Cohen S, et al. Recommendations on Surveillance and Management of Biallelic Mismatch Repair Deficiency (BMMRD) Syndrome: A Consensus Statement by the US Multi-Society Task Force on Colorectal Cancer. Gastroenterology 2017;152(6):1605–14.

44. Latchford AR, Neale K, Phillips RKS, et al. Juvenile polyposis syndrome: a study of genotype, phenotype, and long-term outcome. Dis Colon Rectum 2012;55(10): 1038–43.

45. MacFarland SP, Ebrahimzadeh JE, Zelley K, et al. Phenotypic Differences in Juvenile Polyposis Syndrome with or Without a Disease-causing SMAD4/BMPR1A Variant. Cancer Prev Res (Phila) 2021;14(2):215–22.

46. Attard TM, Burke CA, Hyer W, et al. ACG Clinical Report and Recommendations on Transition of Care in Children and Adolescents with Hereditary Polyposis Syndromes. Am J Gastroenterol 2021;116(4):638–46.

47. Durno CA, Wong J, Berk T, et al. Quality of life and functional outcome for individuals who underwent very early colectomy for familial adenomatous polyposis. Dis Colon Rectum 2012;55(4):436–43.

48. Hagiwara S, Nakayama Y, Tagawa M, et al. Pediatric Patient and Parental Anxiety and Impressions Related to Initial Gastrointestinal Endoscopy: A Japanese Multi-center Questionnaire Study. Scientifica (Cairo) 2015;2015:797564.

49. Ruan W, Fishman DS, Lerner DG, et al. Evolution of International Pediatric Endoscopic Practice Changes During the Coronavirus Disease 2019 Pandemic. J Pediatr Gastroenterol Nutr 2022;74(6):e138.

50. Ruan W, Fishman DS, Lerner DG, et al. Changes in Pediatric Endoscopic Practice During the Coronavirus Disease 2019 Pandemic: Results from an International Survey. Gastroenterology 2020;159(4):1547.

51. Koskenvuo L, Pitkaniemi J, Rantanen M, et al. Impact of Screening on Survival in Familial Adenomatous Polyposis. J Clin Gastroenterol 2016;50(1):40–4.

52. Kakembo N, Kisa P, Fitzgerald T, et al. Colonic polyposis in a 15 year-old boy: Challenges and lessons from a rural resource-poor area. Ann Med Surg 2016; 7:75.

53. Lightdale JR. Measuring Quality in Pediatric Endoscopy. Gastrointest Endosc Clin N Am 2016;26(1):47–62.

54. Cohen J, Pike IM. Defining and measuring quality in endoscopy. Gastrointest Endosc 2015;81(1):1–2.

55. Corley DA, Jensen CD, Marks AR, et al. Adenoma detection rate and risk of colorectal cancer and death. N Engl J Med 2014;370(14):1298–306.

56. Patel Rv, Barsuk JH, Cohen ER, et al. Simulation-based training improves polypectomy skills among practicing endoscopists. Endosc Int Open 2021;9(11): E1633–9.

57. Walsh CM, Lightdale JR, Fishman DS, et al. Pediatric Endoscopy Quality Improvement Network Pediatric Endoscopy Reporting Elements: A Joint NASP-GHAN/ESPGHAN Guideline. J Pediatr Gastroenterol Nutr 2022;74(S1 Suppl 1): S53–62.

58. Gutierrez Sanchez LH, Alsawas M, Stephens M, et al. Upper GI involvement in children with familial adenomatous polyposis syndrome: single-center experience and meta-analysis of the literature. Gastrointest Endosc 2018;87(3): 648–56, e3.

59. Martin I, Hawkins J, Hyer W, et al. Upper GI in patients with FAP—the need for formal research. Gastrointest Endosc 2020;91(1):206–7.

60. de Brabander J, Eskens FALM, Korsse SE, et al. Chemoprevention in Patients with Peutz-Jeghers Syndrome: Lessons Learned. Oncologist 2018; 23(4):399.
61. Taylor H, Yerlioglu D, Phen C, et al. MTOR inhibitors reduce enteropathy, intestinal bleeding and colectomy rate in patients with juvenile polyposis of infancy with PTEN-BMPR1A deletion. Hum Mol Genet 2021;30(14):1273–82.

Moving?

Make sure your subscription moves with you!

To notify us of your new address, find your **Clinics Account Number** (located on your mailing label above your name), and contact customer service at:

Email: journalscustomerservice-usa@elsevier.com

800-654-2452 (subscribers in the U.S. & Canada)
314-447-8871 (subscribers outside of the U.S. & Canada)

Fax number: 314-447-8029

Elsevier Health Sciences Division
Subscription Customer Service
3251 Riverport Lane
Maryland Heights, MO 63043

*To ensure uninterrupted delivery of your subscription, please notify us at least 4 weeks in advance of move.

Printed and bound by CPI Group (UK) Ltd, Croydon, CR0 4YY

08/05/2025

01864715-0002